It's Great! Oops, No It Isn't

Ronald R. Gauch

It's Great! Oops, No It Isn't

Why Clinical Research Can't Guarantee
the Right Medical Answers

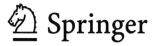 Springer

Ronald R. Gauch, Ph.D.
Marist College
3399 North Road
Poughkeepsie, NY 12601
USA

ISBN 978-1-4020-8906-0   e-ISBN 978-1-4020-8907-7

Library of Congress Control Number: 2008934289

For Sarah, Christine and John

The greatest gift a man can receive
is his children.

Preface

The truth is, few people know the first thing about clinical research. The public reads about a medical research project that announces unbelievable results for a miraculous drug. Some years later, another investigation completely wipes out those initial favorable findings.

Hormones Cut Women's Risk of Heart Disease (San Francisco Chronicle, 1994)

Hormones Don't Protect Women from Heart Disease, Study Says (Washington Post, 2001)

The people are confused because we do not understand the process behind these conflicting results. Our health, and in fact, our very lives are dependent on clinical trials, but we know little about them.

This book explains the issues the public needs to be aware of when it comes to clinical research. It uncovers the problems in medical investigations that can not be overcome no matter how much care and diligence medical researchers bring to a research project. The basic premise that drives the writing is that it is impossible for medical researchers to guarantee that they can get all the right answers from a single study. No matter how good the investigators are, no matter how well a study is planned, no matter how carefully the plans are executed and no matter how conscientiously the results are analyzed and interpreted – the answer may still be wrong. The deck is stacked against medical researchers and the public – you – should be skeptical of the results no matter how impressive they seem on the surface.

Do not, however, think that a trial cannot come up with an accurate answer. Many trials have found the correct answer, but there's never certainty that that will happen. Getting a correct result requires a combination of skill and luck. And furthermore, the correct result from a single study is almost always a narrow finding. The drug is proven effective, but its safety still needs to be established. Or perhaps the drug, given in a fixed regimen does not cause kidney damage, but its effect on other systems (heart, liver, lungs etc.) remains unanswered and the results when a different regimen is given may be very different. Note that I emphasize the evaluation of drugs throughout the book because drug testing is the dominant form of medical research and provides many valuable examples of the kind of problems that can be encountered.

From this book you'll also appreciate the building block approach required when evaluating clinical treatments. The results produced by a single study are only fragmentary evidence about a drug's true potential. A full understanding of what a new medical treatment can do relies on an accumulation of evidence from multiple sources and the use of all the different research methodologies available. The process of multiple testing serves to validate or invalidate the earlier research and that body of knowledge is in a constant state of revision as new data becomes available – or at least it should be.

Don't assume that the problems with clinical research lie with the individuals conducting the studies as tempting as that may be. Some of the most dedicated, smart and hard working scientists perform medical research. They are ethical, inventive and inspired professionals. The trouble is that the process they must use is inherently flawed. The things they must know are unknown. The things they must control are uncontrollable. And yes, in addition to these fatal defects, sometimes the problem is exaggerated by incompetence, deceit and bad luck.

Perhaps the greatest handicap the public faces is that what they learn about medical research does not come directly from the research community. What they are given comes from the popular media – newspapers and TV news in particular. Medical researchers may share their concerns and point out flaws in their research practices with their colleagues, but these limitations rarely trickle down to the millions of people who prescribe, dispense or use medications. The public is frequently awed by what is involved – biology, chemistry, pharmacology and statistics – they fear their lack of understanding about these subjects means they could never understand the research process. But here they are wrong – it is not that complicated. Most of the issues can be comprehended by better understanding the research process and by just using common sense. I've written this book to prove that that last statement is true.

Aimed at a broad general audience, this is not a technical book. There is not a single formula in it. Whenever possible, I have used familiar terms to describe procedures or conditions, such as heart attacks rather than myocardial infarctions, strokes rather than cerebrovascular accidents and heart disease rather than cardiovascular disease. In the end the reader will come away with a deeper appreciation and understanding of the complex nature of medical research. Each of us has a rightful interest in what medical investigations should be pursued and what new discoveries should be promoted for our use. But to be more than bystanders people must be informed, knowledgeable and confident so that their concerns can he expressed and listened to. This book provides people with the wherewithal to better understand and appreciate the research enterprise, but at the same time to be aware of its problems and vulnerabilities.

Contents

Part I
Medical Research Explained

Chapter 1
Medical Research – Searching for Answers

Abstract The book begins by enumerating the many accomplishments achieved by medical research, but also notes its failures and tendency to raise hopes that are not met. The difficulties researchers face and some of the major challenges that must be met are presented. Major research methods are introduced and briefly described. Included are the case report, case-control trial, cohort trial, medical survey and clinical trial. The chapter concludes with a case study of how the connection between smoking and lung cancer was established.

Keywords Epidemiology research · lung cancer · medical survey · research methods · smoking risk

Most of the public is well aware of the major advances in medical practices that have taken place because of valuable medical research. Illnesses that once were feared are now almost eradicated or under control. You need only to look back 25 years ago and see that the accomplishments are staggering. AIDS was essentially untreatable, many patients with depression were told to live with their illness, targeted chemotherapy for cancer was only a theory, and the U.S. death rate from heart disease was significantly higher than it is today.

Looking back we see that medical research produces true miracles and contributes to our higher standard of life as well as man's increased longevity. However, the record of clinical research is littered with false hopes and major failures as well. There is a long history of drugs that caused disastrous harmful effects and others that were not even effective. Many medical practices remain locked in controversy. For example, male circumcision, one of the oldest operations that is still performed, began as a religious rite. It became routine medical practice 100 years ago because doctors believed it prevented disease. However, there is now evidence that advantages such as lower risk of inflammation, infection, transmitting of a sexually disease and cancer may be overstated. Likewise the disadvantages, surgical complications, sexual dysfunction and pain experienced by a newborn male, may be overstated as well. The report card may be mixed – circumcision may be useful in places with poor sanitary conditions, but a liability in areas with good sanitary practices.

Men are confused on whether PSA screening for prostate cancer is worth it or not. Women are perplexed about whether they should or should not have a mammogram. Hormone replacement therapy is good for women. Oops – no it isn't. Breast implants are fine. Oops – no they aren't. Oops – they're great after all.

Some of the advances claimed for medical research may be exaggerated. Streptomycin, whose benefits were demonstrated in a classical clinical trial published in 1948, may get far too much credit for the control of tuberculosis. If we go back in history we will see that most of the decline in tuberculosis occurred before streptomycin even became available. By the time streptomycin was introduced the disease had already been well on its way to elimination.

We are also inundated with premature, if not false claims. A major breakthrough is heralded in the newspaper as capable of reducing the symptoms of Alzheimer's disease. A newscast announces that a Chinese herb has been found to greatly reduce arthritic symptoms. A magazine article totes a new indication for an older drug that will improve eyesight. Such headline claims are frequently based on a single report and require years of substantiation before ever becoming a true medical advance.

Scientific research is not itself a science, it is an art or craft. (W.H. George, *The Scientist in Action; A Scientific Study of His Methods*)

Make no mistake about it, doing medical research is a tough assignment. Look at a physical science such as physics or chemistry and compare their research environment to that of clinical medicine. A physical science provides all sorts of ways to produce identical experimental conditions that are impossible to replicate in the clinical setting. In the physical sciences all the relevant variables can be held constant (heat, light, temperature, etc.), but there is no such control for the clinical trial. We can also move from basic science to that of a biological laboratory experiment and see how more difficult a clinical investigation compares to that endeavor.

Consider a typical example of a well-controlled experiment in the lab, testing the effect of a diuretic versus a placebo in rats. Select 10 rats and randomly allocate them to the diuretic or placebo group. The rats are inbred, identically reared and handled. Furthermore, they do not vary significantly in their pharmacological responses. They are housed, fed and manipulated in an identical manner. The biologist compares the outcome variable, urine output, between the rats in the two groups. If the diuretic is effective, there will be no overlap in the result for the groups. All the rats receiving the diuretic will excrete more urine than any of the placebo rats.

This answer comes about because all relevant variables are held constant and the results in the diuretic and placebo treatment groups will either be very similar (if the diuretic is no good) or distinct (if the diuretic is effective). When conducting trials, control of all relevant variables is a goal in clinical research, but it is unreasonable to expect a researcher to even come very close to that objective. No matter how hard researchers try, holding constant all the relevant variables of the experiment is not going to happen. Quite simply, the idealized experimental conditions are not possible in clinical research. This does not mean that researchers cannot get a truthful right answer, but it does mean they have to be very lucky to avoid all the pitfalls that are lurking in the shadows. When it comes to conducting clinical trials even the best researcher cannot overcome an uncooperative environment.

Nothing is more demanding, more difficult, more frustrating, more time consuming, and requiring more creativity than clinical research. (J. Vaitukaitis, Director of the National Center for Research Resources in S. Lindahl, *Lancet*)

A Paradox

In one breath, consumers express their high regard for researchers, wholeheartedly support their work and swear by the treatments they receive because of those efforts. In another breath, they ignore medical science and trust their own evaluations when it comes to their health care. The widespread use of unapproved over-the-counter health remedies, with little or no scientific evidence to back up their claims, is a clear sign that the public does not feel medical research is always necessary to find useful medicines. The public is quick to pounce on testimonials and unproven claims for vitamins, herbs, nutrients, animal extracts and natural occurring enzymes. Celebrities such as Tom Cruise and Dr. Phil proudly endorse health products that have never undergone vigorous testing. The market for such unproven remedies exceeds $15 billion annually. The popularity of these products is a reflection of lack of respect the public has for medical research to be the sole source for judging medications.

It is not that people do not believe medical research results – if anything they are too gullible, accepting on faith results that may be wrong. Although they know there's been an outbreak of wrong answers, they are still more than willing to accept any promise of help when it comes to their health. The snake oil salesman of the past can still enjoy lucrative profits in today's marketplace.

Even so, medical investigators command respect and admiration from all parts of society, which is their due. By and large they are dedicated, intelligent and often relentless in their quest for knowledge. Most do their very best and they should not be faulted for their efforts. Unfortunately, the truth of the matter is that the task they face is a daunting one. No matter how sincere their commitment, how well they plan and hard they work, there is no assurance that they will end up with the correct result from any one study.

Challenges Facing Medical Research

Research is critical to all fields: biology, sociology, economics and even comparative religions. It resolves taxing problems and provides greater clarity to poorly understood issues. Through research new ways are discovered that enhance and improve the quality of life. Research uncovers novel methods that can control and reduce pain and suffering. Although there is no one way to carry out research, almost always it begins with a question or problem. Plans differ depending on the problem to be investigated and the research discipline involved. In some cases, the research is essentially chemical experiments performed in a laboratory, but in other cases, it involves repetitive animal tests that can predict what drugs may be harmful to people. However, the research that is the most challenging and problematic involves investigations in human beings and a number of different research designs are regularly used.

The medical research process is reasonably well programmed and can be found in the many textbooks written on the subject. Identifying the steps in a research plan is easy. The tough part is filling in the details. For example, a plan for a clinical trial needs to contain the following information:

> Treatments to be given (how much and for how long).
> Kind of subjects to be used (their disease, age, condition, medications they can or cannot take).
> Measurements to be made to evaluate efficacy and safety (how often and at what times).
> Statistical evaluations of test results (what tests should be used and what constitutes a significant treatment difference).

Make a mistake in answering these questions, or others that must be addressed, and the conclusions of the entire study may be of little value.

It is also not enough to give all the specifics – the plan has to be executed properly. For instance, inappropriate subjects must not slip through the screening process and poor compliance by subjects must be recognized and steps taken to ensure they follow the treatment schedule. Subjects must be prodded to show up for required tests and examinations, and the proposed analysis plans adjusted when trial execution fails. No question, human testing is a Herculean task requiring a relentless effort on the part of clinical investigators and their staffs.

A medical research project is not a one-man show, a team approach is required. A project may include physicians with different specializations, personnel with training in basic sciences, nurses, statisticians, epidemiologists, pathologists, laboratory technicians and administrative personnel. Not only do these staffs have to be recruited and assembled, they must be managed and supervised. Many times the members of a research team are at entirely different locations and may have different bosses which only puts more pressure on the coordination effort.

People who do research are not secluded scientists working in a remote laboratory or isolated library. For many physicians who become clinical investigators, the demands of their medical training left little room for in-depth courses in research methodology. Hence, they learn their trade through post-doctoral programs, mentors or by on-the-job training. Technical knowledge is also not enough. Researchers need to know how to plan programs, how to run projects and how to manage people all of which require interpersonal, communication and leadership skills – attributes not taught in medical school. Their backgrounds must make them qualified in the specific medical field being investigated, and knowledgeable about the unique drug or drugs under study. They must ensure the health and safety of the subjects enrolled in a trial, institute polices that protect the records and reports generated and work with other external groups that have a role in clinical research (e.g. the FDA and outside committees established by law to be sure the patients are willing participants who are not subject to unnecessary risks).

The lead investigator(s) are responsible for their research, but it also must be remembered that they work for some organization that is paying for the research. The research sponsor is frequently a pharmaceutical company, but it can also be a governmental entity (e.g. the National Institutes of Health) or, on rare occasions, an independent healthcare organization. The size and complexity of medical research comes at a sizeable cost. The NIH is a good barometer of that cost with a budget approaching $30 billion a year. The cost per patient for the drug trials that leads to an eventual marketing approval is estimated to be $26,000 by the Association of Clinical Research Organizations. That's not the total trial cost – it is the cost for each patient in a trial. Clinical research has become a major investment in the U.S. and the art and science behind that investment deserves close scrutiny.

Research Methods

Researchers using human beings as subjects have distinct choices as to how they will plan and organize their research. They can just observe people, or review medical records or conduct clinical trials.

The four primary options for medical research are listed below.

1. Case report
2. Case – control study
3. Cohort study
4. Clinical trial

The case report is a description of a patient or group of patients who have an unusual condition or response that a health professional believes should be brought to the attention of others. Frequently there is little evidence presented to explain why the problem occurred or what to do about it. The case report, usually published in a medical journal, can stimulate a discussion about possible explanations for the unusual finding presented and lead to the use of one of the higher levels of research.

A case-control study is often employed to identify possible causes for a disease by using past medical records of people. It begins by finding patients with a disease and looks back through their past records to find possible causes. Investigators try to find reliable and complete records, but that cannot be guaranteed. In this approach, the histories of a group of patients with a disease or condition of interest (the cases) are compared to another group (the controls) who do not have the disease or condition. Factors that show a difference between the groups represent possible causes of the disease.

A cohort study does not have to rely on past records and manufactures the necessary research information in a systematic fashion as the study progresses.

Investigators begin by recording the health status of subjects who then have follow-up assessments made over a period of time. Some of the people get an illness, and others do not. Investigators form two groups that are as similar as possible, but one group has the targeted disease, which is not present in the other group. In a comparison of the groups, researchers look for factors that distinguish the two sets of subjects, and therefore may be the cause of the disease.

The case-control study, along with the cohort study are frequently lumped together and called observational studies. However, the term "observational" can be misleading because you also make observations with the case report and clinical trial. I believe a more accurate title would be "exploratory" because these methods do extremely well when looking for possible effects from medical treatments, but they do not provide strong enough evidence to be totally convincing. Clinical trials are in the best position to get correct medical answers.

In a clinical trial, a group of volunteers having a certain disease is assembled and receive either an experimental treatment or a control treatment. Researchers want the groups to be as similar as possible at the start of the trial,and they strive to keep al the factors that could affect the outcome the same during the trial, so that the only important difference is the treatment the subjects receive. This approach therefore resembles a true experiment, which is not achievable with the other methods. At the end of the trial, the experimental and control patients are then compared in order to assess the safety and effectiveness of the treatments.

The clinical trial is considered the best method followed by the cohort study, case-control study and finally the case report. Although the methods can be ranked, it does not mean one is always better than another. Different circumstances (time, cost, resources, etc.) may make a lower rated method the best choice or even the only option for the researcher. No one study can be trusted to give all the right answers so in the end, medical research relies on accumulated results from different studies to come up with convincing findings.

Medical Surveys

I've covered four research methods, but there is a tool available to researchers that merits comment as well. Researchers use medical surveys to gain valuable information about diseases and their treatment. For example, researchers may survey a group of people to see what diseases they have. They may want to know how many people in New York have a sleep disturbance or how many premature births occur in southern cities.

One of the major uses of surveys is to identify disease prevalence. By prevalence I mean how many people have a given disease at the present time. In fact, a survey is sometimes called a prevalence study or a cross-sectional study. Whatever term is used, the method can provide researchers with very useful information. As an example, there was a time when nobody quite knew what was going on with AIDS – who was contracting the disease, where did they live, etc. It was the medical survey that helped identify people most at risk. Surveys showed that the highest rates for the disease were (1) among young men in certain high risk cities (e.g. San Francisco), (2) people who had multiple blood transfusions and (3) hemophiliacs. Now the research could be focused on these types of patients.

Make no mistake though; there are weaknesses and major limitations with surveys. One devastating disadvantage has to do with cause and effect. It may not be possible through a survey to determine the time between (1) the exposure to the possible cause of the disease and (2) the actual onset of the disease. For example, a survey could show that over-weight people were more likely to have arthritis. However, it would be wrong to conclude that the excess weigh caused the arthritis because it isn't clear if the excess weight preceded or followed the arthritis. If the arthritis came first, people may have become very inactive with less exercise and that was the true cause of the extra weight.

Unfortunately, it is also well recognized that surveys can be intentionally manipulated by the way a question is asked. However, even if there is no attempt to deceive, answers from surveys can be misinterpreted easily, and research based on surveys can be seriously flawed.

An example of a flawed survey is the one conducted on the relationship between sleep and longevity that appeared in the *Archives of General Psychiatry*. Researchers conducted a survey and reported that adults live longer if they get six or seven hours of sleep a night rather than the usual eight hours. The survey was massive. It included over 1 million U.S. adults. Those who slept five hours or less and those who slept eight hours or more a night, were more likely to die than those who got 6.5–7.5 hours of sleep. Sleep experts noted, however, that the survey had several flaws. It relied on participants' recollection of their sleep habits and did not ask if they took naps. It did not look at the quality of people's sleep or whether they felt drowsy all day. Furthermore, participants who got little sleep or slept eight hours or more may have had medical problems that would explain their increased death rate. The survey process didn't get at nuances, a potential shortcoming of all surveys.

Smoking and Lung Cancer

I'll close this chapter with a case study that shows how medical researchers used various approaches to link smoking to lung cancer.

The question: does smoking cause lung cancer? Would you be surprised to open your morning newspaper one day and read this startling headline?

Smoking Does Not Cause Lung Cancer

Could you ever imagine such a headline? Sounds ridiculous doesn't it? Isn't everyone convinced that smoking is a cause of lung cancer? And yet there is just the smallest, slightest, infinitesimal possibility that it is not. But it's been proven you might protest. Unfortunately, "proven" is a most difficult standard to reach in medical research. The term is too absolute and requires every conceivable possibility to be ruled out leaving no room for the slightest doubt.

But let's go back to the beginning. People have smoked for centuries. The Mayans burned leaves and inhaled the smoke over 2,000 years ago. When tobacco was first brought to Europe it was thought to have medicinal value. It was chewed, taken nasally and even applied to the skin to treat cough, asthma, headaches, stomach cramps gout and even malignant tumors. At first tobacco was smoked in pipes – cigarette and cigars came later. We can thank Sir Walter Raleigh for making it a socially accepted practice.

Early evidence that smoking caused lung cancer was based on the case report method of research. Reports of lip cancer among pipe smokers appeared in medical communications as far back as the late 1700s. Nonetheless, the connection wasn't taken seriously and written off as a result of the heat produced by the pipe. In the early 1900s lung cancer, which had been a rare disease, was seen much more often. Cigarette smoking was identified as a possible cause. But since nonsmokers also developed lung cancer this possibility received little support. In fact, most people who smoked did not even get lung cancer.

Early Signs of a Problem

There were a few reports, suggesting a possible connection between smoking and lung cancer in the 1920s and 1930s. However, a 1939 German study is often considered the first research study to show a link between lung cancer and cigarette smoking. Questionnaires were sent to relatives of people who had died of lung cancer. Based on the data sent in, the German researchers concluded that tobacco use caused lung cancer. Unfortunately, the study was apparently quite sloppy and received little attention by the greater medical community.

In the 1940s smoking was fine from an environmental, social and medical perspective. Cigarettes were advertised using sport stars and movie idols (including future President Ronald Reagan). An ad claimed over 10,000 physicians smoked Lucky Strikes and another proclaimed that while smoking Camels, throat specialists never have throat irritation. However, at this time there was also a growing body of evidence – infrequently reaching the public – that linked cigarette smoking to lung cancer.

During the 1950s the situation changed dramatically following publication of a number of investigational studies based on the case-control technique. With this method, patients who already had lung cancer were identified and their medical records examined to see likely causes of the disease. A group similar to the group of lung cancer cases, except they did not have the disease, was also established. Identical information was gathered on both sets of patients. Researchers use the term "cases" for the people with the disease and those without the disease are called the "controls". Comparisons were then made between the cases and controls to see if there were characteristics (i.e. likely causes of the disease) in one group and not in the other. Smoking was discovered to be present in a larger proportion of cases than controls making it a prime suspect as being responsible for the illness.

There was general agreement among the case-control studies done at that time, that there was an association between cigarette smoking and lung cancer. However, a major weakness of the case–control method was that it could not rule out other causes for the people who developed lung cancer. Obviously, if data were not collected on a possible cause of lung cancer, then it would be impossible to incriminate that presumed cause in an analysis. For example, maybe the cause of lung cancer was, in fact, air pollution. However, if no data on polluted air had been obtained then the air pollution – lung cancer relationship could not be uncovered. Therefore, while there was general agreement that the studies showed that there was an association between smoking and lung cancer, that did not mean that cigarette smoking was definitely a cause of lung cancer.

Case reports and case-control studies were useful but researchers, who sincerely thought there was a link between smoking and lung cancer, decided that they needed a different research methodology to support their position. The cohort research method was called for and researchers from Great Britain led the way in the use of this method. As noted above, a cohort trial often observes two sets of people (those with and those without a presumed cause of a disease). After a reasonable amount of time, the two groups are compared to see what group has the highest proportion of patients with the disease.

The researchers, in the smoking case, chose to study doctors in Great Britain who did not have lung cancer. They identified physicians on a governmental list that included almost 70 percent of the physicians in the country. Next they identified, among these physicians, those who were smokers and those who were not smokers. The two groups were then observed to see which one ended up with the most cases of lung cancer. The study lasted 2 ½ years and produced findings similar to those of the case-control method: lung cancer was again more common among smokers. A subsequent U.S. cohort study that was even larger and longer – about 200,000 men for almost four years – also showed a higher rate of lung cancer among smokers.

Still, in spite of the growing body of evidence against smoking, the methods of research used did not permit universal condemnation of tobacco. The case-control and the cohort methods still had serious drawbacks. Most importantly, when these methods were employed, it was impossible to be sure that the treatment and control groups were comparable. People who smoked could be very different from people who didn't smoke. They could drink more or sleep less. There could be a preponderance of males or an under-representation of white-collar workers. Even if researchers tried to get the groups to have similar traits there could be subtle differences that researchers weren't aware of that resulted in dissimilar groups. And if there were factors that were dissimilar between the groups, could one of those factors account for the higher number of lung cancer cases?

There was one way to answer this challenge or so it seemed. The objection could best be resolved by using the gold standard of research methods – the clinical trial.

On paper all you had to do was design a study in which half the volunteers would be randomized to a smokers group and the other half would not be allowed to smoke. Then wait and see which group developed the most cases of lung cancer. Of course, such a study was impossible – (1) you could not require people to smoke and (2) you'd have major problems keeping others from smoking.

Governmental Action

Without data from the strongest research method, clinical trial evidence, cohort and case-control studies would have to be the main offensive weapon and they continued to appear in the late 1950s and into the 1960s. The research involved different settings and countries – Denmark, France and Japan. The period of observation was also extended reaching upwards of 10 years. All studies came to the same conclusion – smoking tobacco increased the risk of getting lung cancer. In addition, other conditions were found to occur more often with those who smoked including heart disease and different types of cancer. Studies consistently showed that the more a person smoked, the greater the risk of lung cancer. They also demonstrated that the longer a person smoked, the greater the chance that they'd get lung cancer. Statistical methods were used to adjust results based on any differences between the characteristics of the smoker and non-smoker groups. After the adjustment, the higher rate of lung cancer held up. The weight of the evidence became overwhelming placing pressure on governments to act.

Without a clinical trial, scientists had to make do with the weaker case-control and cohort studies which benefited cigarette manufacturers. The tobacco industry now under attack, received help from an unusual place. A major scientist in the U.K., held in high esteem all over the world, raised serious doubts about the smoking and cancer connection. Ronald Fisher, knighted for his research work and considered the "father" of modern day statistics, had reservations. His basic argument was that there could be a genetic factor that caused both a desire to smoke and a predisposition to lung cancer. Those with this genetic factor would likely take up smoking and when they did they could come down with lung cancer. However, the cause of the cancer would be the genetic factor, not smoking.

However, even before the Fisher controversy was resolved, major research organizations in the U.S., U.K. and Canada concluded that there was a casual relationship between smoking and lung cancer. In 1962 the Surgeon General of the U.S. also found that smoking was a major cause of lung cancer and announced the momentous decision requiring warning labels on cigarette packages. In spite of that decision the tobacco industry continued to argue that a precise link from smoking to cancer had not been established. They noted that no study of smokers had ruled out all other factors that could be the cause of the cancer.

Eventually, even the concern expressed by Fisher was laid to rest when the results from studies of identical twins became available. The twins had the same genetic make-up, but for each twin pair, one was a smoker and the other wasn't.

The results of the study, published in *Social Science Medicine*, showed that the twin who smoked was much more likely to develop lung cancer than the twin who didn't. The evidence greatly weakened the force of Fisher's criticism.

The condemnation of smoking continued to mount and by the end of the 20th century the evidence against cigarettes had become overwhelming and even a major tobacco company said cigarettes were harmful to a person's health. Yet that smallest, slightest, infinitesimal possibility that cigarette is not a cause of lung cancer can not be totally eradicated even today. In part this is because the "gold standard test", a comparative clinical trial of smokers and non-smokers, has never been conducted.

Even if a clinical trial had been conducted, there is always the possibility that it would produce a contested result for reasons that will be explained later. Furthermore, let's re-examine the concern expressed by Fisher that a genetic factor causes both a desire to smoke and lung cancer. Replace the genetic connection with some event in a person's life that triggers a physiological or anatomical change in some people. The change has two effects. One it makes smoking a desirable habit and two it causes lung cancer. Yes, this idea is far-fetched, most unlikely and it's even fair to say I'm grasping at straws. However, even if the likelihood of such an event is one chance in a million or a billion or a trillion, it is not absolutely impossible either. But it is fair to say that smoking as a cause of lung cancer has been proven beyond a reasonable doubt. And note the qualifier, "beyond a reasonable doubt", is essential.

Chapter 2
The Case-Control Method – Looking Backwards

Abstract The process used in a case-control trial is examined and the strengths of the method described, especially its speed and flexibility. However, the obstacles and reservations associated with the technique are also discussed. The fact it only uncovers association rather than cause-and-effect relationships is highlighted. Ways to enhance the case-control method are provided. Based on the available evidence a conclusion is reached that the case-control method can lead researchers in the right direction, but not guarantee a definitive answer to a medical research question.

Keywords Association · case-control study · cause-and-effect · selection bias · treatment evaluation

The case-control method played a prime role in examining the link between smoking and lung cancer and gained a great deal of respect with researchers worldwide. However, much of that research took place in the 1950s and today it would be fair to say that the case-control method has more of a mixed reputation. There are still circumstances where it may be the only reasonable approach available, but if there are options, one of the higher ranked techniques will usually be preferred by research teams. Why? Because the case-control method may be relatively easy to do, it is very hard to do correctly.

As noted in the last chapter, a case-control study starts with an outcome and looks retrospectively for a cause. In a typical case-control study then, the histories of a group of patients with a disease or condition of interest (the cases) are compared to another group (the controls) who do not have the disease or condition.

Epidemiologists, who study factors affecting the health and illness of people, are trained to use the case-control and cohort trial methods. In fact, an exploratory research trial is sometimes referred to as an epidemiological study. The technique has been used to find possible risk factors or causes for a wide variety of diseases. As pointed out in the last chapter, the case-control design was instrumental in showing the link between smoking and lung cancer. Case-control studies also found heavy alcohol consumption was a risk factor for Alzheimer's disease. Epidemiologists have also used case-control trials to investigate other mental illnesses such as schizophrenia and manic-depression. In addition, a case-control study can also clear an accused agent of harm. It was largely responsible for showing that an alleged connection between artificial sweeteners and bladder cancer did not exist.

The Process

In a case-control study, you always begin at the end. Let us go back to the research on smoking and lung cancer. By "end" I mean you begin by identifying the people who already have the disease (i.e. lung cancer). Note that lung cancer is the result of a presumed causative agent (i.e. smoking). This method, therefore, starts by finding a group of people with lung cancer. As noted earlier, the lung cancer group is referred to as the "cases". Researchers look at the history of the cases to see if they have any characteristics in common that could be the cause of their disease.

But it's not sufficient in a case control study to look only at the cases. If we did, we'd find some smoked, but there would also be a group of non-smokers. To make sense out of those numbers we need a reference group and that's where the controls come in – they are the comparison group for the cases. The goal is to have the controls and the cases look alike except for one critical factor. The one requirement is obvious: the controls cannot have the disease under investigation; they must not have lung cancer.

The next step is to determine what the cases have in their backgrounds that are missing in the controls or visa versa. Did more people with lung cancer do some things that people without lung cancer did? For instance, we might find an unusually large number of lung cancer patients have stained yellow fingers compared to the controls. Could yellow fingers be the cause of lung cancer? No, logic tells us that yellow fingers cannot cause cancer. We may have found a relationship, but that doesn't make it a cause and effect relationship.

Obstacles and Reservations

Epidemiologists call the relationship found between lung cancer and yellow fingers an association. An association is based on a numerical connection between two variables. If one variable goes up and the second variable also goes up, they are said to be associated. If the price of tea goes up and the price of coffee goes up, there is an association between tea and coffee prices. But association does not mean cause and effect. The increase in the price of tea does not necessarily cause the increase in the price of coffee. There may be another factor that produces a rise in tea prices and a rise in coffee prices. Perhaps a harsh environment affected both tea and coffee production causing a shortage of these products and a consequential rise in the price of both tea and coffee.

There is an obvious factor that could account for the larger proportion of lung cancer patients with yellow fingers – people with stained yellow fingers are smokers. Heavy cigarette smoking can leave a yellow residue on the smoker's fingers. In addition smokers are more likely to develop lung cancer. Thus, it is the common factor, smoking, that causes a positive association between yellow fingers and lung cancer. Yellow fingers must be exonerated as a possible cause of lung cancer.

Epidemiologists recognize that association does not mean causation. They are well aware that the factors identified in a case-control project may not be the true cause of the disease. However, the likelihood that the exposure identified is the real cause can be strengthened if a dose response relationship is present. Let's go back to our smoking and lung cancer case.

Studies showed that the risk of having lung cancer was related to the number of cigarettes smoked each day, the age at which smoking began, and the number of years a person smoked. Furthermore, the risk of having lung cancer can be reduced by quitting, and the younger the person is when they stop smoking, the greater their health benefits. These findings provided strong support for the argument that prolonged exposure to smoking was a cause of lung cancer.

There are naturally difficulties with any research method and I'll briefly touch on some of the more important ones that apply to the case-control technique. When identifying who will be the cases, epidemiologists look for medical facilities that have records on a large number of patients with the target disease. There may be many possible places that have the desired information, such as hospitals, health maintenance organization, etc. Assume epidemiologists set out to conduct a case-control study about the cause of a fairly new illness and they locate a medical research center that has accumulated a large pool of medical records on people with the illness. As it turns out, the center is in the heart of a major city and is considered the best choice for trauma care and emergency room services. Having access to so many records will make the job easier the researchers reason. It appears that the researchers have selected an ideal setting for a case-control study. But no, that is not the case for several reasons.

First, think about the facility itself. Chances are that many of the potential cases may have arrived at the center through the emergency room and were very likely pretty sick at the time they entered the facility. As a result, there's a good chance that they are a unique set of patients that doesn't resemble the "typical" patient with the same illness. This means that these cases are almost assuredly a special subset of the total population of patients. Whatever finding results from the case study, it may not apply to all the people with the target disease.

Second, it's also important that all the cases have the same target disease, but at a large health care facility patient records are based on input from many different doctors who probably do not follow a consistent and rigorous definition for the same disease. If the target disease involves mental, emotional or behavioral disorders this also complicates a diagnosis since it's harder to have consensus among physicians when it comes to these psychological conditions. Unless strict parameters are applied to defining a disease, the selected patients at such a large health facility may represent a heterogeneous cadre of cases, and that can lead to misleading findings.

Selecting subjects for the control group can also be a problem in any setting. Controls often come from similar sources as the cases whether it is a hospital, clinic or medical research center. Epidemiologists want to end up with a control group that comes from the same general population as the cases. The goal is to have two equivalent groups with a major exception – the controls can not have the disease being investigated.

To illustrate the importance of selecting the right control group considers the implication from a case-control study in which aspirin is found to be one of the unusual exposures in the study of a particular disease. A very different conclusion would result if the controls used in such a study were ulcer patients or arthritic patients. The use of aspirin in ulcer patients would be very low since ulcer patients are told to avoid aspirin because it can cause bleeding. On the other hand, an opposite outcome would occur if the control group consists of patients with arthritis. Aspirin use would be unusually high among these patients because they take aspirin to offset the pain and inflammation associated with their disease. As a result, it would be very easy to implicate aspirin when the controls were ulcer patients because aspirin use among these patients is so low. However, it would be almost impossible to incriminate aspirin when the controls were arthritic patients because of the unusually heavy use of aspirin in this group of patients.

It is also possible to show how the selection of cases and controls can produce misleading results by using our smoking example. Suppose a naïve investigator undertakes a case-control investigation on whether smoking causes cataracts. He selects as his cases, patients with cataracts from a major eye clinic in Nevada. For controls, he picks people from an eye clinic in neighboring Utah that does not treat cataract patients. An unusually strong association between smoking and cataract development is found because the proportion of cases who smoke is much larger than the proportion of controls who smoke. The investigator prepares a paper on the fascinating result. However, a colleague reads the paper and saves him from a major blunder. She notes that most people in Utah belong to one religious group – they're Mormons. And, what is the Mormon church's position on smoking – the use of tobacco in any form is forbidden. The low proportion of smokers in the control group appears to be due primarily to the Mormon ban on smoking. Selection bias has affected the control group results and has almost assuredly caused the "fascinating" result.

When collecting data for a case-control study, especially data related to possible causes, there is the possibility that the thoroughness of the medical records may differ between the cases and the controls. If the information on cases is more extensive than that of the controls, then an overestimate for the number of cases with any exposure will occur. Obviously, the artificially higher rate of exposures in the cases will produce an incorrect conclusion. This problem is especially likely if the cases and controls come from two different places (e.g. two different hospitals or a walk-in medical facility in the suburbs versus an outpatient service at a metropolitan clinic).

Even if the records of the cases and controls are in the same institution, the recording process may not be the same throughout the facility. Because of their training, and the demands of their profession, different medical specialties may record information about a patient in a different fashion. Perhaps the doctors treating cardiac patients are more thorough recorders than those treating cancer patients. On the other hand, it could be the other way around. It doesn't matter because it's the inconsistency that's the problem.

In addition to collecting data from medical records, the case-control method may also gather information from interviews or questionnaires. All sorts of people have troubles remembering things, and participants in a case-control study are no different. However, many people cover up their forgetfulness by guessing. Worse yet their answers may be motivated by what the individual thinks the researchers wants to hear. In either case, the tainted information becomes part of the research evidence and incorrect data are deadly in any research project.

Strange as it may seem, patients' memories may differ between the cases and the controls. Cases often remember "better" than controls. When individuals are sick they may do a little research. They try to remember events such as: how could I have gotten this illness? How long will it last? They may ask friends or go to the Internet to learn more about their problem. They try to find out possible causes, recommended treatment, the prognosis and other signs and symptoms that may occur. From this kind of investigation, people may realize that they were exposed to a substance that our research says could be a precipitating cause for the illness. They can become unusually knowledgeable about their sickness. If the illness becomes the subject of a case-control study and they're included as a case, they can provide all sorts of information based on their research. A comparable control subject in the study, who by definition does not have the illness, is much less informed. The person could have had the identical substance exposure a case had, but there's no recall. It was no big event so he or she simply forgot it, but the case didn't. This type of recall inequality has a particularly negative effect on case-control studies. The control subject provides an erroneous answer and the suspected cause for the illness is under-reported.

Another potential problem with case-control studies is the untimely death issue. Let's assume there are data available on the relationship between heart attacks and smoking. The percentage of heart attack victims who smoked is compared to the percent of heart attack victims who did not smoke. The data are broken out by three age groups: 40–49, 50–59 and 60–69. In this hypothetical example, the results show a large difference for the youngest group. Most heart attack victims smoked (the cases) and only a relatively small percentage of those without a heart attack smoked (the controls). This is just what would be expected – so far so good. In the middle age group there is still a difference between cases and controls but it's much smaller. Finally, in the oldest group there is no difference at all between the case and controls. What's the conclusion?

On the surface it looks like smoking is bad for the younger people, but things improve with age. That doesn't seem right, but that's what the data appear to show. What's going on here? Why does it look like the effects of smoking become less damaging as people age? The answer is death. The 40–49 year old smokers who die never make it to the next age bracket. Many of the smokers who do make it to the 50–59 age grouping subsequently die as well, and they can't be included in the 60–69 age bracket. As a result, in the higher age groups, the people who died from their lung cancer can't be included; they don't count anymore. Their omission wrongly created the incorrect impression that developing lung cancer in smokers levels off with age.

Finally there is another major problem that can never be ignored in the case-control study. It's called selection bias. Assume epidemiologists did a case-control trial to find what might be the cause of an unusual kind of skin rash. The results point to a relatively new drug since a much larger percentage of the cases (those with the rash) took the drug compared to the controls (those without the rash). It certainly looks like the drug is responsible for the onset of the rash. However, always lurking in the background is the fact that the cases took the drug for some reason and the controls didn't need the drug. We are therefore always left to wonder if the reason for taking the drug, and not the drug itself, is the cause of the rash. Here's what could happen. What if the drug with the excessive number of rashes was used to treat allergies? Furthermore, in the past it was some of the allergies that produced the rash being studied. Consequently, the drug didn't cause the rash; the rash was an allergic reaction and then the drug was used to treat the rash.

Now it's easy to see what happened in this case because it's well known that allergies can cause rashes. Any epidemiologist involved in the trial would have collected information on allergies and not been misled when a drug to treat allergies came up as a possible cause. However, it is only possible to recognize the selection problem and control for it when the factors (e.g. allergy) that could cause an outcome (rash) are known. If that information doesn't exist, selection bias can wreak havoc with any case-control study.

Note that in this discussion the term bias has a special meaning. Researchers like to use the term bias to refer to an element in a research study that may lead to a wrong conclusion. For instance they may say the study groups are biased because the groups being compared are not equivalent and the inequality causes one group to end up with more positive (or negative) results. Note that the observed result is a consequence of the composition of the groups rather than the treatments administered. Here's an example. One group has a greater proportion of females and the disease under study is tougher to treat in females. Consequently the treatment group with more females is penalized, but not because a treatment is less effective. It's because the group has a larger proportion of females.

The Advantage of Speed and Flexibility

Since I was quick to pick out flaws, let's be fair and close on a positive note by citing the advantages of the case-control method. Number one: it can yield important medical results within a short period of time. It doesn't cost a lot of money compared to other research methods. It doesn't require as much effort either.

Use of the case-control technique is an ideal way to obtain initial ideas on possible causes of a disease. It is very efficient. All, or at least most of the data already exists – unlike the cohort or experiential study, it doesn't have to be manufactured. Medical centers have an abundant number of patients with all sorts of diseases. The records containing historical and current information about the patient are there for the asking. If the investigators don't get all the information they need they might have to do some interviewing or sending out a questionnaire, but that's a lot less costly than generating all the data from scratch.

The method is also extremely versatile. Case-control studies are particularly useful in studying multiple causes of a single disease. Several different potential causes can be identified when comparing the data from the same set of cases and controls. In addition, the case-control methodology can be used to find the potential cause of other entities besides disease. It can be used to find the cause of accidents, deaths, major adverse drug reactions or just about anything a researcher wants to investigate. Its flexibility is nicely demonstrated by the diversity of outcomes examined (from earthquakes to racehorse injuries) and exposures tested (ranging from pickled vegetables to pig farming).

When researching a rare disease, the case-control approach may be the only choice. The cohort method could require extremely large number of participants and possibly a very long period of time before the disease appeared in enough patients to provide useful data. The experimental clinical study could have a difficult recruitment process and could also be subject to a long observation period before results would be available. In terms of time and cost, the case-control study is often the clear winner. There are also definite ways to strengthen the case-control method.

Enhancing the Case-Control Study

An important enhancement is to use more than one control group to help overcome the selection of controls problem. With a second or third control group, researchers can obtain substantiation or rejection of the findings that surfaced with an initial control group. Here's how this could work. Assume the disease in question is colon cancer and the epidemiologist uses hospitalized patients with other cancers for the initial control group. It's possible to create a second control group consisting of people who are neighbors of the cases. The neighbors would be about the same in terms of socio-economic status, but they would not have colon cancer. If the control group of neighbors gives similar results to that of the hospital controls, we have a form of confirmation, strengthening the study conclusions.

Because a lack of equivalence between cases and controls is such a problem, here's a technique researchers use to get around it. Match the patients in the two groups. Matching involves setting up categories such as age and gender and then making sure that for every case there is a control person of the same gender and approximate age. Race and socioeconomic status are other popular matching criteria. Researchers can use whatever categories they want, but they have to be careful. As they add categories they make it more difficult to find a control who matches a case on all factors. If there's not an abundance of potential controls, the matching scheme may not work.

The case-control study plays a critical role in medical research. By and large the investigators who use the method are unusually talented, creative and careful. They deliver extremely valuable information and are well aware of the limitations of this research method. When case-control trials are well designed and carefully executed, they provide invaluable medical information. Nevertheless, they, as all research techniques, have flaws. Good epidemiologists are aware of these pitfalls. They need do all they can to overcome the obstacles, and carefully qualify their results when they believe a possible problem was not adequately addressed.

Unfortunately, as the news of their research wends its way through the media, the results can be overstated and the cautions understated. If you read a story of a major finding (good or bad; positive or negative) from a case-control study be skeptical. It is clear, and researchers would agree, that there are always reservations associated with a case-control study. The truth is when it comes to case-control trials, it is best to treat the conclusions from these studies as hypotheses. Hypotheses that need to be supported or refuted by additional research.

There is one qualification to this recommendation. If there are no other decent studies on hand for a health problems that demands attention and all health officials have is a well designed and executed case-control trial, then it should be used. The chances are much more likely that it has correct rather than incorrect answers. Ignoring the results would be irresponsible. But use the results with caution, don't overly interpret them, be sure your audience is aware of the study's qualifications and continue to support continuing research on the subject.

Chapter 3
The Cohort Study – Watchful Waiting

Abstract The cohort study, a natural and straight-forward approach to medical research offers investigators another tool to evaluate medical treatments. All sorts of heath data are collected on a set of people who are then followed to see what happens to them over time. Background data on participants who develop a disease are compared to those without the disease in hopes of findings what may be the cause of the ailment. Two successful major cohort studies, the Framingham Heart Study and the Nurses Health Study are described so readers can appreciate the cohort technique. Disadvantages such as cost and possible bias because of participant dropouts are also covered.

Keywords Cohort study · Framingham Heart Study · Nurses Health Study · prospective research · retrospective research

The degree of confidence in the answers from a medical study depends heavily on the research method applied so we now need to look more closely at another research design available to investigators – the cohort study. This method is intuitively appealing – a group of people are carefully followed and observations are made about what happens to them. However, even when epidemiologists apply this method flawlessly and ingeniously, there's still no guarantee that their answers will be absolutely correct.

The cohort study is another exploratory research method with many aliases. Sometimes it is called a follow-up study, at other times a longitudinal study. The term "cohort" may be the best choice (and it is most often used in medical communications) because it refers to a group of people that will be or have been followed over a period of time.

As an illustration, suppose a case report suggests that drug X protects people from the inevitable decline in physical and mental health as they age. A health maintenance organization (HMO) agrees to use its patients in a study to see if drug X really works. The researchers create cohorts with people who have the same disease (one with people who are taking drug X and another for people who do not take drug X) and follow them to see how their health status changes over time.

Assume that after a number of years a difference in the health status of the two groups appears. The group on the drug is healthier. There appears to be a relationship between the drug and better health. But remember, there is only an association – there may not be a cause and effect connection.

What could explain the result? The finding could be due to other reasons besides having an effective drug. The drug group could have received better medical care, the non-drug group could have had more subjects with a poor prognosis. If the subjects who took the drug also tended to be better off financially, they could easily have had better access to health care. Perhaps that superior access was what kept them healthier – not the drug they were taking, There are all sorts of possible explanations and each one needs to be examined by the researchers and information produced to see if it should be eliminated as a possible causative factor. Identifying and tracking down the evidence is an enormous task.

A cohort investigation does not have to begin by targeting a drug for study. It may begin with a group of people without a disease who are monitored to see what diseases develop over time. Baseline information is collected such as their ages, weights, blood pressures, drugs they're taking, illness they had, etc. At periodic intervals the participants are re-examined to see what has changed. The data is collected according to preset standards. Still the epidemiologists have to worry about whether the association they have found is a true cause and effect relationships or just an irrelevant correlation.

The cohort studies can be described as the crème de crème of the exploratory research methods although many of the issues that plague the case-control study can also undermine the cohort study. Nevertheless, the cohort approach usually has fewer problems because the data is better organized than that for a case-control study and is collected in a more consistent manner. We don't have to rely so much on "old" records that are loosely organized.

An important feature of the cohort method is that epidemiologists can use the data collected on a cohort trial that has run for a long time to research a new question. The valuable information accumulated in a cohort study may also be used to learn more about a second disease. Many patients in the database will not have the new disease, but some will have subsequently acquired it while others remained disease free. Epidemiologists can now see how the backgrounds differ among people with and without the new disease. For instance, in addition to lung cancer a cohort that includes smokers and non-smokers could determine smoking's association with such conditions as emphysema or heart disease.

Excellent data sources for cohort trials are the large databases health insurance plans have. As an example, the records of Kaiser-Permanente, an HMO, have been used as the data source for a number of important cohort studies such as the effect of coffee on cirrhosis of the liver and whether obesity increases dementia later in life. Within Kaiser-Permanente, there is a division dedicated to research with over 80 published scientific papers to its credit.

Adding Up the Advantages

The cohort study has a number of distinct advantages compared to a case-control trial. Here are some of the most important ones. In a cohort study, researchers can lay down strict rules so the information is collected in a uniform manner, and that results in more consistent and better quality data. Cohort investigators do not have to worry as much about how well the controls remember important events compared to the cases because in a cohort study the research information is collected before the disease occurs. Therefore, differences in what "sick" and "well" people remember are nullified in the cohort method.

To be legitimate, a possible cause must precede the development of the disease. With a cohort study it is generally clear what came first – the possible cause or the disease because the data are collected on am ongoing basis. The case-control method is more vulnerable to the possibility that the sequence of the two events could be reversed because all the data are obtained from past records that may not contain accurate information on the onset of a treatment or disease.

Cohort studies also provide a disease rate which is not possible in a case-control study. This is so because to calculate a disease rate, two numbers are needed – the number of people with the disease and the number of people at risk for the disease. A disease rate is not possible in a case-control trial because the number of people at risk is not known. Obtaining a disease rate for a cohort study is straightforward. Suppose a cohort study starts with 1,000 people who do not have arthritis. Over time, 14 of the subjects developed the disease. There is both the number with arthritis (14) and the number at risk (1,000) and for this cohort, arthritis developed in 1.4 percent of the people. In a case-control study, epidemiologists know all the cases have arthritis, and also that all the controls do not have arthritis. However, they do not collect information on the number of people at risk for arthritis because such information isn't necessary in the comparison between the cases and controls.

Disadvantages

In spite of its advantages however, the cohort study doesn't escape criticism. Selection bias, cost and dropouts all contribute to its vulnerability. Self-selection bias is perhaps the most serious failing of the cohort study, a flaw that it shares with the case-control methodology. Self-selection bias can lead to an imbalance in the type of subjects that make up the treatment and control groups. In a cohort study, the individual patients along with their physician, select what treatment he or she will take. The patients also decide whether they'll consume alcoholic beverages, drink lots of milk, avoid coffee, etc. For instance, cohorts could be created for coffee and non-coffee drinkers. If a cohort study finds that a disease is much more common among the people who drink coffee, it may indeed be because of the coffee. However, people who drink coffee may differ from the non-coffee drinker in a number of ways. They may smoke more, consume more alcohol, eat fewer vegetables, etc. Maybe one of these factors is the cause of the disease and as a result coffee should be exonerated. The truth is that we do not know for sure if coffee is the culprit or not.

A serious challenge to the soundness of a cohort study occurs when a significant number of participants drop out: they move away, they lose interest or they die. Each loss is a threat to the value of the study because it reduces the number of participants in the database, but more importantly it, could introduce a bias into the study itself. Bias occurs if the losses are related to the disease being studied. For example, assume epidemiologists use an ongoing cohort study to learn more about causes of a lung disease in the local community. However, shortly after the study begins a major employer in the area closes its factory and relocates workers to another state. Unfortunately (for the researchers), one of the causes of the lung illness is the use of toxic material dispensed at the plant in question. With the relocations, the cohort loses a disproportionate number of subjects who will develop the disease. Had they not dropped out of the trial, the toxic substances at the plant might well have been identified as the likely disease cause. That is less likely to happen now because those subjects are no longer part of the cohort. The cause of the lung disease is under-reported and any relationship may be missed.

Cohort studies are also costly. They run a long time and the required medical tests are expensive. Consequently, a disease that takes a long time to develop is hard to research in a cohort trial. A 20 or 30 year wait to find the possible causes of a disease that takes a long time to develop may be intolerable. For example, stomach and pancreatic cancers tend to develop over a relatively long period of time. It may take decades after a cohort is assembled until there are enough cases of these kinds of cancer to have an adequately sized data set and the search for potential causes begins. The cost and time problem is exaggerated when the disease of interest has a low occurrence rate. In this situation, a large number of people must be followed up before useful results become available. For example, diseases such as childhood cancers are unusual and not a good disease to study using the cohort approach. The longer the study, the greater the risk of losing a high percentage of the patients for a variety of reasons and that, as we saw in the discussion on dropouts, bodes poorly for a successful trial.

No one can dispute the fact that categorizing a smoker as a non-smoker or visa versa can make a really mess of a study on the causes of lung disease. However, classifying possible causes of a disease isn't as straightforward as it may appear. Here's where the problem lies. Whenever people stop doing something they were doing regularly or start doing something they hardly ever did before, a cohort study has a big problem, especially when the change goes undetected. Suppose epidemiologists set out to find risk factors for liver disease. When a subject joined the cohort trial, he rarely drank and was placed in the non-drinker category. His habits then changed – he now enjoys a glass of wine with his dinner meal and a cordial after dinner. The original classification is wrong. We no longer have a teetotaler, but the researcher may have no way of knowing this. Fads come and go, but they can leave in their wake a great deal of confusion for researchers doing a cohort study. The latest diet craze may help an overweight woman take off a few pounds (a good effect). But if she is in a cohort trial, that's looking into the causes of obesity, and she started out as a case in the overweight group, should she stay there? Even if she's no longer obese, she's probably been obese most of her life and besides, maybe she'll put those pounds back on pretty soon anyway. But what if she wasn't always heavy and doesn't put the weight back on? The epidemiologist faces a tough decision on whether she should be considered a study case, be re-classified as a control or be disqualified.

Although misclassification is a problem in any kind of medical research, it is a greater issue for cohort trials due to their extended length. There's simply more time for subjects to modify their behavior.

Framingham Heart Study

It will be worthwhile to next examine a couple of well know cohort studies and see how the technique works in practice. Case studies nicely illustrate how the cohort method can advanced medical sciences as well as stymie it.

Almost daily, we are warned that certain behaviors and lifestyle choices, may be dangerous to our health. In the Framingham Heart Study (FHS), the goal was to learn more about cardiovascular disease, what factors were associated with heart and blood vessel abnormalities. Much of what is known today about risk factors for heart disease: high blood pressure, high cholesterol, overweight, physical inactivity, smoking and diabetes was a mystery before the FHS shed light on these subjects.

The FHS got its name from a small New England town, Framingham, Massachusetts. Researchers formed the initial cohort in 1948 using the town residents. The cohort was selected in a random fashion and consisted of just over 5,000 men and women. In 1971, another 5,000 plus residents were added – they were the children of the original group plus the children's spouses.

At the time the study was conceived, it was already known that cardiovascular disease was the leading cause of death among men. But little was known about how the disease developed. The original participants, who were between 30 and 60 years of age when they joined the study, underwent detailed physical examinations every two years, including an electrocardiogram, chest X-ray, and laboratory tests. They took dozens of other medical tests and answered detailed questions about their personal habits. Eventually the epidemiologists collected a diverse set of data. It included all sorts of information. For example, the use of estrogens, age at menopause, smoking history and alcohol consumption. After the researchers collected their data, they waited and watched looking for connections between the diseases the people contracted and the background information that had been assembled. It took over 10 years before the most significant results began to be recognized. Time had been required for diseases to develop.

The FHS is now considered a landmark research trial – one of the most important medical studies in history. The cost exceeds $40 million, paid by the study sponsors, the National Institutes of Health (NIH), and is considered a wise investment. In the 1960s, the study demonstrated the role cigarette smoking plays in the development of heart disease. Those findings helped to fuel the first anti-smoking campaigns of that era. Data gathered from the participants also showed how elevated blood pressure contributes to the risk of heart attack and stroke. Engaging in physical activity was found to reduce the risk of heart attacks. Obesity was discovered to be one of the important risk factors for heart attacks.

However, in spite of all the positive news, the weaknesses of the cohort approach are also present. Not all its results can be applied to the general public. After all 5,000 residents in a New England village may not be all that similar to 5,000 people who live in a sleepy hamlet in the South. Furthermore, the participants who receive regular health exams, are more aware of heart disease risk factors and have their medical problems noticed a lot sooner than the people who reside in a remote dessert town in the Southwest.

One noticeable FHS finding that has been questioned dealt with cholesterol levels. In 1961 the FHS found that high cholesterol levels increased the risk of heart disease. In 1988 the finding was refined when the FHS reported that high levels of HDL cholesterol (often called the "good" cholesterol) actually reduced the risk of death due to heart disease. It was LDL (the "bad" cholesterol) that was the problem.

An NIH sponsored committee established guidelines on recommended levels of HDL and LDL (in large part based on the FHS results) that would be needed to begin a treatment program. Treatment options included losing excess weight, exercising regularly, and following a diet low in saturated fat and cholesterol as well as taking cholesterol-lowering drugs.

However, the standards for the HDL and LDL levels took a hit in 2004 when the results of a clinical trial were reported in the *New England Journal of Medicine*. The trialists treated patients with a class of drugs called statins, even though the subjects had LDL levels below the recommended values set by the NIH committee. In theory, there wasn't much to be gained by treating these patients with cholesterol lowering drugs. Surprisingly, the patients treated with Lipitor, one of the study drugs, had large decreases in their LDL and there was a major bonus – they also had fewer heart attacks and deaths. Their healthier status was also supported by the fact that fewer remedial procedures (bypass surgery and angioplasty) were needed. Had the FHS missed the boat on how best to protect people?

A second finding also reflected poorly on the Framingham cholesterol recommendations. This time it had to do with the good cholesterol, HDL. The Framingham based recommendation essentially allowed high levels of HDL to offset some of the negative result from a high LDL level. But, based on the experimental study mentioned above, the benefit of lowering LDL was the same whether HDL levels were high or low.

There is no guarantee that the experimental clinical study got it right and Framingham's cohort study had it wrong. Maybe they are both off the mark. Perhaps when best to begin treatment is based on a totally different set of HDL and LDL levels. It's too early to tell, but the point is that you can never be sure what the correct answer is to a medical problem from a single study,

Several new Framingham initiatives are under way, including research into what genes are responsible for heart disease. Researchers from around the world have access to the data that's been accumulated on FHS research topics such as osteoporosis, nutrition, as well as eye and lung diseases. When others use the

Framingham database for a research project they frequently employ the retrospective cohort study design. For example, there exists over 50 years of information on Framingham participants' alcohol consumption and frequency of bone fractures. Using this database researchers concluded that alcohol consumption was associated with a significant increase in the risk of a fracture. Another study found that post-menopausal use of estrogens protected women against hip fractures. We'll see later that the value of estrogens in women who went through menopause became very controversial, but the reduction in hip fractures has remained a positive finding for estrogen users.

> *In the little more than 50 years of its existence, the Framingham Heart Study has yielded many of the central insights that support our current approach to assessing risk for cardiovascular disease. The investigators' high standards have consistently led to observations of enduring value.* (Vaccarino V, Krumholz H., *Annals of Internal Medicine*)

Nurses' Health Study

Another major cohort study is the Nurses' Health Study (NHS). It began in 1976, also funded by the National Institutes of Health. The primary purpose in starting the study was to investigate the long term use of oral contraceptives. In 1976 the "pill" had become a very popular method to prevent an unwanted pregnancy. Women, who did not want to become pregnant, planned to stay on the pill for decades. They felt passionately about this means of contraception, but there was a looming problem. There was considerable uncertainty about whether the pill was safe. In smaller trials, taking the pill was shown to increase the risk of blood clots, heart attacks and stroke. A link with breast cancer was also suspected.

The epidemiologists selected nurses for the study and for good reason. Due to their education, they could accurately answer technically worded questions. In addition, their medical background motivated them to join and fully participate in the long-term study. The subjects, married registered nurses aged 30–55 and living in the 11 most populous states, enrolled in the cohort after they answered a baseline questionnaire. Approximately 120,000 nurses out of the 170,000 nurses to whom the questionnaire was mailed, responded.

Every two years cohort members received a follow-up questionnaire about diseases and health-related topics such as smoking, hormone use, child bearing and menopausal status. Information about other health areas, added in later years, included diet habits, exercise programs and quality of life issues. Response rates to the questionnaires were high – around 90 percent for each two-year cycle.

The thoroughness of this project is impressive. Because certain aspects of diet, such as minerals that come from the food a person eats, cannot be measured by a questionnaire, the nurses submitted 68,000 sets of toenail samples between the 1982 and 1984 surveys so that quantitative measures of mineral intake could be calculated. Similarly, to identify hormone levels and genetic markers the researchers collected over 30,000 blood samples in 1989 and almost 20,000 in 2001.

A second cohort project, with the descriptive but unimaginative name of Nurses' Health Study II, began in 1989. The purpose of this study was to examine reproductive health issues that could not be addressed by the original study. For example, birth control pills contained substantially lower doses of hormones in 1989 then they did when the women in the NHS began taking them. The researchers also wanted more data on younger women. The study organizers mailed questionnaires, similar to the ones used in the original NHS, to the target population – 117,000 nurses between the ages of 25 and 42 years. Response rates for this cohort also were very high, about 90 percent.

The NHS helped to identify many of the factors that affect women's health. A partial list of the impressive findings appears in Table 3.1.

Table 3.1 Finding from the Nurses' Health Study

Health behavior	Result
Oral contraceptives	Taking the pill lowered ovarian cancer risk
Pain pills (i.e. aspirin)	Taking large amount of aspirin doubled the stroke risk
Alcohol	Drinking small amounts of alcohol decreased heart disease risk
Fats	Using vegetable oil rather than animal fats lowered heart attack risk
Fiber	More fiber in the diet decreased heart disease risk
Meat	The more meat eaten, the higher the colon cancer risk
Nuts	Eating nuts lowered heart attack risk
Physical activity	Brisk walking lowered heart disease risk
Fractures	Estrogens after menopause lowered hip fracture risk
Smoking	Smoking increased heart disease and lung cancer risks

For our purposes the major finding had to do with the effect that hormone replacement therapy (HRT) had on the heart in post menopausal women. The initial report of the NHS, published in 1985 after nurses had been observed for almost 10 years, found that the hormones reduced the risk of heart disease in postmenopausal women. This remarkable finding was expanded in a NHS 1996 report to add that estrogen and progestin in combination reduced the risk of heart disease by essentially the same degree as estrogens alone. According to the NHS data, postmenopausal women, who used estrogen or the hormone combination, had about a 40 percent lower risk for heart disease compared with women who never used hormones. Many other studies using the exploratory research method had come up with a similar result, but the finding by the NHS was the most impressive. It was large (over 70,000 postmenopausal women), it was methodologically sound, it covered a long period of observation (20 years) and it was conducted by a prestigious university (Harvard University School of Public Health).

> *(The Nurses Health Study) – One of the most significant studies ever conducted on the health of women.* (Donna Shalala, Secretary, U.S. Department of Health and Human Services)

The cohort trial can be a powerful tool for medical research. It has uncovered innumerable truths about medical matters, but it has also had its share of failures. Medical science looks to the cohort trial to continue to play a crucial role in gaining insights into diseases and the best treatment for illnesses. A later chapter, devoted to the use of HRT in women, revisits the optimistic results from the NHS.

Chapter 4
The Clinical Trial – The Gold Standard

Abstract The clinical trial, the most highly regarded research method is evaluated and a brief history of the clinical trial is included. Considered the gold standard for medical research, the clinical trial is held in such high regard because it is based on the simple but remarkable principles of a scientific experiment. Randomization of subjects to treatments, double blinding and the use of contemporaneous control groups add to its appeal. Nevertheless, in spite of it lofty position it can't guarantee that it's found all the correct answer in any single trial. No matter how well planned and executed a study's conclusions may still be wrong.

Keywords Clinical trial · control group · double-blind · randomization · scientific method

The clinical trial is the sine qua non in clinical research. It is the most highly regarded and popular design for advancing medial science. It could more accurately be called an "experimental trial", but that expression is rarely if ever used in the medical literature. Medical researchers usually use the term "clinical trial" or "clinical study" as synonyms and I will also use those terms to refer to the experimental approach. In part, the aversion to the expression "experimental study" can be traced to the horrific and immoral medical experiments performed by the Nazi's in World War II. Modern day researchers do not want to be connected in any way to that dreadful period. Still, experimental study is a very descriptive term because it exemplifies how science discovers the truth about unknown phenomena. The ability to conduct experiments is the incredible advantage that this method has over exploratory studies.

Due to its popularity and importance, I devote many chapters to the clinical trial. But first let me set forth its main features and place it in historical context.

The experimental approach allows a researcher to intervene and design a study to overcome the biases that undermine the exploratory approach. Researchers can assign patients to treatments so that the selection bias, that threatens and frequently defeats the validity of the case-control and cohort trials, is in principal held in check. As we saw, with the exploratory research methods, the control and treated groups may be quite different because researchers cannot be assured that they placed subjects in these groups in an unbiased fashion. Furthermore, a clinical trial tries to keep everything, except the treatment the subjects receive, the same. This includes what the patients are told about the trial, what other drugs they can or cannot take, what tests they must have performed, when they must have an examination, etc. In contrast, there are few, if any, restrictions on study participants in exploratory studies. For example, they may start or stop other medications, change their diet, etc. As we have seen, the lack of control allows outside factors, and not just the comparison treatments, to influence the outcomes of an exploratory trial.

The Scientific Method

Disciplines that consider themselves "sciences" follow a common approach to research referred to as the scientific method. The clinical trial seeks to emulate this approach. In brief, the scientific method consists of four basic steps:

1. Identify an issue or problem
2. Form a hypothesis
3. Test the hypothesis – perform an experiment
4. Draw conclusions

The scientific method assumes that the event or condition that a scientist is interested in has a cause or causes. It is also implied that the cause(s) can be discovered. The process begins by being alert, observing, by noticing something that is unusual, unexpected, a problem that needs to be investigated.

All scientific disciplines use the scientific method as their paradigm. However, each field must adapt the method to the subject matter with which they work, and along the way, they face formidable problems. Each discipline relies on inquisitive professionals to overcome the obstacles and produce explanations and answers. The challenges vary from one field to the next and require the development of special skills, tools and methodology. The clinical trial serves as the primary means for medical researchers to get at the answers they desire.

It's useful to see how this process works. For an example, I'll go back to the end of the 18th century before the cause of scurvy was identified. A member of the British Royal Navy observes that there is an unacceptable level of scurvy on naval ships. A possible cause, he surmises, is the lack of fresh fruit eaten by the sailors. This possibility is framed as a question: will eating fresh fruit protect sailors from developing scurvy? An experiment is designed in which some sailors on board a ship are given fresh oranges and limes (the experimental group) and others are not (the control group). The number of sailors is the same for each group and outside of the difference in fruit, the diets are the same. The number of sailors in each group who develop scurvy are noted. If the number with scurvy is much lower in the group that eats fresh fruit, we conclude that fresh fruit prevents scurvy.

This simple example and conclusion is just that – too simple. The conclusion may be absolutely correct, but then again it may not. A little more thought is called for. Even if there is less scurvy among the sailors eating fruit, could there be other causes for the observed difference? Were the two groups equivalent at the start of the trial? If one group was younger, could that result in a lower rate of scurvy? There must also be a level of operational control that can rule out other causes besides the treatment (eating fresh fruit) as the cause of the scurvy. Did one group have light work duties with less exposure to the elements? If so, could that have been the cause of the lower number of scurvy cases? There are a plethora of other questions that could be asked as well. A look at the qualities of the clinical trial will help us understand what else could have influenced the scurvy trial results.

Clinical Trial Features

In designing the study a vital step was omitted. The planners correctly included a treatment and a control group, but they should have assigned the sailors to the two groups based on a random assignment process. They could have picked their names out of a hat and assigned the first sailor chosen to one treatment and the second to the alternative treatment. They could repeat this selection process until all sailors had been assigned to one of the treatments. This step, called random treatment allocation, would have increased the possibility that the two groups were equivalent for factors such as age, work duties, etc.

In medicine, the acronym RCT is often used to refer to a most popular form of a clinical trial. RCT stands for randomized controlled trial. The R clearly identifies the need for randomization and the C the need for controls, which are essential features of a sound clinical study. The T simply stands for trial. However, even the initials expose an important omission – the best clinical trial uses blinding and there is no initial for that feature. Most clinical trials are called double blind studies, which means that two parties, the patient and the researcher, are unaware of the treatment assigned to the patient. Blinding eliminates prejudice on the part of the subjects and the individuals who make the assessments in a clinical trial. They cannot modify their observations and assessments based on the assigned treatment because they are unaware of that treatment assignment. If only one party (the investigator or the subject) is unaware of the assigned treatment, the expression "single blind" is used, but few trials are run in this fashion. From now one, the term blinding will be used to refer to double blind trials since this is the preferred and most common approach.

The omission of a reference to blinding is a serious oversight and in this book the acronym RABCOT (RAndomized Blinded COntrolled Trial) rather than RCT is used to represent the best kind of clinical trial. The essential components of the RABCOT are listed below along with a comparative look at the exploratory studies.

1. Allocating treatments fairly. The way to avoid an unfair result is to assign subjects to the control and treatment groups so any inequality is minimized. Case-control and cohort studies are unable to randomize subjects to treatments so the clinical trial is far superior in respect to this attribute.
2. Providing a frame of reference to judge the result. The best way to evaluate an experimental treatment is to compare its results to those from a carefully assigned control group. Clinical trials can include control groups that are superior to those used in the case-control and cohort method.
3. Keeping personal preferences from influencing the result. Through the blinding process researchers control the risk that one of the treatments in a clinical trial may be favored over the other one. This feature is not possible in the case-control approach nor is it feasible in a cohort trial.

The First Clinical Trial

The earliest recorded clinical trial, documented in the Old Testament, describes how Daniel proposed an experiment to King Nebuchadnezzar. For 10 days servants would be fed a diet of legumes (vegetables such as peas, beans, etc.) and water. The appearance of the servants would then be compared to youths who ate the "King's food". At the end of the 10-day trial the servants looked better and healthier than the youths who ate the King's food. Because of the "experiment", the young people's diet was switched to legumes and water. Perhaps, motivated by the move to a healthier diet, the King also ordered a reduction in wine.

Although this biblical experiment is extraordinary for its time, there are some obvious flaws. Among the most egregious sins is a clear lack of comparability between the experimental (servants) and control (young people) groups. In addition, the measurement was quite subjective (how they looked) and in an unblinded trial that spells trouble. It also would be nice to know the number of people participating in the trial. It would make a big difference in our confidence in the results if there were three people per group versus 50.

The first clinical trial of a novel therapy is usually attributed to a Renaissance surgeon. In 1537 Ambroise Paré, who was the official surgeon for the Kings of France, served as a military surgeon during the French campaign in Italy. To prevent battlefield wounds from becoming infected, the customary practice was to pour boiling oil on the wound. When the oil ran out one day, Paré prepared an ancient Roman remedy containing egg yolk, oil of roses, and turpentine to treat the wounds. When he compared the results of the turpentine mixture to the standard boiling oil method, he found, much to his delight, that the new treatment was more effective than the traditional formula he had been using.

This trial, just as our biblical story, lacks the qualities required by a RABCOT. There is no control group, no randomization and no blinding and yet the result seems very believable. You clearly don't need to conduct a RABCOT to find a reasonable answer to an important medical question. But by today's standards,

Dr. Paré mini-experiment would require a lot of verification by RABCOTs before his turpentine mixture became a battlefield staple.

A number of more current examples show how clinical trials continue to enrich medical research. Today, a new drug will not enter the U.S. marketplace until its efficacy is demonstrated in clinical trials. However, the clinical trial can do much more than find effective products. It is also extremely good when it comes to exposing ineffective treatments. Here is one example.

The use of bone marrow transplants seemed to make sense as a treatment option for women with advanced breast cancer. Bone marrow taken from a patient would be re-infused to replace the cells damages and destroyed after high dose chemotherapy. Other treatments were only minimally effective and, therefore, the bone marrow transplants were, on theoretical grounds, a promising alternative. Unfortunately, there were no conclusive clinical trials showing that the transplants were effective and it became very difficult to conduct a controlled trial. The bottleneck was trying to recruit subjects. Physicians did not want their patient randomly assigned to the group that would not receive the bone marrow. It took decades before researchers performed several clinical studies and, in 1999, the preliminary results started to come in with disappointing findings. By 2001, the results failed to improve and bone marrow transplant appeared to be no better than the other minimally effective treatments. Unfortunately, by the time the clinical trials showed that bone marrow transplants were ineffective, more than 30,000 women had received the costly but useless treatment.

The clinical trial can also be instrumental in finding the cause of baffling medical catastrophes. The contribution of the clinical trial was especially noteworthy in the case involving the use of oxygen in premature babies, which is beautifully illustrated by a report in *The Braille Monitor*. The use of oxygen to treat underdeveloped newborns was first tried back in 1780. By the early 1940s, supplemental oxygen was standard treatment for premature infants in the best-equipped hospitals. Oxygen saved the lives of countless babies. Unfortunately, a physical improvement turned this laudable scene into an unbelievable calamity. In the mid-1940s, a new manufacturing process produced airtight incubators. No longer would pumped-in oxygen leak out. Shortly thereafter, an epidemic of blindness struck premature newborns and baffled scientists for a decade. What made the solution so difficult was that the blindness was not quickly recognized. Children could be one or two years old before the parents discovered something was wrong with their child's sight.

Finding a cause for the loss of sight was no easy task because when the loss occurred was not known. The research to find the cause began with a case series publication in a medical journal about five blind children. All five babies had been born prematurely. Even if the blindness could be related to a premature birth, it was important to know when it occurred. If the blindness occurred in the gestational period the use of incubators would not be relevant. Proof that babies weren't born blind came from a look at past records at Johns Hopkins Hospital. A research team found no cases of child blindness from 1935 to 1944, but five after 1945. The five cases all occurred in premature infants, but all five had normal eyes at birth. A giant step forward, but no one still knew what was causing the blindness. Then two doctors had a novel thought – was it the high level of oxygen given to premature infants? They tested their theory in a small clinical trial run in the wards of a hospital in Washington. They published their work incriminating excess oxygen as the cause of blindness, but nothing happened. Their trial was small and the world didn't believe them. They designed a second, bigger experiment conducted at more than a dozen American hospitals. When this large trial confirmed the earlier report, physicians paid attention. A lower level of oxygen could still save babies lives, and their sight as well.

But the study's results did something else equally important and historic. They convinced many in the American medical profession of the usefulness of the clinical trial. The lesson learned was that you should never assume that what seemed like a good idea (better oxygen delivery), would necessarily lead to a successful outcome. The cost was significant. An estimated 10,000 children around the world are blind from too much oxygen. Perhaps the most famous is Stevie Wonder, born prematurely in Michigan in 1950.

The record is clear – clinical trials are the most valuable technique in the medical research arsenal. The medical community is convinced that the clinical trial has earned its place as the gold standard when it comes to evaluating new medical products. It is the principle method to demonstrate what works (and what doesn't) in medicine. New drugs and medical devices cannot be made available to the public until clinical trails satisfy FDA's requirements for safety and efficacy. And a clinical trial that disproves the effectiveness of a treatment, while disappointing, is just as important as a trial that proves the effectiveness of a new treatment.

Nonetheless, the clinical trial is a complex and demanding research method in which there are many opportunities for error. Part II of this book explores the workings of the clinical trial more thoroughly and provides convincing evidence that even the best researchers cannot guarantee that their clinical trial has come up with all the correct answers. But first, there will be the next chapter, which compares the clinical trial to the other research methods.

In general it will be seen that the essence of a successful controlled clinical trial lies in its minutiae – in a painstaking, and sometimes very dull, attention to every detail. (A.B. Hill British Medical Bulletin)

Chapter 5
Comparing the Methods – Qualitative Differences

Abstract A comparison of the three major research methods, discussed in the preceding chapters, begins by demonstrating how the techniques could be used to investigate the same medical problem. The methods are also judged in terms of three goals that drive medical research: efficiency, generalizability and validity. In addition, the methods are also compared in terms of the most crucial standard of all, causation – is the result likely to be true? For the sake of completeness, the chapter also touches on qualitative research, a novel and totally different way to examine medical issues.

Keywords Causation · efficiency · generalizability · qualitative research · validity

Each (research) method should flourish, because each has features that overcome the limitations of the others when confronted with questions they cannot reliably answer.
(D. Sackett and J. Wennberg, *British Medical Journal*)

This chapter compares the leading research methods studied so far and, for the sake of completeness, touches on a novel and totally different way to examine medical issues called qualitative research. I begin by demonstrating how the three major research techniques could be used to research the same kind of problem. The contrast will be based on researching the identical question – does vitamin C prevents colds. All three research methods will use the same definition of a cold, a common standard for an effective vitamin C dosage and a consistent outcome measurement to judge the result.

Case-Control Study

The case-control study begins by searching through the medical records of a large number of people at a major medical center and identifying all those that report having had a cold in the past winter season. These people become the cases. Next it's necessary to find controls. There is again an examination of medical records, but this time epidemiologists only identify people who did not have a cold in the last winter season. Next, trained interviewers ask the people in both groups to give an exhaustive accounting of all medicines or alternative products they take based on a standard list of prescriptions drugs, health foods products, over-the-counter medications, etc. Most importantly, for each group it's important to record how many took a proper dose of vitamin C prior to the onset of a cold.

First, epidemiologists look at the proportion of cases that took vitamin C prior to coming down with a cold. Assume half of the cases took vitamin C and half didn't have vitamin C. They then determine the proportion of controls that took vitamin C. If it also is about a 50-50 split they would conclude that this study did not produce evidence that vitamin C prevented colds. However, if among the controls, a great many more took vitamin C, then that would indicate that vitamin C prevented a cold. The last possibility, there is only a small minority of the controls taking vitamin C, would indicate that vitamin C actually increases the possibility of a cold.

Cohort Study

The cohort study begins just before the winter season starts. At a clinic of the same major medical facility, epidemiologists request all patients to have an examination to determine if they have a cold. If they do, they are excluded from further involvement since it makes no sense to include people who already have the outcome of interest (i.e. a cold). Epidemiologists want to see how many develop a cold and that rules out people who already have a cold.

The participants in the study are asked to keep a diary of all the medicines and related preparations they take based on the same product list used in the case-control study. At the end of the winter season, they are interviewed to determine how many came down with a cold. The diaries of those with a cold will be reviewed and all those taking vitamin C at the appropriate dosage during the winter months will be placed in one group (treated patients). Those remaining will not have taken any or only a small amount of vitamin C, and will be placed in a second group (control patients). Epidemiologists compare the two groups in terms of the proportion of people catching a cold. As was true for the case-control example, three answers are possible. If a smaller proportion of people in the vitamin C group developed a cold, that would mean vitamin C had a protective effect. On the other hand, if the group on vitamin C and the group without vitamin C have the same incidence of colds, it would appear that vitamin C does not prevent colds. The last possibility, vitamin C causes colds, will be accepted if a large proportion of people who took vitamin C end up with a cold.

Clinical Trial

The clinical trial starts by lining up people for a study; this well might be done at the same medical facility used in the case-control and cohort studies. Researchers explain what is going to happen during the study and identify the risks and benefits of participation. The participants are also told they may not take vitamin C on their own during the study. Those who agree to the terms of the trial become the study subjects.

Next researchers randomly assign the participants to one of two groups. One set of subjects receives pills that contain vitamin C, but they are not told what is inside the pills. They take the pills as directed and continue to take them throughout the winter. That they may not take any supplements containing vitamin C is reinforced. The second group, who will receive dummy pills that do not contain the vitamin C (only a placebo), will be told the same thing.

At the end of the winter researchers bring all the patients back and find out how many had a cold. The same standard used in the other cases is employed to decide if vitamin C is effective, ineffective or a product that may increase the chance of a cold.

Comparing the Methods

Ask doctors and they will tell you that the clinical trial is the flagship for medical research – it's not perfect, but it's the best that they have. Yet it's fair to ask: if the clinical trial is so great, why do medical researchers use other kinds of designs: the case report and exploratory trial? The case report and the exploratory methods (case–control and cohort trials) can be the preferred approach – it all depends on the objectives of the research program. This proposition is supported by examining the three goals that drive medical research:

1. Efficiency. Is the result obtained with minimal time, cost and resources (e.g. number of subjects required)?
2. Generalizability. Is the result widely applicable?
3. Validity. Is the result likely to be true?

When it comes to efficiency, the case report is clearly the winner. Researchers collect the required information for a study during the normal process of treating patients. The major expenditure is the process of writing up the report. The case-control method does well in terms of efficiency because it is a relatively inexpensive research method and it can produce results in a very timely fashion. Remember all of the cases in a case-control trial already have the disease the researcher interested in. The cohort trial is not as efficient as the case-control approach because it must follow many subjects over a relatively long period of time and the costs to take the required assessments can make it relatively expensive. However, it is the clinical trial that tends to be the least efficient. The expenses to run these studies are high, to get the best results many subjects are usually required and there is an increasing emphasis on long term trials.

Generalizability asks the question: can the research result be applied to other patients and situations? Generalizability is quite low for case reports since the information presented is based on unusual patients. The patients presented in a case report represent exceptional cases rather than typical ones. The case-control method is much better, but still has a problem because the cases and controls are usually selected from institutions with large databases and there is no assurance that these patients are similar to the patients in the broader population. Contrast this to the cohort study where researchers observe people whose medical care is essentially provided in a typical medical care setting. The patient's behavior is not interfered with nor restricted. They may be given extra tests and exams, but they still are a very close match to what happens to the "average" patient. Most clinical trials do not get high ratings for generalizability. Selecting only certain kinds of participants, placing restrictions on dosing schedules and requiring protocol adherence reduces generalizability. Furthermore, in an attempt to be more efficient by reducing the number of required subjects, clinical trials often enter relatively high-risk patients since they can show the greatest degree of improvement and thereby reduce the number of subjects needed for a trial. However, these steps have a negative effect – they lower generalizability.

Validity, coming up with the right answer, has become the nonnegotiable demand placed on medical research. Case reports do very poorly when it comes to this trait. In their defense, case reports do not pretend to be providing answers to medical questions, they mainly are asking questions and raising awareness. How good the exploratory techniques (case-control and cohort trials) are debatable in respect to validity. They have been useful in important areas, the case-control method uncovering the smoking-lung cancer link and the Framingham cohort study that identified important risk factors for heart disease. Nonetheless, there is little argument anymore that for validity, they are inferior to the clinical trial. The clinical trial is the hands-down champion when it comes to validity. The opportunity to utilize randomization, blinding and control over the research environment places it at the head of the class.

What is interesting about this analysis is that no one method is always superior. Each medical research technique can claim a victory using the criteria of efficiency, generalizability and validity. Each method has a place in the modalities available to medical researchers.

The Ultimate Test – Causality

It should be clear that nothing about medical research – as knowledgeable and earnest the researchers may be – is easy. Efficiency, generalizability and validity are valuable qualities, but to get at the truth, medical researchers should be able to determine if agent X causes outcome A. The ability to find cause and effect relationships is a prerequisite goal of any research endeavor. How good is a method at showing that an agent has an effect? That, above all, is the decisive question.

Case reports are very weak when it comes to causality. They are only descriptive renditions and cannot link a result with a cause in a definitive fashion. Even if the report implies a cause, it offers little or no evidence to rule out other agents or conditions as alternative explanations for an outcome. As noted in an earlier chapter, exploratory trials (both the case-control and the cohort) find associations, but an association does not prove causality. The exploratory methods are immensely valuable in pointing out relationships that could represent cause and effect relationships, but they cannot rule out other possibilities for the interaction. It is the experimental clinical trial that has the greatest potential to identify causation. In a clinical trial, the researchers manipulate the factors that they think causes a specific outcome.

Granted the clinical trial is best at showing causality, but the does not mean it is always successful. There is no guarantee that there can't be mistakes in the planning, execution and interpretation of a clinical trial and that can lead to an error about a cause and effect relationship. With a single clinical trial there could be multiple factors operating individually or in combination that could have a significant effect on a perceived relationship. Generally, a causality claim requires that an effect from an agent be strong, consistent, specific, follow a logical time sequence and show an increased effect with higher levels of the agent. This is quite a set of demands and it's virtually impossible to satisfy them with a single study. Multiple trials in different settings and circumstances are needed to establish causation.

Qualitative Research

Compared to the research methods we have discussed so far, qualitative research (QR) is a totally different approach to studying health issues. The major techniques we've presented (case-control, cohort and clinical trial) are considered quantitative research methods. The label is reasonable because their findings are usually expressed numerically – a 32 percent mortality reduction or an average improvement of 16 percent. Critics note that a quantitative conclusion is not suitable for all types of medical discoveries and QR is offered as a better research approach in some instances.

Quantitative studies aim to test well-specified hypotheses and investigators start out by selecting predetermined variables for evaluation. These studies answer questions such as how much weight was lost? Or what was the percentage change in cholesterol levels? Advocates of QR argue that medicine is not only a mechanistic and quantitative science, but it is also an interpretive art. Interpretive research delves into interactions that cannot be addressed using quantitative methods. For example, a QR study could examine the social interaction among multiple parties: the patient, family members, nurses, social workers, clergy, and physician. Note the QR focus is on understanding human behavior and the reasons that people act as they do.

Qualitative research attempts to provide insight into social, emotional, and experiential phenomena in health care. Examples include inquiry about the meaning of illness to patients, their loved ones, and their families. Qualitative research questions tend not to ask whether or how much. Instead they explore what, how, and why. Qualitative reports do not typically generate Yes/No type of answers. Instead they generate narrative accounts or conceptual frameworks.

The methodological differences between qualitative research and the more conventional quantitative approach we've discussed are remarkable. The exploratory nature of QR typically requires investigators not to pre-specify a study population in strict terms. They fear that an important person, variable, or unit of analysis could be overlooked. It's just the other way around for the quantitative school that wants a carefully defined sample of people to study. Qualitative researchers readily avoid the "typical" patient favored by the quantitative investigators.

A QR study will select a small but focused sample rather than large random samples used in a clinical trial. The QR researcher may select unusual cases, critical cases or medically important cases. Subject selection criteria often evolve over the course of a study, and QR investigators return repeatedly to the data to explore new leads or find new angles to pursue.

A good illustration of the difficulties faced by the quantitative approach concern the evaluation of treatments used in complimentary alternative medicine (CAM). A quantitative orientation focuses on a very specific treatment (e.g. a specific drug), but CAM research often involves complex and multiple treatments – e.g. naturopathy (an eclectic system of care that promotes the body's self-healing mechanism) or a combination of herbal Chinese medicines. The treatments are not standardized and require individual and flexible dosage adjustments. The outcome measurements are frequently non-specific and involve multiple conditions (e.g. stress and lack of energy). In addition, the outcome is relatively vague (e.g. "restoring balance") in contrast to conventional science that requires a strict definition for an outcome. Randomization is often impossible because of participant refusal to be part of a control group.

Finding an appropriate placebo treatment for a CAM treatment (e.g., acupuncture or massage therapy) is often difficult or impossible. Keeping the treatment hidden from the patients and researchers is also frequently impractical. The conventional medical study generally tries to minimize or exclude the impact of the patient-physician relationship, but in CAM research the therapeutic effect of the patient-physician relationship is considered a crucial part of the intervention. Many of these challenges are not unique to CAM and apply equally to several conventional interventions, such as physiotherapy, psychotherapy, surgery, and nursing care.

It's no wonder that QR is seen as unscientific and anecdotal to some medical researchers. However, from the practicing physician's point of view, QR has appealing features because it involves the same skill set they apply with each patient: – personal observation, reflection, and judgment. When it comes to treating a patient, doctors can't rely on the simple application of scientific rules, but rely instead on their experience and insight to find the appropriate treatment.

In the end, whether QR should be used may depend on the question being investigated. If the question is "what is the best way to treat an enlarged prostate in men" then a quantitative approach using a clinical trial would be the design of choice. If the question is "whether effective care is being given to men with an enlarged prostate and are the men benefiting from that care" then another type of quantitative method, the case-control or cohort design would be favored. But if the question is "what is the importance of patient preferences in the choice of treatment for enlarged prostate" then the qualitative approach could be the best way to conduct the research.

The type of issues that could be studied with QR methods is appealing. Yet, the weakness of the approach in terms of conventional scientific rigor reduces its acceptability. However, there is an interest in merging the two approaches on the assumption that the addition of qualitative techniques can enhance quantitative approaches. How that merger could occur is pretty unclear. For the present, the medical community will continue to speculate on the uses and value of QR. There seems to be a growing interest in QR for health care research, but it has a long way to go before there's general acceptance.

Part II
Understanding the Clinical Trial

Chapter 6
The Protocol – The Guiding Light

Abstract This chapter on the protocol, and the six that follow it, take a closer look at the clinical trial, the most popular and revered research method. The protocol lays down the rules and regulations that must be followed in a clinical trial. It is a comprehensive document and preparing it is an immensely difficult chore. Many of the elements contained in a protocol, such as identifying the control group and determining the assessments to be made, become the subject matter for future chapters. A trial still needs to be carried out according to the protocol specifications, and the choices a researcher makes in designing a study plus the decisions required in the execution of a trial, have an enormous impact on the kind of the result that will be found. Consequentially, the same medical treatment evaluated by two different research teams can easily end up with conflicting results.

Keywords Clinical research protocol · disease definition · experimental treatment · research design · subject selection

To fully understand a clinical trial, it is essential to examine the principal elements that serve as its foundation. Arguably, the most important being the protocol, the document that sets down the rules and regulations that govern a clinical trial.

The protocol must be comprehensive, unambiguous and thorough – leave something out and there's a good chance the trial will fail. It may seem to a nonprofessional that a protocol is easy to write – after all the researchers know the disease they want to treat, the drugs they want to use, the test they want to make, etc. Nevertheless, preparing the protocol is an immensely difficult and hazardous chore. Perhaps that is one of the reasons why D. Fredrickson, who would become Director of the NIH, described a clinical trial as an "indispensable ordeal."

A protocol is the blueprint for a medical trial; it is the instruction manual for all those involved in the research project from the nurses to the technicians. If it is flawed the trial will be flawed. If for example there are concerns about bias in a trial, it is the protocol that will be used first to find the sources of the bias. If two trials give conflicting results, evaluators begin looking at the protocols to find an explanation for the likely cause of the differences.

There is no set format for research protocols. They vary from one research group to another and although the semantics may vary, they tend to cover the same material. Here are the main sections that you are likely to find in any protocol:

– Introduction
– Criteria for selecting subjects
– Definition of the target disease
– Definition of the experimental treatment
– Identification of the control treatment
– Measurements and observations to be made
– Statistical analysis plans
– Other elements

Introduction

An introductory section usually provides the background, rationale and a summary of prior research for the study. It is likely that as part of the introduction, the study objectives will also be stated.

Selecting Subjects

One of the most vital parts of a protocol lays down the criteria for the inclusion and exclusion of subjects. What characteristics a subject must have and what they must not have, defines the future group of patients that will receive the treatments being compared. Suffice to say at this point that the elements may be as mundane as a subject's age (they must fit into a prescribed age range); to a complex description of an esoteric medical examination done by a specialist.

Defining the Disease

A description of the disease or condition being investigated is essential. There are nice neat names for many diseases such as Parkinson's disease, Alzheimer's disease, and Hodgkin's disease. The terms are very familiar and each is associated with a set of recognizable symptoms, but an accurate diagnosis can be unbelievably illusive.

Verifying the very presence of a medical condition can be tough assignment. Take the case of identifying patients with acute kidney failure. One review of the medical literature appeared in the journal *Critical Care* and identified more than 30 definitions. The one definition a researchers selects for the protocol can produce an outcome that is similar to, but not the same as another choice. Just to make things even more difficult, there are clinical trial protocols that require subjects to have a specified level of a disease. Determining disease severity can offer a greater challenge than coming up with the initial diagnosis. Severity can involve multiple factors so it is often necessary to measure a large number of variables to come up with a rating. Here's a case in point from an article in the journal *Chest*. Board certified allergists were sent medical documents and asked to assign the patients to one of five asthma severity levels. When the results were looked at, it was concluded that there was only a "low level of agreement". This poor showing occurred in spite of the fact that there existed an NIH asthma severity guide to help allergists make the severity assessments.

Any misclassification of the primary disease can hurt an experimental drug's chances of showing it is effective because people without the target disease water down the results. This can lead to finding that a drug is ineffective when it is truly efficacious. The likelihood that there are a large number of incorrect diagnoses may be small, but this kind of problem nevertheless contributes to research errors and makes a careful description of the disease in a protocol essential.

Defining the Experimental Treatment

Researchers clearly know what experimental agent they intend to study, but they must also specify how and when it is to be used. Again, as obvious as it might seem, that decision may not be so easy for new experimental compounds. From medieval days it was known that often what distinguished a medicine from a poison was the dosage. The number of exposures, the actual dose in each exposure, the timing of the doses, and the length of exposure all matter. Even the most benign substance can be toxic when administered in a high enough dose. Look at radiation; in low doses it kills cancer cells, in high doses it kills the patient.

The research leading up to large-scale clinical trials tends to rely on studies with only a small number of patients. The emphasis in early drug research is on establishing the safety of the drug rather than its efficacy. Small safety studies make sense since it is unwise to subject a lot of people to a newly developed drug. An efficacious dose is looked for by performing more small studies until researchers decide that there's sufficient information to allow the new therapy to enter a more vigorous efficacy-testing phase. The planned dosage schedule for these large-scale trials come from the small clinical trials as well as work done in animals. Consequently, there can be a scarcity of information on humans and the wrong clinical dose may be selected and used in the protocols for the rest of the research program.

Another factor that raises the risk of using an inappropriate dose occurs when there is a lot of pressure to quickly find a "cure" for a grave disease. In that circumstance it is understandable that people want access to a new therapy as early as possible. This pressure may result in selecting a suboptimal dose prematurely.

Failure to list the best possible dose in the protocols of investigative studies is well illustrated by the antidepressant drug imipramine. Imipramine was a very successful drug, a market leader, and as a result frequently chosen as the control treatment for new antidepressant drug studies done in the 1960s. However, it turned out that the treatment schedules were often too short and the dose too low. A report in the *American Journal of Psychiatry* found that imipramine dose in those trials was often half of what doctors now consider the optimal dose. Furthermore, the studies often lasted less than four weeks, and it is now recognized that trials must be longer than four weeks to get the most favorable drug effect.

The experimental drug can also be a marketed drug that may have new uses. An example of this is the doctor trials conducted in the U.K. and the U.S. at about the same time. The trials had the same goal, each wanted to see if aspirin could prevent a heart attack. Despite the same goal and the use of male physicians as subjects, plus the fact there was collaboration between the trial designers, their protocols differed markedly in terms of the aspirin dosages. The British physicians received three times the dose of aspirin compared to that used in the American study. Not too surprisingly, the trials ended up with contrasting results. In this instance, however, the difference was not what one would have expected. The higher aspirin does in the U.K. trial was not effective, but the lower dose in the U.S. study was. Perhaps the British researchers overshot the optimal dose and wound up demonstrating that too much of a good thing is no good at all. The lesson from this story is very obvious. Researchers have a great deal of latitude in writing a protocol; they can choose not only what drugs they'll test, but also the dosages to be used. And these decisions can have huge consequences when it comes to results.

As part of the specified dosing schedule noted in a protocol, researchers need to decide when to begin and how long to give a treatment. Two short cases show how these decisions can affect a clinical trial. The first case, described in an intriguing article on the complexity and contradictions in clinical trial research, published in 1987 by the *American Journal of Medicine*, deals with a randomized trial assessing the effects of high-dose steroids in patients who had gone into shock due to blood poisoning. The investigators designed the study to avoid problems noted in previous positive studies. In the earlier trials, there was a concern whether all subjects met the subject acceptance criteria. Under the new protocol, before patients could be enrolled in the study they were monitored in the intensive care unit to make sure they satisfied the subject inclusion standards. In addition, patients in shock were not enrolled until a source of infection was identified. The revised protocol improved the quality of the patients who would be treated and that made sense, but it delayed the onset of treatment and that created a major problem.

At the end of the trial, the treatments looked very similar in terms of benefit. The authors concluded that steroids did not improve the overall survival of patients with shock. However, they also noted that the time from onset of shock to the start of steroid treatment was 17.5 hours (and ranged from 0 to 316 hours). Clearly there was a problem since previous studies demonstrated that early treatment was beneficial. When treatment was delayed, therapeutic efficacy was impaired. Thus, by withholding treatment to be sure subjects were properly qualified, the investigators inadvertently caused a successful treatment to fail.

Studies on rheumatoid arthritis show that the duration of treatment set down in a protocol can turn out to be wrong. Clinical trials are expensive and short trials are much preferred over long ones, but that preference can create problems. An article in 1988 by a Professor at Vanderbilt University School of Medicine, found that almost all experimental trials done on rheumatoid arthritis ran for two years or less. Yet, the disease is a long-term illness. Drugs shown to be effective for a year or two may not maintain that level of response in subsequent years. In fact, when it comes to rheumatoid arthritis, long-term epidemiological studies tend to have poor results and short term clinical trials have good results. There is an apparent loss of efficacy over time, backing up the point that duration of treatment set forth in a protocol is critical, but it can be extremely difficult to know in advance how long a trial should last.

In addition to the experimental drug, the results of clinical trials can be influenced by omitting or permitting other therapies. Drugs that can be taken are frequently limited in clinical trial protocols because their presence could interfere with the actions of the experimental drug. Therefore, protocols spell out what other drugs the subjects can or cannot receive.

The following example, also described in the previously mentioned *American Journal of Medicine* review, shows how concomitant therapies can affect a clinical trial. Two clinical trials studied the same experimental drug, a product similar to nitroglycerin, in individuals who had suffered a heart attack. Both trials were placebo-controlled. One study found fewer deaths from the experimental drug treatment, but the other trial found no difference in mortality between the placebo and the experimental drug. The inconsistent findings were amazing. Why was the test drug better in one trial and no better than placebo in another trial? The contradictory results required an explanation. The answer surfaced after comparing the protocols for the two trials. There was an inconsistency in the use of concomitant diuretics.

The first study required all subjects (i.e. those on both treatments) to receive the same standard medical care. In the other study, the protocol allowed concomitant medications on a discretionary basis and it was up to the attending physician to decide what drugs a subject could receive. As it turned out the physicians in this latter study prescribed diuretics more frequently in the patients on placebo. Almost four times as many placebo treated patients received diuretics than those on the experimental drug. The physicians, concerned about the health of their patients, correctly assumed the diuretics would help. The diuretics apparently provided a lot more help than anticipated because the placebo group ended up with a result similar to that of the experimental treatment. In the other study, where concomitant drugs were consistent between treatment groups, the experimental drug produced a superior finding.

Identifying the Control Treatment

The results for the experimental treatment need to be compared to a standard and that standard is usual a placebo or active drug. Selecting the control treatment is a crucial step when preparing the protocol and later on, I devote a full chapter to this subject.

Measurements and Observations

An essential ingredient of any trial is the choice of measurements and observations that are used to evaluate the treatments. When these assessments occur also has a major influence on the study outcomes. Success or failure may ride on the decisions researchers make and I include a full chapter on the choice and timing of assessments later in the book.

Statistical Analysis Plans

In the best protocols, a section on the proposed method for the statistical analysis becomes a part of the protocol. No one likes to make a priori commitments if they can possible avoid them, but when it comes to the statistical analysis, failure to include the basic analysis plan can be a disaster. Therefore, in addition to the rational for the number of participants chosen and any plans for interim analyses, the protocol should also spell out how the data will be analyzed. I dedicate Part III of this book to statistical and methodological issues because they can have such a profound effect on the results from a clinical trial.

Other Elements

There could also be other items included in a protocol such as the informed consent procedures for the volunteers who will serve as subjects. Any pertinent instructions on the recruitment process for obtaining subjects may also be included. If a special diet or a required assay procedure were necessary, the details for these elements would need to be described. Comments on the method of randomization and information on the technique to ensure blinding may be incorporated into the protocol as well. In the chapter on bias control, I go into some detail explaining why these essential features of a RABCOT sound great, but offer no guarantees. It is also critical that all those participating in a study have a common understanding of the protocol. Many of the most important trials involve multiple research centers, and methods to coordinate the overall research project need to be spelled out. The way in which each of these supplementary elements is written can have a subtle but important effect on the results of a clinical trial.

No matter how careful researchers are, there are places where the protocol may prove to be inadequate and that may lead to inaccurate answers. Asking a researcher to construct a protocol that is thorough, accurate and clear is quite an assignment. There are abundant opportunities for something to go awry due to the complexity and uncertainty of medical research. There are so many decisions to be made and with each decision an unintended effect can compromise a trial's validity.

It should be obvious that it is extremely difficult to write a good protocol. The variety of subject matter that needs to be considered means many specialists are involved. Even then, there are many unknowns that baffle seasoned researchers. It's impossible to know if a protocol has dealt with all the potential problems inherent in clinical research. A given trial may appear to be successful until additional research reveals years later that there were unknown factors that caused the result to be misleading. In a survey done in the 1987, a cross section of individuals from industry, universities and the government who were involved in clinical trials, were asked to judge the quality of protocols. The results, published in the *Journal of International Medical Research*, showed that over 70 percent of this well-rounded group of experts believed that controlled clinical trial protocols were inadequate.

Rigid protocol requirements may, on the surface, look reasonable, but they can produce studies that have very limited application. On the other hand, a protocol that tries to more inclusive can easily end up with findings dissimilar to those from trials with tighter standards.

One of the most remarkable sources of distortion in randomized clinical trials occurs because of rigid requirements of study protocols. (R. Horwitz, *American Journal of Medicine*)

Trial Execution

After a researcher prepares a protocol, it must also be executed and that process offers another set of challenging problem. Human nature being what it is does not guarantee that the protocol specifications will be adhered to. In selecting subjects, a patient history is required. Investigators must often assume the information provided is truthful, but that may not always be the case. Some subjects may slant their answers to improve their chances of gaining entry into the trial. The protocol spells out exactly how the experimental and control medications are to be taken, but that does not mean the subjects will follow those rules. Subject compliance with the required medication schedules offers a good example of problems with protocol execution.

How can an investigator verify that the subjects, in fact, took the study medication as directed? Pill count is probably the most common way to monitor compliance, but there are other alternatives. Blood analyses and urine analyses are also used, but all of these techniques only check on very recent medication intake.

Monitoring by pill count means that a subject receives a precise number of pills at each visit. When the subject returns for the next visit the pills are returned, counted and the balance compared to what the subject was suppose to have taken. Typically, subjects who fail to take the prescribed number of pills are subject to a stern lecture on the importance of taking all their medication. Human nature being what it is means that the way to avoid being criticized for negligence is to destroy the pills for all missed medication. Easy to do and as a bonus the researcher now applauds the subject's performance. They are classified as "perfect compliers" even though they could be consuming little or even none of their medication.

One report, that appeared in *American Medical News*, probably represents an extreme case of the extent of cheating that can go on. The study, designed to evaluate effects of bronchodilators, found that 30 percent of subjects dumped the contents of their inhalers shortly before follow-up visits in an effort to conceal their failure to take the medicine properly. The subjects knew the inhalers would be weighed at each visit, but they did not know a device had been imbedded into the inhaler that recorded the exact date and time of each use. The study organizers discovered that over the course of the first year some subjects dumped all the medication at one time, not knowing the act would be detected.

Even more revealing was the finding that the subjects guilty of "cheating" were otherwise ideal subjects. They got along well with the staff and turned up for visits on time. They were thoughtful people who didn't want to disappoint the investigators. Except for the revelation from the monitoring device, they appeared to be perfect subjects.

An excluded drug may be taken accidentally or on purpose during a trial and the indiscretion never revealed to the researchers. Some measurements require special preparation (fasting, exclusion of certain foods or drugs, etc.) and subjects may violate those provision without informing anyone. They may be late for scheduled visits or miss having crucial tests done because of an illness or travel. In these cases, important data may be lacking and threaten a fair or complete analysis. Worse yet subjects may dropout of the trial prematurely.

Subjects drop out of a trial for both drug-related and legitimate reasons such as leaving the area due to marriage or a job change. Various incentives have been tried to keep subjects enrolled and having all their tests and observations completed. Among them are financial considerations such as offering a monetary bonus to those who remain until the trial is finished. There is even the suggestion that subjects should put down a refundable deposit, which they will receive if they complete the trial. Clearly these kind of techniques appeal to a certain type of individual and while they may improve the retention rate, they also weaken the ability to translate the findings to a broad representative group of patients. Furthermore, there is an ethical problem of coercing subjects to remain in a trial when it would be to their benefit to dropout.

The degree of attrition can vary a great deal. In one clinical trial over half of the subjects dropped out. The trial tested calcitonin, a product used to prevent bone fractures in osteoarthritis patients. In retrospect, the high dropout rate was in large part attributed to the fact the trial was only partially blinded. The attending physician as well as the patient could see bone density results. When the bone density findings were disappointing, it motivated subjects to withdraw. Also, the attending physicians withdrew patients because they felt it was in the patient's best self-interest. The trial was a success in one respect, it mirrored what happens in the real world, but it was a disaster when it came to the analysis due to the quantity of missing data.

Unquestionably, an incomplete protocol or an inadequate execution of that protocol can cause a biased clinical trial result. D. Sackett, a noted physician and methodologist, came up with 35 different kinds of biases that inhibit medical research. Many items on the list would be applicable to all forms of research methods, but even so, the large number is disturbing because it let's us know the wide variety of things that can go amiss in spite of a carefully developed research plan and thoughtful implementation of that plan.

This chapter focused on the difficulties with writing the protocol and conducting a trial according to that document. A vast amount of information is required and in some cases the information needed to make the right choices may not even exist. Practicalities also require tradeoffs that may introduce flaws in the protocol. Speed and cost consideration almost always require concessions in the design and conduct of a trial as well. In some respect, it is remarkable that there are so many well-written and executed protocols given the environment of uncertainty and impracticality that exist in the medical research world. However, what's important to realize is that the choices a researcher has in designing and carrying out a clinical trial can have an enormous impact on the trial results. As a result, the same medical treatment evaluated by two different research teams can easily end up with conflicting results.

Chapter 7
The Control Group – Leveling the Playing Field

Abstract One of the signature characteristics of a clinical trial is the use of a con-temporaneous control group. The evaluation of a new treatment without a rational comparison group is extremely vulnerable to error. Historical and anecdotal accounts illustrate how the use of control groups became popular in clinical research. Had early physicians only used a control group they would have discovered the futility of blood letting when it came to treating all sorts of diseases. The text highlights the challenging issues involved in the choice of a comparison group for the experimental treatment. Should a researcher use placebos or active drugs? Or if neither is possible, would historical controls or untreated subjects be appropriate? Possible explanations for the placebo effect are also offered.

Keywords Active medicine controls · historical controls · placebo controls · placebo effect · untreated controls

For centuries physicians were sure that blood letting would cure all sorts of dis-eases, and old records contain testimonials espousing the miraculous effect this medical remedy had on sick people. Had they only used a control group they would have discovered the error of their ways. Without a group that would be spared the ordeal of having considerable quantities of blood removed, there was no way to see how futile the surgery was, and the practice continued from the golden age of Greece till the late 19th century.

One of the signature characteristics of a clinical trial is the use of a control group. As noted in the clinical trial chapter there are sound reasons why researchers should include a comparative treatment group. The evaluation of a new treatment without a rational comparison group would be extremely vulnerable to error.

The awareness of the need to make fair treatment group comparisons was present as early as the 18th century. The scurvy example I used in the clinical trial chapter to show how an experiment could be planned was actually a true experi-ment conducted by James Lind, a physician serving in the British Royal Navy. Giving fruits to half of the sick sailors and withholding fruit from the other half is often considered the first controlled clinical trial.

Another interesting example of the value of controls takes place in 1854. Thomas Balfour, a physician at the Royal Military Asylum, faced a raging scarlet fever epidemic. He was aware of a 50-year-old claim that belladonna, a very toxic plant, could in small doses prevent scarlet fever. To find out if belladonna really worked, Balfour identified 151 boys at the institution who did not have scarlet fever. He gave 76 of them belladonna, leaving the other 75 untreated. He then observed the boys to see how they did. Two in each group came down with scarlet fever; the other 147 were disease-free. Given the fact they were in the midst of an epidemic, the four cases were far below the expected number. The result probably disappointed Balfour who was hoping he had a way to combat scarlet fever, but he was astute enough to note that had he not used a control group we would have arrived at the wrong conclusion. Had all the boys taken belladonna, he would have incorrectly attributed the low number of cases as proof of belladonna's effectiveness.

When it comes to selecting control groups, there are a surprising number of options. The most obvious choice is a placebo control group. Unfortunately, for the placebo, it is the proverbial underdog in clinical research since it's not expected to have much, if any, effect and consequently it should turn out inferior to an effective experimental treatment every time. Unfortunately, for researchers, it doesn't always turn out that way.

Another alternative is to use an active drug as the control, especially a well-established product that's been on the market a long time with proven effectiveness. Frequently the term "standard treatment" is used to refer to a control drug that is currently in wide use and considered an effective treatment for a specific disease or condition. Researchers can also use two control groups – placebo and the standard drug. It is also possible to select a treatment group that participated in a previous study to serve as a control group. A final option is to use untreated subjects as a control group. There are distinct advantages and disadvantages in each choice.

Placebo Controls

A placebo is an inactive substance that literally means, "I do nothing" in Latin. To represent its impotency, it is often called a "sugar" or "dummy" pill. In spite of its definition of inactivity, people can be affected when they take one. Indeed, their "placebo effect" is often a positive response because people are conditioned to expect a useful effect from a drug.

Before the 20th century, much of the success physicians obtained when caring for patents was likely due to a placebo response. There just wasn't much in that black bag to help a sick patient. It was the bedside manner and authoritarian figure of the physician that produced the "cure". Medical scientists tried to figure out a plausible explanation for the placebo effect for years. They came up with several possibilities. One is based on Pavlovian conditioning. People who take medication often experience relief and they are "set up" to have that same experience again. A second possibility is that placebos stimulate the release of endorphins, the group of chemicals produced in the brain. The endorphins in turn activate parts of the body to bring about a physiological effect such as pain reduction. A third possibility is that taking a placebo in an atmosphere of hope relieves stress. If stress is related to the condition under investigation, the patient experiences symptomatic relief.

However, the use of placebo groups isn't considered acceptable in studies of life-threatening conditions. Where there are already effective agents, using a placebo group that could jeopardize the subjects' health would be considered unethical. An example of this kind of situation would be a study to evaluate treatments for heart attack victims where anticoagulants, nitroglycerin and beta-blockers are known to be effective treatments. To use a placebo to test a new drug rather than one of these know agents would clearly be improper.

Even if the study involves non-life threatening conditions, some medical ethicists frown upon the use of placebos. Critics cite the Declaration of Helsinki in their opposition to placebo-controlled trials. Created by the World Medical Association, the Declaration of Helsinki sets forth ethical principles to guide medical research involving human subjects. A clause in that document states that patients in a medical study should be assured of the best proven diagnostic and therapeutic methods available. As a result, placebos are contraindicated because they offer little benefit and expose patients to unnecessary risk.

This position can be taken a step further. A study is justified only if the investigator is completely uncertain about which trial treatment would be better for the patient. However, there is plenty of opposition to this controversial position as well. Researchers point out that if taken literally, the statement would bar all clinical trials when effective treatment exists because the patients receiving the investigational treatment are not getting the "best proven" treatment. They argue that placebo-controlled trials may be ethically conducted even when effective therapy exists if the inclusion of the placebo group does not increase the risk for death or irreversible problems.

In practice, placebo control groups are used routinely. When it comes to the patient, how do they justify their participation in a placebo-controlled trial? After all there is usually a 50/50 chance they will be given the placebo rather than the active medication. Therefore, they need to be fully informed about the risks and benefits of their participation. However, since this information primarily comes from the researcher, the same researcher who is strongly motivated to get them into a trial, it presents another ethical dilemma. Will the researcher give complete and honest information to the prospective subject? Fortunately, there is some control over this potential conflict. Researchers must obtain approval from an outside committee on what prospective patients will be told about their participation in a trial.

There is almost universal agreement that placebos are invaluable in RABCOTs because they prevent researchers and subjects from observing and seeing what they think they should observe and see. It is also assumed that placebos by themselves cause significant patient improvement. This latter belief was challenged by Danish researchers in 2001 based on a meta analysis, which combined the results from a number of studies investigating the same research question and provided an overall assessment by integrating the individual study findings. Their review came from a collection of over 100 studies that used three treatment groups – standard drug, placebo, and no treatment. Their analysis focused on the comparison between no treatment and placebo treatment. They found no evidence of a beneficial effect for placebo except for subjective outcomes such as pain. No difference was found between the placebo and the no-treatment groups when the outcome assessment involved objective measurements such as blood pressure. The authors still advocated the use of placebos in double blind trials, but discouraged the use of placebo in medical practice.

In spite of that paper, studies demonstrating that placebos produce an effect continue to appear. One of the most intriguing results came from a study that found that placebo treatment caused a definite change in brain activity. The truth of the matter is that in spite of all the studies using and investigating placebos scientists still do not understand the "placebo effect", but researchers need to take it into consideration in their trials.

Standard Drug Controls

An alternative to placebo is to use an active drug as the comparison treatment. This approach seems to make sense; it certainly provides a tougher test than competing against a placebo. However, it's more complicated than it may appear to be on the surface. The difficulty begins with the next logical question – what active drug should be used? If there is only one drug currently available for the indication under study the answer is easy, but frequently that is not the case. When multiple comparison drugs exist, a rational choice would likely be either the current market leader or the drug that has been available the longest period of time. There are also other options. For example, researchers can select the drug that is chemically most similar, or they can choose the drug they feel the experimental drug can easily beat.

After selecting a control drug, its dosage regimen must also be specified. Surprisingly, the right dosage schedule for many comparison drugs may not be obvious because the drug's published dosage might be extremely flexible giving a researcher a lot of leeway on what dosage to use. This situation was evident in the U.K. and U.S. aspirin trials in doctors, where there was a threefold difference between the two studies in respect to the amount of aspirin given.

Inconsistency of aspirin dosing also takes place in rheumatoid arthritis research. As reported in *Controlled Clinical Trials*, daily doses of aspirin ranged between 1.5 g up to 6.4 g depending on the study. Some studies did not allow a dosage increase and others didn't allow a dosage decrease. Some protocols allowed doses to be titrated, so the dose could be changed based on how the subject was doing, and others did not. There is no doubt that the various researchers had sound reasons for these alternative treatment regimens, but such disparity can cause enormous confusion in terms of how well a treatment performs in a clinical trial.

In addition to amount of drug, the duration of treatment can also vary as well and have a profound effect on the treatment results. Take the case of the popular steroid prednisone, given to patients with liver disease. A review article in the *American Journal of Medicine* pointed out that the prednisone strength varied from as much as 60 mg daily to as little as 15 mg daily in clinical trials. In addition, the duration of treatment ranged from one month to six years. Not surprisingly, the researchers who employed small doses for short intervals reported no benefit for steroids. On the other hand, investigators who administered larger doses for longer intervals noted substantial benefit. The striking difference in treatment schedules illustrates how easy it is to end up with totally opposite results for the same reference drug.

However, there is potentially a substantial risk when using only standard drugs in a clinical trial. How will researchers know if the trial could find an important difference? Maybe the trial is insensitive in that the outcome measurement cannot differentiate a good agent from a bad one. Consequently, if you get a "no difference" result, it could be because both the experimental and control drugs are effective. But it could also occur if the primary measurement in the trial is incapable of showing a treatment difference. A claim of "drug equality" makes no sense in that circumstance. The safer option is to use two controls; one a placebo and the other a standard drug.

Placebo and Standard Drug

Researchers can employ (1) placebos to see if the new drug has any value and (2) a major marketed drug to see how well the new treatment stacks up against the best. Note that the placebo versus standard drug comparison provides invaluable information. It tells a researcher if the trial has the ability to find an important difference. If that contrast does not result in a meaningful treatment difference, the trial is deemed insensitive – it couldn't find the difference between a known effective drug and placebo.

The concern over insensitive trials is especially pertinent when the outcome observations are soft (i.e. they come mainly from subjective rather than objective measures). A review in the *British Medical Journal* illustrates this point. The researchers of a trial relied on subjective patient reports of nausea and vomiting to evaluate the treatments, two active drugs and a placebo. The results indicated that placebo was as effective as one of the standard compounds and better than the other. Clearly something was amiss and it was the placebo arm in the trial that exposed the problem. A placebo doing as well as a successful marketed drug would be unusual and compel the researcher to search for a possible explanation. But, to also have placebo end up better than a second marketed drug would reinforce a conclusion that the method of evaluation was invalid.

The three-treatment trial can also end up with a finding that the new drug is more efficacious than placebo, but not as good as the standard reference drug. This result would not necessarily condemn the new treatment. The finding could still advance medical practice if the new drug had advantages over the marketed agent such as substantial cost savings or a considerable reduction in side effects.

Nothing comes without a price and using the three-treatment design translates into more cost and time. This kind of trial requires at least 50 percent more subjects. More time is needed to conduct the study and analyze the results as well. That's a big investment and it may come as no surprise to find including two control groups isn't a particularly popular design in clinical research.

Historical Controls

So far the type of controls I discussed for clinical trials are concurrent controls. The control subjects participate in the study at the same time as the treatment group subjects. However, an alternative is to use an historical control group. As the name implies, the control group comes from an earlier trial. Imagine an earlier placebo controlled trial used to see if drug A was safe and effective. Two years later researchers want to do the same trial to see if drug B is any good. Why not just run the new trial without a placebo group and, for comparative purposes, use the placebo data from the first trial?

Historical controls make sense when a researcher can't use any kind of a control group in a clinical trial because there is (1) a compelling ethical concern about using a placebo and (2) no acceptable standard treatment is available. In medical research you sometime must make do with what you have available, especially when the ideal is out of reach.

The major drawback with historical controls is that there is little assurance that they are comparable to the subjects receiving the standard treatment. Time plays a major role in medicine. New treatments arrive; old treatments disappear. Patient care acceptable five years ago is now frowned upon. The type of patients doctors treat with a given disease may be quite different as time passes.

Historical controls tend to produce answers that are not the same as the answers from studies using a contemporaneous control group. A 1982 scientific paper exposed the danger of employing historical controls. Medical scientists from Mt. Sinai Hospital in New York identified six different therapies in which some of the studies used historical controls and other studies used contemporaneous controls.

When the scientists combined the results across all six therapeutic areas they had 56 studies with historical controls and 50 studies using current control groups. When they compared the results based on the type of control group, the data revealed a huge difference. Only 20 percent, 10 out of the 50 studies using current controls, found the experimental treatment effective. On the other side of the ledger, with historic controls a whopping 79 percent (44 out of 56 studies) came to this decision. There could only be one conclusion – research studies using historical controls tended to produce a lot more positive results than those using concurrent controls.

The Mt. Sinai scientists also discovered another fascinating fact. All studies, regardless of the type of control used, had a similar success rate for the standard treatment groups. However, the results for the control treatments failed to follow this consistent pattern. If the trial employed an historical control group that group had lower success rates than the concurrent control groups did. This led the Mt Sinai authors to conclude that the outcome of trials with historical controls might irretrievably weight the results in favor of new experimental therapies.

Untreated Subjects as Controls

It is possible to design a study and have one group receive the test drug and the other group receive nothing at all. In a situation where there is no current acceptable treatment, and placebos are deemed inappropriate for practical or ethical reasons, this approach may be the only viable option. In fact, a landmark clinical trial relied on just that approach – an untreated control group.

The historic trial took place in Sweden at the end of the 19th century. The objective was to determine if a serum to treat diphtheria was effective. The researcher, Johannes Fibiger a Danish physician, was not convinced by earlier investigations that gave mixed results over the serum's efficacy. The earlier trials were too few and the important number, the number of deaths, so small that the results could hardly serve as statistical proof of the serum's effectiveness. Also, the researchers allocated patients to treatments based on the personal choice of the researcher. If that wasn't bad enough, there were other problems as well. For example, one study compared patients treated with the serum in one hospital to untreated patients at another hospital. The differences in quality of care and hygiene between the two hospitals could have easily accounted for any difference in the observed results.

The Swedish trial simply allocated the treatment to patients by giving all patients admitted on one day the live serum (the active treatment group) whereas none of those admitted the following day received the active serum (the untreated control group). It would certainly be fair to challenge the trial by today's standards. After all, the treatment assignment was not random nor were the treatments blinded. Still, the methodology used in this trial is remarkable given that the research was done over 100 years ago.

In terms of results, eight out of 239 patients in the serum-treated group and 30 out of 245 in the control group died. No formal statistical analysis was performed, but it would be hard to dispute the strength of these results demonstrating the serum's effectiveness. As a side note Dr. Fibiger received the Nobel Prize in 1927, but not for his diphtheria study. He was awarded the prize for research that indicated a worm (a nematode) was the cause of gastric cancer. Ironically, subsequent research rejected this conclusion.

The importance of controls in any clinical study is best summarized by this assessment from the U.S. Food and Drug Administration's Center for Drug Evaluation and Research:

The choice of control group is always a critical decision in designing a clinical trial. That choice affects the inferences that can be drawn from the trial, the ethical acceptability of the trial, the degree to which bias in conducting and analyzing the study can be minimized, the types of subjects that can be recruited and the pace of recruitment, the kind of endpoints that can be studied, the public and scientific credibility of the results, the acceptability of the results by regulatory authorities, and many other features of the study, its conduct, and its interpretation.

In short, the decision about the control group for a clinical trial can elevate the importance of the trial or destroy it.

Chapter 8
Measurements – They're Never Exact

Abstract Measurements encompasses more than simple quantitative information such as height, weight, volume or frequency. In clinical trials, measurements refer to all the data collected on the subjects including efficacy and safety measures. It's not always clear what measurement should be used and in researching conditions such as schizophrenia, heart attack prevention, cancer, and anorexia nervosa there is a wide assortment of choices. The distinction between objectives versus subjective measurements is drawn and collecting safety data, vitally important in all clinical trials, involves both objective laboratory rests and subjective patient reports. Researchers must also decide when a measurement will be taken and whether to use surrogate and/or composite measurements. Due to the multiplicity of measurement decisions, two research teams may design very different trials and, as a result, obtain very different results.

Keywords Composite measurement · efficacy measurement · safety measurement · subjective measurement · surrogate measurement

The term "measurement" encompasses more than simple quantitative information such as height, weight, volume or frequency. In clinical trials, it refers to all the data collected on the subjects. This includes elementary information such as whether a person smokes, the presence or absence of a disease and a blood pressure reading to more complex data such as the results from a hormone immunoassay,

Again, the right choices are critical. But, given the many options that may be available, it's not always clear what measurement should be used in any given trial. In some research areas such as mental health, it is especially hard to select an appropriate measure. Schizophrenia research reveals the wide choices researcher have when it comes to selecting outcomes. In an investigation of 2,000 schizophrenia trials presented in the *British Medical Journal*, over 600 different rating scales were identified.

Measurement selection can be a major source of contradictory trial results. For example, two studies evaluating the same experimental drug for the treatment of patients with a heart attack, but using different measurements, could end up with different results. In one trial the primary endpoint is a reduction in overall mortality. In the other, the outcome variable is a reduction in irregular and disorganized beating of the heart (i.e. ventricular fibrillation). Because of the difference in the outcome variable, one trial could report no effect of a treatment, but the other could find a significant effect from the same drug. The measurement choice is but one more challenge for research designers.

Technological advances also increase the number of options researchers have on what to measure in order to determine treatment success. Look at cancer, a disease that has received billions of dollars in research support. Considering the enormous investment, many feel the results are disappointing. It is thought that the reliance on x-rays to determine if a cancer drug worked is one of the reasons for the low level of success. If x-rays indicated the tumor had shrunk or stopped growing, researchers assumed that the drug was working. However, it turns out that in some cases tumor size does not matter all that much. Attention is now on new methods (e.g. magnetic imaging, computer tomography and blood tests) to better tell what is actually happening to a cancerous growth.

In most research, investigators select a primary outcome measure and some secondary measures as well. For example, in an assessment of treatment for pulmonary edema the primary assessment could be a clinical score based on the shortness of breath a patient experiences due to fluid accumulation in the lungs. The secondary measurement might be the number of times a patient had to have a tube inserted in the trachea to improve breathing. Given that there are innumerable measurement choices to assess pulmonary edema (one study identified 21 different outcome measurements that could be used) there are many choices available to a research team. Depending on the choices made by different researchers, the effectiveness of an experimental treatment could vary significantly.

An example of the confusion that different outcome measures can create is illustrated by a trial, which appeared in the *American Journal of Psychiatry*, comparing three treatments for their effectiveness in treating anorexia nervosa. Four outcomes measures were used and one, the Global Assessment of Functioning score (GAF), was designated the primary test. The GAF found significant differences between some of the treatments, but two of the other measurements failed to find any important treatments differences at all. The other test, an eating disorder inventory (EDI) found a treatment difference, but for only one of four dimensions that made up the test. In addition, the treatment differences identified by the EDI were not totally consistent with those found for the GAF.

Nonetheless, no matter what measurement a researcher selects, the result for that measurement should be accurate. Replication of a measurement is a well-known method to insure its accuracy. However, the time pressures and cost of a clinical study are not conducive to repeating a measurement to be sure it's right. Most time a single measurement is taken and no attempt is made to repeat it to see if it is in fact correct.

Objective Versus Subjective Measurements

Objective data such as a woman's weight or a man's PSA (prostrate specific antigen) score are preferred in clinical research because of their reliability and accuracy. However, they are frequently more difficult to carry out, and the process of collecting objective data is usually more time-consuming and costly. In contrast, subjective data are viewed as less objective, and patients can be very erratic when reporting subjective information such as how they feel. Experience leads us to believe that too many subjects want to tell the investigator what they believe he or she wants to hear. On the other hand, they may become totally silent when it comes to information about personal experiences they deem embarrassing or detrimental to a healthy life style.

Despite the apparent benefits of objective measurement, the real question remains – are objective measurements more valid than subjective ones? In some cases the answer is no. In many studies the patient's personal opinions and preferences are essential in evaluating a treatment and these assessments are subjective in nature. Take the treatment for osteoporosis where the objective bone density test is often viewed as the definitive way to measure bone mass. If a treatment was shown to increase bone density, but patients didn't report any gain in their daily lives such as less back pain or fewer fractures, should the treatment be considered a success? Bone density might not be the critical factor that signals the effects of osteoporosis for a given patient. While the objective measurement may well indicate treatment success, the subjective measurement may be the more appropriate assessment. No question, relying on objective tests alone can mean a study will end up with an impressive quantitative answer, but it might not be the answer to the more relevant question regarding the ultimate effectiveness of the treatment from the patient's perspective.

In addition to measuring major efficacy variables, collecting safety data is vitally important in clinical trials. Safety information comes from two primary sources – laboratory rests and patient reports. The objective laboratory tests, based on urine and blood samples from subjects, provide invaluable data on how the drug affects the functioning of organs such as the kidney and liver. On the other hand, there aren't standardized tests for side effect information. Patient's volunteer the information and that means much of what they report are subjective personal assessments.

Unfortunately, there is also no standard way to collect information on patient reports about a drug's harmful adverse effects. A researcher can accept volunteered statements by subjects, they can specifically ask if the subject is encountering any side effects, or they can use a check list to record specify types of side effects. Furthermore, just the presence of a side effect may be noted or the degree of the side effect can be required. The many variations for recording adverse events produces large differences in the incidence of side effects for the same drug from one study to the next. Sadly, even the method to chronicle adverse experiences used is too often omitted when researchers publish their clinical trial results.

The journal *Controlled Clinical Trials* published a survey of rheumatoid arthritis trials conduced from 1959–1984 and noted that the method to record side effects was not mentioned in over 50 percent of the trials. That dismal result is probably not a whole lot better today. Given he current state of affairs, it's not reasonable to know what the side effect incidence figures mean based on reports produced for too many clinical trials.

Timing

When to take measurements may, on the surface, look like an easy question to answer. Experimental designs require measurements to be made before, during and at the end of the treatment period. But, in reality, "when" may be a very difficult question for the research team and one that could have major repercussions on the soundness of medical research projects. Timing of measurements is based on pre-determined endpoints specified in the protocol. When a drug's action on the various assessment made in a trial are not fully understood, the time specified in the protocol may be too early or too late. In either case vital information is lost and incorrect conclusions is a likely result.

There are treatments that have a long latency before their effect is demonstrated in a patient. Cancer treatment offers a good example since the emergence of a good effect may take several years before it is apparent. Failure to continue treatment and make assessments for at least two years may well miss a useful therapeutic agent.

This timing issue is also a concern when it comes to patient safety. It may take months or even years before there is recognition of a very harmful drug-related side effect. For instance, with many chemotherapeutic agents, fertility problems can be a delayed side effect. However, due to cost and time constraints, clinical trials are not long-term ventures. As a consequence, there is an obvious disconnect between finding unusual side effects that could be lethal and the length of clinical trials. The consequences of this discrepancy is one of the greatest challenges facing the medical research enterprise.

It is important to point out that frequently research teams develop a model to test drugs for the same indication. The model uses the same assessments that are taken the same way and done on a set schedule. There are many sound reasons to praise this approach. Repetition reduces errors, increases performance and provides a reasonable basis to compare different drugs that go through the process. However, there are drawbacks. Flaws in the design of the basic model are repeated over and over. Furthermore, a novel drug may be unfairly penalized because the standard assessments fail to pick out its advantages. The reverse can also be true. Due to a standard schedule of safety tests and observations, that is carried out too infrequently, negative effects can be missed repeatedly.

Surrogate Measures

A surrogate measurement is one that replaces the clinically meaningful endpoint because it is thought to be a suitable alternative. In an experimental study there is always a major clinically important outcome that is the primary measurement in the trial (e.g. preventing a death, curing a disease or eliminating an infection). Typically, the primary endpoint matters most to the patient, but it takes a long time to appear. A surrogate endpoint measurement is expected to reflect the state of the primary endpoint. For example, a test confirming an antibody response to a flu vaccine is a surrogate endpoint for the primary outcome, prevention of flu. Substituting surrogate measurements for primary outcomes appeals to researchers because they allow shorter and smaller trials.

If researchers wanted to do a clinical trial to see if a new drug could reduce the incidence of deaths from a stroke, they would face an onerous task. The number of subjects needed would be very large; the length of the trial would be very long. The delay in completing the trial would also deny patients access to an exciting and promising new therapy. A way out of this dilemma is to use a surrogate rather than the primary measurement, stroke. Keeping the blood pressure under control reduces the risk of a stroke so blood pressure is an acceptable surrogate measurement. Typically, a blood pressure study would involve less than 100 patients could last only two or three months. A stroke study on the other hand would require four or five thousand patients and take four or five years. The alternative of using blood pressure rather than stroke as the endpoint is quite appealing in this setting.

Today blood pressure is considered a surrogate measure for a number of other illnesses related to heart and blood vessel abnormalities. It hasn't always been that way. Back in the 1960s, whether it was worth medicating people who had a mild or even a moderate elevation of blood pressure, was in question. Ten years later the results of various clinical trials provided convincing evidence that lowering blood pressure prevented heart attacks and saved lives. Finding drugs that keep the blood pressure in check is one of the greatest success stories in clinical research.

However, introduction of a surrogate measurement requires precise knowledge of its relationship to the primary outcome. Without careful selection, it could skew the entire study if it proves not to be a valid endpoint. Also, since a surrogate measure reduces the size and length of a clinical trial, there is less safety data due to the reduced incidence of treatment exposure and accumulation of data.

Unfortunately, relying on a surrogate measurement can indeed fail. First, as suggested, the surrogate may not be a valid endpoint – it doesn't measure what scientists think it is measuring. An example of what can go wrong was brought to the attention of cardiologists by articles in the *New England Journal of Medicine* on the cardiac arrhythmia suppression trial. It had been hypothesized that suppressing irregular heart rhythms (i.e. an arrhythmia) would reduce the rate of death in patients who had had a heart attack. The primary endpoint was avoiding a heart related death and the prevention of abnormal heart rhythms was the surrogate measure. Researchers designed a brilliant trial to test the surrogate by including measurements for both the surrogate and the primary end points. The treatments included placebo and three drugs that had been marketed because they controlled irregular heart rhythms. The subjects were patients who survived a heart attack, but now had irregular heart rhythms so their lives were at risk for further attacks.

The study came up with a startling finding. Early into the trial, two of the "effective" drugs turned out to be associated with more deaths than the placebo treatment. The death rates were almost double and, understandably, the two drugs were removed from the trial. Eventually it was also discovered that the third drug was associated with more deaths than the placebo. The active drugs had their expected effect and abnormal rhythms decreased, but, the drugs also had secondary effects on the heart and they led to an increase in overall deaths.

Another surrogate, used in HIV (Human Immunodeficiency Virus) trials, didn't work out either. A blood cell type (CD4) is present in patients with HIV and cell counts could be readily measured from a blood sample. It made biological sense to use the CD4 counts as a surrogate since CD4 cells helped fight infections. If there were low counts, it implied that the disease was overwhelming the body's defenses. In the end however, CD4 counts did not accurately predict the effect of treatment on the ultimate endpoint – time till death.

When they work, surrogate markers represent a fantastic tool in clinical research. They provide a result about a drug's effectiveness that is obtained sooner, at less cost and with less inconvenience to the subject than the true endpoint of interest. However, they can be inappropriate substitutes and when that happens the penalty is severe: incorrect results and conclusions. In addition, an ironic drawback of a surrogate is that one of its strengths becomes a liability. It reduces the size and length of a clinical trial, but that means there is less safety data due to the reduced drug exposure.

Composite Measurements

A composite measurement combines multiple endpoints into a single measurement. There are several benefits to using composite measurements. Visualize a research effort in which the ultimate endpoint is a reduction in deaths. It will take a long time to accumulate enough deaths so there would be a valid test of effectiveness. Researchers can design a shorter trial by creating a composite endpoint that counts subjects who have outcomes that relate to the same basic problem. For example, a cardiac death, a heart attack and hospitalization for a heart-related event all related to an abnormal heart condition. In a trial of a treatment intended to protect patients from adverse cardiac effects, a subject who experienced one of these events would be counted as a treatment failure.

The use of a composite endpoint is risky because it is based on an assumption that may not be true. The assumption made is that all the components of a composite are equally relevant. But this is not always the case. A death is at a different level of importance than a non-fatal event such as a hospitalization. In fact, it is rare when all components of a composite endpoint are of equal importance. As a result, unless the composite and all its elements give a relatively consistent finding there is an interpretation problem. If there is an inconsistency, the result for the composite could be misinterpreted to mean that it applies to each of its element, but that may not be the case. To avoid this trap, each event type could be analyzed separately, but that raises its own set of problems. It creates a problem of multiple testing in the statistical analysis which is discussed in a later chapter. It also raises the question of why create a composite if each event is going to be analyzed separately anyway?

> *Measurement is never exact; observations and inferences drawn from them are subject to various errors.* (K. Rothman, *Annals Internal Medicine*)

Measurement decisions play a critical role in designing clinical trials – this fact cannot be undervalued. It's not unusual for investigators to have a number of choices, but whether few or many, the choice they make may spell the difference between showing a new agent is effective or ineffective, safe or unsafe. This kind of inconsistency should make anyone hesitant to accept the results from any one clinical trial because another trial that uses different measurements may come up with a conflicting result.

Chapter 9
Bias Control – A Closer Look at Blinding and Randomization

Abstract There are many uncontrolled factors in clinical studies and, in order to make sound treatment assessments, researchers need to impede their influence. The two pillars of the clinical trial that deter bias are blinding and randomization. Blinding keeps the subjects and researchers honest by concealing the mediation a subject takes and randomization is designed to produce equivalent treatment groups. But blinding isn't fool proof – treatment identification may be exposed to researchers and/or subjects because of the unique action (e.g. dry mouth) of a drug and there are also many examples of deliberate attempts to un-blind clinical studies. Without randomization researchers would decide who gets a new treatment and who gets a control treatment t (e.g. placebo) and those choices would almost assuredly biased a study's results. Allowing treatment assignments to be made by a random process is a major way to overcome that possibility, but, there is no guarantee that randomization has succeeded in creating unbiased treatment groups.

Keywords Bias · blinding · equivalent groups · randomization · treatment code concealment

Many people believe they can tell if a treatment is any good just by trying it. They certainly know if it is helping them or causing a problem. If this were true, all researchers would need to do is give the experimental treatment to people and keep track of what happens to them until a trend is established. That logic is simple and easy to follow. But, it's not sound reasoning. How patients respond to medications is complex and can be effected by little known or even unknown factors so investigators can be easily fooled by merely giving a drug and relying solely on patient evaluations. To counter the many uncontrolled factors and in order to make sound treatment assessments, researchers need to build in ways to subdue the factors that could bias the study.

No question, the two pillars of the clinical trial that serve to limit bias are blinding and randomization: The goal of blinding is to keep the subjects and researchers objective by concealing the medication a subject takes while the purpose of randomization is to produce equivalent treatment groups.

R.R. Gauch, *It's Great! Oops, No It Isn't,*
© Springer Science+Business Media B.V. 2009

Blinding

Blinding means more than just keeping the name of the treatment hidden. In a double blind trial, the treatments must be identical in every way so neither the patient nor the researcher is aware of the treatment assignment. Patients may well see the treatment being given to patients in the other treatment group(s), and the appearance of the drug used in the study could give a clue to its identity. Differences in taste, smell, or mode of delivery may also influence patient response, so these aspects should be identical for each treatment as well. It's been shown that even the color of a medication can influence efficacy so the treatments must also be matched on color.

When using a placebo control group the experimental medication and the placebo are prepared to they look and taste exactly alike. However, if the study is designed to test two active medications, it may be necessary to use the "double dummy" method to achieve blinding. For example, if researchers want to compare two medicines, one that comes as a green tablet and one as a pink capsule, they could also prepare green placebo tablets and pink placebo capsules. Now the subjects in one treatment group take a green active tablet and a pink placebo capsule. The other treatment group receives the pink active capsule and the green placebo tablet.

Another problem researchers need to overcome is the possibility that an active drug will produce a unique reaction (e.g. dry mouth). Subjects who experience that reaction and associate it with the active drug have clearly broken the blind. Subjects may also recognize a 'medicated' state, particularly when they have received an active drug in the past. Definitely, protecting the blind in a clinical trial can be formidable task. In antidepressant research, a review article in the *Journal of Nervous and Mental Disease* speculated that the results in favor of an active drug may be due entirely to biases linked to unblinding.

If a subject inadvertently breaks the blind, the harm is more likely to affect observations reported by the subject. Consequently, the frequency of adverse reactions, which are usually based on self-reported complaints, may be biased more than an objective measurement such as the subject's weight. It is also believed that the blind is easily broken in psychiatric drug studies because these drugs have specific adverse effects (e.g. dry mouth, constipation and sexual dysfunction). The results of a review done in 1993 by scientists at the SUNY Health Science Center, Syracuse, NY offers strong evidence that blinds are vulnerable in psychiatric research. Twenty of the 23 psychotropic studies examined, produced evidence that both clinicians and patients knew well beyond chance whether real drugs or placebos were being administered.

Patient feedback to an investigator can also defeat blinding. Even if the clues given off by a drug are subtle, without realizing it the investigator may become aware of the treatment a subject is on. For example, the effects produced by an active medication may clearly expose its identity when there is a clear sign (e.g. flushing) present in a large proportion of the cases taking an active drug, but absent among the placebo-control subjects.

Researchers, aware of the unique reaction problem, can try to retain the blind by adding a chemical to the other comparison agent so that it also causes the same reaction. This method helps retain the double blind, but it does alter the control preparation. It's probably a wise trade-off, but one shouldn't lose sight of the fact that the ingredient added to the placebo medication may have other properties that could influence the way people react.

It thus emerges that the double-blind trial is in itself no guarantee of absolute reliability and uniformity of results. (P. Martini in J. Klotter, *Townsend Letter for Doctors and Patients*)

Some research advocates take blinding to a new level by introducing the notion of triple blinding. With triple blinding the statisticians in charge of the data analysis are also blinded so they only know there is a treatment A and a treatment B, but A and B are not identified. The rationale in this instance is that statisticians have a number of options, when it comes to choosing and performing the statistical analysis, and knowledge of the treatments can result in biased decision-making.

History

Blinding is not a new concept – it has a rich 200 year-old history. Benjamin Franklin introduced blinding in the late 18th century to test claims made for Mesmerism, a treatment based on the belief that magnetism could heal people.

The adoption of blind assessment as a regular part of drug testing is linked to the 19th century struggle between mainstream medicine and alternative approaches such as homeopathy. Mainstream medicine held the high ground. It was generally believed that their medicines worked so they did not have to produce prove that they were effective. But, that meant the more "unorthodox" sciences had to show that their agents were effective as well. Consequently, advocates of homeopathy remedies decided it would be important to test their medicines against inactive preparation in a blind fashion. The results of one of the earliest and most carefully designed experiments using this approach appeared in an 1880 homeopathic journal. The study compared sugar pellets containing a miniscule amount of a homeopathic product against pellets without the homeopathic agent. Physicians, knowledgeable about homeopathy, served as "provers", they would take both preparations and see if they could tell which one contained the active homeopathic agent. A minister who also served as a Bowdoin College professor coded and dispensed the test preparations. The trial originally planned to use 100 provers, but just 25 turned up on the day of the test and in the end only 9 rendered a choice as to which preparation had the active material and which one didn't. In every single case they were wrong. Conventional medicine supporters couldn't be more pleased and noted that the negative result did not come from the opponents of homeopathy; it came from its adherents. Nevertheless, by 1900 homeopathic medicine had adopted blinding as a routine procedure for evaluating its products.

In modern times, 1954 is often used to mark the time when belief in the use of the double blind method took hold in medical research. That year an influential physician, and the organizer of a medical conference on how to evaluate new drugs, presented a paper that showed that in a double blind study there was no difference between an active drug for angina and a placebo. That result contradicted a previous unblinded study showing there was an effect by the identical drug. In this case, it is clear that the prestige of the conference leader carried the day; the drug was considered ineffective and study blinding was seen as a critical component of clinical research.

Blinding is important – even essential – but it is not always possible. An authority, no less than the National Cancer Institute, notes that in a trial comparing surgery with cancer chemotherapy, blinding would be impossible. Think of a study to test a new surgical technique that is compared to the current choice of treatment which relies on drug therapy. You can blind the medication by having one group take an active preparation and the other group identical-appearing placebos. It's true that sham surgery could be instituted as well, but then the trial would totally fail ethical standards. Subjecting a subject to the risks of anesthesia only increases the ethical burden. Needless to say, the risk of major surgery for those who don't need it represents irresponsible professional behavior.

Fortunately, some types of sham surgery represent minimal risk to subjects as illustrated by the following example that appeared in the *New York Times*. Operating on an arthritic knee had become an accepted practice to relieve the pain patients experienced. There were theoretical reasons to believe that the knee operations would relieve the pain and many patients reported relief after their operations. In a clinical trial to test this assumption, patients suffering from an arthritic knee were given either a real knee operation or a sham one where they were sedated, but only skin incisions were made. A physician, other than the surgeon, made the treatment assessments. As a result, the patients and those assessing them were blinded. Outcomes, assessed over a two-year period, showed that at no time did the group receiving the true surgery do better than those who had the placebo procedure. If anything, the results were worse for those having the real surgery. The research was invaluable; it showed that a costly procedure was useless.

Randomization

One way to avoid an unfair result from a clinical study is to assign subjects to the control and treatment groups so any inequality between the groups is minimized. Today the most (and for some the only) acceptable method to do this is to use a random process to make the treatment assignment. In a randomized trial the subjects don't get to choose what group they will be assigned to, and neither does the study team. They are assigned to either the control group or the experimental group on the basis of chance. To accomplish this researchers rely on mathematical devices that produce the random allocation. Perhaps the most common method is to use random numbers that are generated by a computer. In this method, patients are assigned a random number after they are admitted to a trial. Odd numbers could place the subject in the experimental group and even numbers in the control group.

The first random number on the list applies to the first individual entering the study, the second number the second person, etc. Thus, if the first two numbers were 37 and 84, the first subject would be in the experimental group and the second one in the control group.

The history of randomization is a bit murky. It includes early descriptions, unsubstantiated claims and the application of a transitional approach called alternation. In the 17th century a Flemish physician wrote that between 200 and 500 poor people that have fevers, pleurisy, and other such diseases should be identified and then divided in half. By lot, half of them would fall under his care where there was no blood letting. The other half would go to another physician who practiced blood letting. The "contest" would be decided by who had to attend fewer funerals. Unfortunately, his challenge was not accepted so in medical annals our Flemish doctor can not get credit for being the first to use randomization in medical research.

Bloodletting again appears in what may be the earliest account of using an alternating treatment assignment method. An 1816 doctoral thesis at the University of Edinburgh describes how patients were allocated to three military surgeons. There were 366 soldiers requiring treatment and they were assigned alternatively to the physicians. The soldiers received equivalent care, but one of the physicians practiced blood letting as part of his treatment and the others didn't. The blood-letting physician wound up with 35 deaths compared to an average of 3 deaths for the other two physicians who did not practice blood letting. The amazing result was so strong it did not require a sophisticated statistical analysis to be convincing.

A 1918 report by the German scientist, Adolph Bingel, described his investigation of an old versus a new serum for diphtheria immunization. The research started out poorly – almost all patients were given the active serum. Fortunately, Bingel revised the study and substituted an allocation process called alternation whereby alternative subjects received either an active or a control serum. This trial is also an early example of the use of blinding. The pharmacy prepared the control serum so it was indistinguishable from the active serum and apparently the deception worked because the staff could not detect a visual difference between the two treatments. Furthermore, other physicians on the ward who were not involved in the study, were asked their opinions of a patient's outcome without telling them what treatment a patient received.

The study most often cited as ushering in the use of randomization as we know it today was a 1948 trial by the British Medical Research Council. The trial was a test to see if the drug Streptomycin could cure tuberculosis. Whether a patient would be treated by Streptomycin or not was made by reference to a statistical set of randomly generated numbers. The details of the numerical series were unknown to any of the investigators or others medical staff. The treatment group for a subject was contained in a set of sealed envelopes, each bearing on the outside only the name of the hospital and a sequential number. After acceptance of a patient, and before admission to the study, the appropriate numbered envelope was opened. The card inside noted if the subject was to receive Streptomycin or the control agent.

A good method to see the value of randomization is to compare the results of randomized versus nonrandomized clinical trials for the same indications and treatments. These days randomization is so well established that it's hard to locate examples where the same drug is tested in both randomized and non-randomized trials. However, in an article evaluating clinical trials that appeared in the *Journal of the American Academy of Dermatology*, the authors noted that non-randomized studies were much more likely to show larger treatment differences than randomized trials. And those positive results for non-randomized trials were more likely to be repudiated at a later time. A typical example cited in the article involved a claim that a cancer drug, azathioprine, could reduce the dose of steroids necessary to treat skin blisters. Several non-randomized studies supported that belief. However, a randomized trial of the drug showed that it had zero or at best negligible effects.

Due to a lack of head to head comparisons, analysts use an alternative way to investigate the effect of randomization. They look at the results of randomized trials compared to those from exploratory trials where randomization was impossible. In 2001, an extensive analysis appeared in *JAMA* and found that non-random allocation studies over-estimated as well as under-estimated treatment effects. However, the over-estimation was on average quite a bit higher than the under-estimation indicating that lack of randomization, on average, exaggerated treatment effects. A second investigation, published in 2006 in the *American Journal of Epidemiology*, scrutinized randomized clinical trials versus case-control and cohort studies that investigated the same treatment comparison. All tolled, there were 45 treatment comparisons involved and a total of 240 randomized trials and 168 exploratory studies. There was a high correlation between the randomized trials and nonrandomized studies in their estimates of what treatment did better. However, the randomized and nonrandomized studies often disagreed substantially on the size of the difference. Larger treatment effects were more likely to occur in the nonrandomized studies supporting the *JAMA* finding that non-randomized studies bias results by overestimating a treatment effect.

The concept of randomization may sound straightforward, but it is not all that easy to describe to prospective subjects. This observation is supported by an amazing review of researcher's explanation of the concept to parents, whose children were potential subjects in a randomized clinical trial. The review appeared in a 2004 article in *JAMA*. In 137 sessions involving written and oral explanations, half of the parents still did not understand randomization. Some of the problem clearly had to do with the physician's explanation of the concept. Here are two examples of what was said:

> *The computer will assign him a regimen and they will pick it instead of me. Cause I don't know which one of these things is the best.*
> *And then she would get randomized by a computer to be on one of those four arms. And we don't decide. It's the computer who decides.*

Clearly parents were confused.

Preoccupation with randomization's goal, group equivalence, is a legitimate concern for the conscientious researcher. It has been shown that imbalances can exert a strong influence on the observed result of a trial. However, it appears some researchers never check to see if the groups are, in fact, comparable. It is also disconcerting to learn that published clinical trial reports that claim to be randomized, tend not to report the randomization methods. According to the review in the *American Journal of Epidemiology* mention previously, only about one in three trials provide an adequate description.

There is also concern that investigators are not sufficiently diligent when it comes to concealing the treatment assignments for a study. This uneasiness is reinforced by the revelation that too many publications fail to include a description of the allocation concealment method. A 2005 review in the *British Medical Journal* examined clinical trial reports appearing in various medical journals and found that 40 percent of the time, the description of the concealment procedures was absent or inadequate.

An imposing article in *JAMA* revealed many examples of deliberate attempts to expose the treatment code. Envelopes that contained the treatment designation were held up to the light by researchers to reveal the code. If the code was in an opaque envelope, special lights available in the radiology department, were used to find the treatment assignment. The ransacking of an office of the person holding the code has also been documented. In addition, the code can be broken by securing one pill from a subject and having it analyzed for its chemical properties.

Patients themselves wonder about the treatment assigned to them. Some may try to find out the treatment group they're in by opening and tasting the capsules thereby nullifying the protection of the double blind. Obviously, code concealment fails on an individual subject level when the blind is broken. It is not surprising, therefore, to find that investigators have been asked to provide detailed reports on the steps they took to blind studies, including results of analyses they used to detect if the blind was broken.

The unblinding of a trial by investigators may be for no better reason than their wanting the trial results to confirm their personal beliefs about the test treatments. Another reason is to insure they obtain the result the study's sponsor want so the researcher will be used for future trials. They may also just want a certain patient to benefit from the active treatment and avoid the possibility the person would be assigned the control treatment. Still, invalidating a trial by exposing the randomization schedule or unblinding it is a disheartening judgment about the integrity of researchers, others on their staff or the subjects who commit these acts.

Patients may also be inappropriately randomized into clinical trials because of human error. Often study personnel work in chaotic clinical environments. Many clinical trials involve acutely ill patients who require urgent interventions. Determination of patients' eligibility for inclusion in these studies must be made quickly with consent and randomization arranged expediently. In these settings, patients who do not meet the predetermined eligibility criteria may, nevertheless, be included in the trial. In addition, simple misunderstandings or inadequate interrogation may also allow unacceptable patients to enter a trial.

In spite of randomization, treatment group equivalence can also be suspect because the data from some subjects may be unusable. Subjects may drop out of a trial because they no longer wish to or can no longer participate. The researcher may also have to expel subjects who do not comply with the protocol requirements such as failing to take the study medication, taking drugs that invalidate the required assessments or not showing up for critically important examinations and tests. Consequently, the dropouts and incorrectly admitted subjects can cause a satisfactory treatment allocation to become unbalanced and biased in favor of one treatment or the other. This problem of unqualified subjects and those with inadequate data also becomes a major concern when it comes to the statistical analysis of the study data. Options on how to deal with this situation are presented in a later chapter on analysis issues.

> There is no way to guarantee that the randomizing process for subjects has created group equivalence on all relevant unforeseen variables. (M. Walizer, *Research Methods and Analysis Searching for Relationships*)

In concluding this chapter, it should be emphasized that randomized and blinded clinical trials are essential to good medical research practice. They are the best insurance for gathering unbiased evidence about new medical treatments. However, the most methodically rigorous trials may still not completely eliminate bias. Problems such as intentional or unintentional unblinding, randomization schedules that do not produce equivalent groups, and unconcealed treatment allocation assignments can occur and cause misleading results.

Chapter 10
Utility – Are Clinical Trial Results Useful?

Abstract The utility of a trial raises the question – how broadly can the study results be applied? Researchers create very strict requirements for selecting trial participants and then they demand that they follow very exacting procedures during the study. These steps make sense – they optimize the effectiveness of a treatment, but, they also have an undesirable downside. The results only apply to those specially selected subjects – and that most likely will be a tiny proportion of the patients in the more broadly based society. Furthermore, only volunteers who give their written informed consent can become research subjects, which has a crippling effect on the usefulness of all clinical trials. The results of a clinical trial may not apply to the people unwilling to take the risks inherent in a clinical trial. In addition subjects often have to be recruited and each recruitment method (newspaper advertisements, appeals by the investigators, payment offers, etc.) may draw a unique set of people. In fact, it's possible to describe most volunteers as the "UN" people. They tend to be unemployed, uninsured, unhealthy and unselfish.

Keywords External validity · generalizability · informed consent · subject selection · study volunteers

> *At its best a trial shows what can be accomplished with a medicine under careful observation and certain restricted conditions. The same results will not invariably or necessarily be observed when the medicine passes into general use.*
> (A. Hill in R. Horton, *Statistics in Medicine*)

The utility of clinical trials raises the question: how valuable are the results from a clinical trial? What is the worth of a clinical trial that generates correct answers if that information isn't useful? How good are the results of a clinical trial if they do not apply to a broad range of settings and situations? Are the results relevant to many different kinds of people and locations or are they confined to a narrow range of people and places?

We know that clinical research uses a sample to tell how well a medical treatment will work. If the sample is composed of very diverse people, the results apply to a broad population. If the sample is very homogenous, then the results apply to a smaller and more restrictive set of people. In theory, enrolled clinical trial subjects should adequately represent a trial's target population. In other words, if two-thirds of the patients with the illness under study are females, the recruitment process should end up with that approximate male:female ratio. Inferring results to groups other than those participating in a clinical trial should not be done without considerable thought, rational and supporting evidence.

In the academic world, the term "external validity" is used to refer to the utility of a study and the term "generalizability" is frequently used as well. I prefer a more descriptive term – usefulness. No matter what term is used, the place to begin this discussion is with the composition of the type of subjects who participate in clinical trials.

Volunteers

Let's begin the discussion on volunteers with a simple but critical question: who would be willing to participate in a medical research experiment? The answer raises a conspicuous problem that has a crippling effect on the usefulness of all clinical trials. Only volunteers become research subjects. The millions of people who do not wish to accept the risks associated with a clinical trial never participate and the results for clinical trials can never directly apply to them. This restriction wouldn't matter if informed volunteers were like everyone else, but that's not necessarily the case.

Much of the research on the type of individual who volunteers for clinical research comes from early trials that use healthy individuals. The aim of these early investigations is to get a better understanding of the clinical pharmacology of new drugs – i.e. how do people's bodies react to a drug. Investigations about the uniqueness of volunteers consistently report that volunteers are a special set of individuals. Even though not all of the research is current, the findings are nevertheless impressive. A 2003 article in *Perspectives in Biology and Medicine* reviewed three investigations (two of which occurred before 1970) that looked into medical conditions of volunteers who participated in early clinical pharmacology trials. The authors concluded that a large proportion of the volunteers had a history of psychiatric illness, plus other medical conditions and temperaments that differed from the general population. In addition, a report in the *British Journal of Pharmacology* on Dutch student volunteers, also used in clinical pharmacology research, found the volunteers to be more extroverted, as well as tolerant, self-confident and optimistic compared to the "average" person.

The results leave a rather confused picture about just what kind of person a volunteer is, but there is a common theme from the research that examined this question – volunteers are different. Still, when it comes to usefulness, the finding that volunteers and non-volunteers are different is relevant only if the difference influences trial outcomes. Readers should keep this qualification in mind as they read the rest of this discussion.

In addition to the early trial in healthy subjects, it is also important to examine the larger trials that use subjects with the target illness and ask the question: do these volunteers resemble the population they are suppose to represent? To this end, one study under the direction of S. Woods, a researcher from Yale University's School of Medicine, compiled demographic characteristics of patients who participated in schizophrenia trials. The same information was collected on other patients in the clinical population from which the trial participants had been selected. This latter group represents the target population. When comparing the two groups, the participants in the clinical trials differed substantially from the non-participants. There was a larger proportion of trial participants who were male and had never married. Since these factors were associated with relatively poor treatment outcomes, it is possible that the trial results had a bias. The subjects participating in the trials also had a higher proportion of three other characteristics. Compared to the non-participants they were younger, more likely to be high school graduates and have full time jobs. This time those three traits were associated with better treatment outcomes so again a biased result was likely, but this time the bias was in the opposite direction.

A second report in the journal *Advances in Psychiatric Treatment* also dealt with psychiatric research and it noted that people with certain demographic characteristics were harder to recruit. The principle traits that adversely affected recruitment were age, gender, race and residence. More specifically, people who are older, male, non-white and living in an urban setting tend to be under-represented in psychiatric research according to this article.

Recruiting Subjects

Volunteers willing to join a clinical trial still have to be recruited. There are many ways to do this and not surprisingly, each method has a bearing on the usefulness of a trial. Investigators may use advertisements, post information about the trial on a Website, utilize their institution's database of potential volunteers, contact colleagues and ask for their support, approach their own patients or use the services of professional recruiting agencies. They could also seek subjects by contacting other sources such as employees where they work or students at a medical school or a nearby college.

The usefulness problem in this instance has to do with the methods employed to attract (some believe the word should be coerce) subjects. Each method can favor one type of subject over another. That preference can distort a clinical trial sample so it fails to represent the target population. For example, a popular inducement, especially in the clinical pharmacology-testing phase, is money. People motivated by a financial inducement are more likely to be poorer than the general population and that also translates into a larger proportion of younger people volunteering and participating in these early clinical trials.

Researchers who approach their own patients or employees at the institution where they work to join their medical trial can apply a great deal of pressure on these individuals. Even if the doctor assures them that participation is their choice, they may fear rejection if they fail to sign-up. It is felt that women are more vulnerable to this kind of inducement than men and, if true, these trials can end up with an excessive number of women. Another source of pressure comes from professional recruitment organizations, employed to recruit volunteers. The recruiting agency earns its money based on the number of people they enroll and they can be quite forceful in convincing people to become subjects. Giving in to pressure is frequently seen as a function of immaturity. Hence, people who join a trial as a result of a recruitment organization are frequently young and tend to tilt the distribution of study subjects in that direction.

People who are seriously ill often search out clinical research studies and try to become subjects. If they have limited financial means, this may be their only chance to obtain treatment for their particular illness. For example, people with a condition such as AIDS may find participation in a clinical trial an especially appealing opportunity. A clinical trial relying on this incentive for their subjects will end up with a lopsided number of subjects in poor health.

The Internet has opened up new avenues for both researchers looking for subjects and patients looking to become subjects. For example, the NIH has a site where healthy volunteers can register their names so they can take part in clinical research studies. Pharmaceutical companies, universities and hospitals all support sites on the Internet that lists experimental studies that may be of interest to potential subjects. The people who actively search out and find clinical trials are more assertive, concerned about their health and competent (computer literate anyway) than the "average" citizen. They may well be overrepresented in clinical trials. On the other hand, patients who do not speak English and who cannot afford a computer will almost certainly be under represented in clinical studies.

Advertisements in newspapers or on the radio are frequently used to obtain volunteers for the large-scale phase III trials. This approach tends to attract better-educated people who may maintain better healthcare practices. Thus, using this set of subjects also becomes a problem since any study findings would apply more particularly to this special segment of society.

Based on recruiting strategies it's tempting to describe volunteers as the "UN" people. They tend to be unemployed, uninsured, unhealthy and unselfish. If you're not working and don't have health insurance, a clinical trial may be quite attractive. Unfortunately, the unemployed and uninsured combination may also mean subjects are in poor health generally. On the other hand, individuals may be motivated to join a trial for commendable reasons. They believe their service will help find cures or alleviate suffering. Their unselfish, altruistic justification also means they are likely to be especially good research subjects. They may accept all protocol restrictions and their behavior increases the chances of a positive result. However, too many subjects like this can also create a bias because such dedication is lacking in the general population. Any thing that causes the sample chosen for a clinical trial to be different from the population of interest reduces study usefulness and should be considered when interpreting the findings from clinical research.

The complexity of a clinical trial can also be a major issue when it comes to the usefulness question. Individuals who will participate in a clinical trial must first give informed consent, which is obtained by their reading and signing a document describing the study and identifying the risks a participant will face. It's been found that the informed consent documents frequently contain language far too difficult for many people to understand. One investigation, published in the *New England Journal of Medicine*, looked at medical schools doing clinical research. It was found that the average consent form was written at a 10th grade level. However, about 50 percent of adults only read at the eighth grade level. Certainly, in this setting, if the educational training of potential subjects is weak, the chances they can understand a consent form is questionable. Technically, people who do not understand the risks of a clinical trial should not be allowed into a trial. However, safeguarding the informed consent requirement by eliminating subjects who do not truly understand the dangers of a clinical trial, threatens the usefulness of a study. Conversely, omitting a group of people based on their reading and comprehension levels, would also reduce the usefulness of clinical trials.

Trial Design

Recruitment and volunteerism are not the only usability issues. A major measure of usefulness involves comparable performance of a drug in clinical trials and in medical practice. In other words, a critical component of usefulness asks the question whether the research findings can be generalized to medical practices. Usefulness would be high if the effectiveness and safety of a drug, demonstrated in a major research study stood up when it entered general use. It is time to take a tour of the protocol and identify additional restrictions that end up impeding a trial's usefulness.

The narrow composition of the subjects selected for the trial, the demands on those subjects to meet all protocol requirements and the specific way the drug must be administered can cripple the usefulness of a study. The strictness set down in a clinical trial protocol can mean the results for a new treatment, obtained from a pivotal clinical trial, may not be repeated when that treatment passes into broader use.

As previously noted, medical researchers carefully select a defined group of subjects for their trial hoping to limit opportunities for error and end up with a group for which the experimental drug will be particularly efficacious. It makes sense to place restrictions on study subjects, but there is also a down side. By being very strict in selecting subjects, researchers hamper their ability to generalize the results of a clinical trial to an array of demographic groups. Often the protocol exclusion criteria are so restrictive that the patients who are eligible for a trial represent only a small proportion of the patients that will be treated when the drug is marketed.

Here is an illustration of what can happen when investigators use only highly selective subjects. A research team at the Department of Medicine, Duke University, looked at the patients currently having bypass surgery using a special technique and published their results in the *Journal of the American College of Cardiology*. They also examined the protocols that were used in the research program that demonstrated the safety and effectiveness of the surgery. Only four percent of the patients currently undergoing the surgery would have satisfied the subject selection criteria stated in the research protocols. That means that 96 percent of the patients now receiving the technique were at some level of risk because the technique had not been proven safe and effective for them.

There are always restrictions on the kind of patient allowed to enter a clinical trial, and rejecting complex patients from clinical trials is common. Patients who have a condition that could interfere with the demonstration of effectiveness (e.g. persons who have a drug addiction) are most unlikely to be accepted into a clinical trial. The lack of compliance with the protocol, as well as other complications related to the addiction, are understandable reasons for the rejection. Yet their exclusion raises an ethical question – why shouldn't these people have a chance to benefit from an effective drug? Shouldn't all types of patients be able to participate in a drug trial even if they risk complicating the demonstration of effectiveness?

It's also true that the behavior of a private patient is far less restricted than that of a subject in a trial. Researchers love subjects who are willing and able to comply with the demands placed on them by the protocol, but that behavior is atypical and when the drug is used by the more cavalier and less compulsive patients found in a typical doctor's practice, the clinical trial result can be quite different in the new setting. Good protocol compliers may be heroes when it comes to clinical studies, but they are saboteurs when it comes to study usefulness. If rigid compliance with a diet, taking a drug exactly on the prescribed schedule and faithful exercising helped a new treatment become successful, all bets might be off when the drug is given to less disciplined patients treated by a family physician.

A study protocol carefully controls how experimental drugs are given and what other drugs must be forbidden in order to increase the likelihood that the experimental drug will be declared effective. However, this level of control is often not reproducible in medical practice. In a physician's private practice, patients are more likely to miss doses, lose their medication, have prescriptions held up by insurance companies, stop taking their medication all together and to consume all sorts of prescription and non-prescription agents that were forbidden during clinical trials. The impact of the new environment can lower or in rare instances raise the effectiveness of a drug established in the more controlled clinical trial. Drug combinations commonly seen in a medical practice can also make patients more or less sensitive to side effects and produce a very different safety profile than that reported in a protocol-controlled clinical trial.

In a clinical trial, taking the drug on a full stomach or in a fasting state may be the way the drug has to be given to reduce troublesome side effects or improve absorption of the drug. The protocol dictates this. In general practice however, these stipulations may not be understood or honored by the patient. In short, drugs that performed well in clinical trials may be unable to meet the challenges of a looser environment.

The usefulness of a clinical trial also depends on whether the outcome measures specified in a protocol are clinically relevant. Many trials use surrogate and composite measures which, as indicated earlier, are often misleading indicators and a trial using them would have low usability as a result.

Generalizability is also affected by the cost of clinical trials because studies can only be run for a limited period of time yet there are many conditions such as diabetes, arthritis and high blood pressure that require people to take a drug for a lifetime. In these cases, there can be no information gleaned from clinical trials to accurately predict what may happen to the patients on long-term treatment.

Trial Setting

An appreciation for the setting of a trial is also essential in assessing usefulness. The results of a trial conducted in one location may not produce similar results when used in an alternative location. Findings may be influenced by customs and behaviors that differ from country to country or even within regions of the same country. Life styles, risk taking behavior, religious practices, etc. all may vary and have an impact on a study. Climate differences can also shape a study result – would you get the same result for a dermatological preparation in a cold dry environment as a hot humid one? Also, consider the variation in results one might get in a stressful city environment versus one in a bucolic country setting that is stress-free.

Health care systems differ and when the care is delivered, who delivers the case, and how the care is delivered can influence the expected actions of a drug. Results from trials done in the industrialized world may not transfer well to third-world countries because of a difference in health-care systems. As an example, trials of acupuncture conducted in East Asia are consistently positive, but those in the industrialized nations are positive only about half the time.

Many of the researchers selected to conduct clinical trials have outstanding credentials, skills and experience. These attributes can affect the efficacy of a drug and cannot be matched by many physicians in private practice. The result can be less effectiveness when a drug is used by the general practitioners. A researcher's ability to recognize patient problems, make judgments about outcome variables (especially those that are subjective) and perform sensitive laboratory tests carefully all can influence a trial's sensitivity to tell a good drug from a bad one.

How a researcher manages a trial can also affect a trial's outcome. Consider the researcher who uses aggressive methods to ensure subjects take their medication. This rigorous approach may ensure better medication compliance and a better result in a medical trial. However, there may be a different result in a medical practice with looser demands on a patient's medication taking.

Researchers also have a preference for doing their research in a hospital setting. That makes sense; in a hospital they have confidence that the experimental drugs are properly administered and the right amount of drug is given at the right time.

There is also the advantage of a relatively aseptic environment and three healthy (not necessarily tasty) meals every day. A treatment found effective in that environment might perform differently in the less constrained atmosphere that outpatients experience.

> Randomized controlled trials carried out in specialised units by expert care givers, designed to determine whether an intervention does more good than harm under ideal conditions, cannot tell us how experimental treatments will fare in general use, nor can they identify rare side effects. (D. Sackett and J. Wennberg, British Medical Journal)

Note that the information in this chapter highlights an ironic conflict. Clinical trials are designed to improve the chances of showing a drug's effectiveness, but this goal reduces a trial's usefulness. As a result, at the end of a research program there may be drug approval, but there will remain many unanswered questions about how the drug will do in the hands of a private practitioner. How much or even whether an individual patient will be helped by a recently FDA approved drug should not be assumed. There are simply too many untested factors associated with a newly approved drug because usefulness is not a priority in designing clinical trials.

Once again, it becomes abundantly clear that it is extremely dangerous to overly rely on the results from a single clinical study. Results from even the best study require affirmation from additional trials because it probably has a low level of usefulness. The obvious consequence is that rarely should one study ever bring about a major change in disease treatment or prevention. Different kinds of studies (not just replication of the same study) introduce different kinds of patients in different settings using a variety of measurements and include other factors that were not present in the initial trial. The usefulness of this set of studies would be invaluable in the practice of medicine, but it's rare to have a variety of clinical studies completed before a drug begins to be sold in the marketplace.

These concerns do not necessarily mean the current approval standards are wrong. As valuable as usefulness is, in most cases it would be impractical and even irresponsible to withhold a drug approval until it was tested in more diverse situations. While the expanded testing program was underway, it would be ridiculous to deny patients like the ones used in the completed trials access to an important drug. However, the unanswered questions about usefulness should not be ignored. Efforts to bolster usefulness need to be carried out in the post-marketing period. Unfortunately, currently there is inadequate emphasis on performing such studies.

Chapter 11
Research Discrimination – Inadequately Tested Populations

Abstract The under-representation of any group in a research program amounts, not only to a decrease in study usefulness, it also represents a form of discrimination against the excluded groups. The neglected groups are deprived and disadvantaged because the overall results from a clinical trial probably do not apply to them. The deprivation is especially focused on demographic attributes such as gender, age, ethnicity and cultural background. Based on these criteria, clinical trials have enlisted volunteers in disproportionate numbers for years and, as a result, their findings apply mainly to a single race (white), a single sex (male) and a single age group (21–55). Consequently, the under-represented groups are left in the dark about the value of new treatments that could help them and the risks they will face from taking recently introduced cannot be adequately understood. Although in recent years, important improvements have been made, the omission of these groups in the past reflects poorly on the medical research community and its passivity to remedy the problem. There is a continuing need to emphasize diversity in clinical trials. The medical research community should work with the FDA and Congress to come up with innovative ways to obtain that diversity.

Keywords Children · diversity · elderly · minorities · subject selection

The last chapter showed there were many factors that conspired to reduce the relative value of clinical trials for large segments of the population. The under-representation of any group in a research program amounts not only to a decrease in usefulness, but also to a form of discrimination against that group. The neglected groups are deprived and disadvantaged because the overall results from a clinical trial probably do not apply to them. In the U.S. the deprivation is especially focused on people who differ because of gender, age, and biological make-up, ethnic or cultural background and as a result they may well have different medical outcomes than that reported for the trial. The under-represented groups are left in the dark about the value of new treatments that could help them. The risks they will face from taking recently introduced cannot be adequately understood.

In this chapter I identify the major segments of society that are most affected by the failure to include them in medical research programs. Although in recent years important improvements have been made, the omission of these groups in the past reflects poorly on the medical research community and its passivity to remedy the problem.

Gender

One of the best and most dramatic illustrations of the lack of inclusion and representation of target populations in clinical trials was the common practice of excluding women subjects. The oversight was especially damaging because the pharmacology of drugs is frequently different in women compared to men. Indeed, the effective dose in males may be dangerously too strong for females. Yet, historically, clinical trials were mostly confined to the male sex because researchers were reticent to include a population that could be destabilized by child bearing and related issues. As a result, once a drug was marketed, an unexpected but important result could appear in women who took the drug. For instance, research confined to male subjects had shown that aspirin cut the rate of a second heart attack, but whether this beneficial effect could be achieved in women could only be assumed. Then, in 2005, a health study under the direction of researchers affiliated with the Harvard Medical School and Brigham and Women's Hospital in Boston showed that aspirin didn't prevent heart attacks at the same rate it did in men.

There are many other pharmaceutical products that have a different effect depending on a person's gender. For instance, Diazepam, a muscle relaxant that is often used to treat epilepsy, impairs the psychomotor skills (control of voluntary movements) of women more than men. In addition, Verapamil, a drug prescribed for high blood pressure, and the antibiotic erythromycin appear to be more effective in women than men.

A primary reason for female censorship in medical research was due to governmental regulations. Until 1993 an FDA policy all but prohibited women of childbearing potential from participating in early phases of drug research. These restrictions excluded almost all women except those who had had their female organs removed or were through menopause. The rationale for their exclusion was reasonable. It was based on a desire to avoid risking the health of a fetus. Since it could take some time to determine if a woman was pregnant, it was safer to avoid the use of an experimental drug in all women who were capable of becoming pregnant. But this practice also meant that physicians knew almost nothing about how to use newly approved drugs in women regardless of their childbearing potential. Actually, according to the regulations, women could be included in a clinical trial if animal reproductive studies showed there was no harm to a fetus, but these reproductive studies occurred late in the drug development process and, as a result, drugs were approved with a dearth of information on their effects in women.

The desire to protect a human fetus was heavily influenced by damage done to the human fetus by the experimental drug thalidomide, and led to the 1962 changes to the laws governing drug research. Even before the thalidomide disaster, subject stability was an important attribute when it came to picking subjects for a clinical trial. Then, and to a lesser extent today, investigators were averse to enroll women because they felt they were less stable than men. Researchers saw shifting hormonal levels as a major contributor to female instability. There was menopause and pregnancy, plus the use of contraceptive pills and estrogen replacement medication, all of which researchers saw contributing to that instability.

There is no question that exclusion of any demographic group from clinical studies can result in substantial gaps in knowledge regarding treatment effects in the excluded group. For instance, it is likely that the female hormones that regulate enzymes break a drug down in one way, while in men, male hormones regulate enzymes in a different fashion. For example, a major antihypertensive drug, propranolol, is metabolized more slowly in women than in men. Other reasons for variation between men and women are the size difference between the sexes and the lower relative fat content in males compared to females.

Excluding women from clinical trials can be equated to a denial of care because clinical trials provide the rationale for drug treatment. By not permitting female participation in clinical research, it essentially meant that the research on the drug's effect in them commenced at the same time a drug appeared in the marketplace. This translated into having women serve as guinea pigs in an uncontrolled setting – no volunteerism or consent required.

Elderly

There have been far too many examples illustrating how clinical research has also neglected the elderly by limiting their participating in clinical trials. Examine almost any protocol and it will contain an age restriction and in most cases that limit will eliminate older patients from the clinical trial. Because patients with an advanced age tend to have many medical problems (hypertension, diabetes, colon cancer, etc.), researchers feel they are less desirable than younger subjects. In addition, older patients are felt to be less reliable about taking their medications and can complicate a study due to their frequent illnesses which lead to high dropout rates. In a word, researchers feel older patients are risky study candidates and it's better not to use them. Obviously, not allowing elderly individuals to participate results in an under-representation of this segment of the population in clinical trials.

And yet, in real life, some of the most likely candidates for a newly marketed drug are the older generation. The elderly, which is the most rapidly growing segment of the population, take a disproportionate amount of the drugs used in this country, but their presence in the research that allowed the drug to enter the marketplace in the first place tends to be overlooked. For instance, in a *USA Today* report over 25 percent of patients treated for a common type of heart attack are older than 75, yet 75-year-olds account for only 15 percent of those in clinical trials of drugs designed to minimize damage to the heart. In addition, an editorial in *JAMA* referred to a study that found 50 percent of the trials to prevent heart attacks excluded patients over 65. Yet more than half of those hospitalized for a heart attack are in the older age groups.

Older people often have biological problems that younger patients don't. Their kidneys don't work as efficiently, and drugs may build up in their blood. Their hearts don't pump as well, their memory is fading and they are more prone to lung disease. It is also true that a drug can be broken down in the body and absorbed into tissues at different rates depending on a person's age. As a result, drug efficacy and safety can vary greatly among younger and older adults.

Even when a trial is designed for "elderly" people an age range could appear in a protocol that is unusually narrow. The protocol could call for people between the ages of 50–65, which excludes all people over 65 even though they clearly meet the definition of "elderly". If the drug turns out to be effective and enters the marketplace, it could be given to someone who is 66 with reasonable confidence. But how about someone 70, or 75 or 80? Would the positive results be expected in all these cases? In the 80-year-old, the drug may not just be ineffective; it could be harmful because it's possible that some of the patient's systems simply can not tolerate the drug.

Ironically, an investigation reported in the *American Journal of Geriatric Cardiology* examined study volunteers and found that older people tend to be more willing than younger people to participate in clinical trials. Older people generally have fewer time constraints and a greater desire to help the next generation by advancing medical research. Nevertheless, elderly subjects usually are under-represented, especially in certain research areas. For example, trials of NSAIDs (Non-steroidal anti-inflammatory drugs) often include an under-representation of elderly subjects. Yet these drugs are commonly used in older people because of the high number of arthritic disorders they have. A report in the *Canadian Medical Association Journal* found that in the major drug trials evaluating NSAIDs only about two percent of patients were 65 years of age or over and less than one tenth of one percent were over 75. The report pointed out that, in practice, elderly people were among the largest users of this class of drugs and had the highest incidence of serious drug-related side effects.

In some research areas, poor representation involves both gender and age. Women are more likely to live longer than men and therefore to develop heart and blood vessel problems at an older age. The development of these cardiovascular diseases may be significantly different in this group than a group of similarly aged male subjects. Innate differences in size, weight, and gender-linked conditions contribute to this group's exclusion as well. For all these reasons, when "elderly people" are included in RABCOTs they are generally younger, fitter and predominantly male. But, ironically and significantly, it is the frail elderly females who are more likely to take the drugs that were tested in these trials. To have to assume that what works in a middle-aged male will be effective to the same degree in an older female is a dangerous assumption.

Children

By far, children are the most difficult age group to study. First of all children cannot give informed consent so parental consent must be substituted if they are to be included in a clinical trial. Even then, few parents can see much value in their child's participation in a medical research program unless their child has an illness that is unresponsive to conventional therapy. Additionally, observations and measurements that rely on verbal skills and attentiveness that are used successfully with adults, become unreliable or impossible assessments in children. As a result, children have often been omitted from clinical trials. A 2005 story in *The New Yorker* stated that approximately 75 percent of drugs approved for use in the United State, many of which are given to children, had never been subjected to comprehensive pediatric studies.

Without direct evidence from children, it's necessary to assume what happens in adults is likely to happen in children, but in fact, children are not "little" adults. The organ that breaks down drugs, the liver, takes years to mature. The kidney, critical for the removal of chemicals, also develops over a period of time. The rate of blood flow to the skin and lungs is also higher in children and, as a result they may absorb topical or inhaled agents more rapidly than adults.

In spite of the dearth of information, amazingly physicians are allowed to use any FDA approved drug in children when they believe it will be beneficial. Nor do they need to inform parents if they prescribe their child a drug that hasn't been specifically tested on children. But they are still left with a tough decision – what is the proper dosage? Because of a lack of research and information, there is no single official repository of information about how to calibrate drug dosages for children. In practice, physicians often try to adjust an adult dose based on a child's weight. But such extrapolations cannot account for the differences in the biology of children. The growing teen-agers, who weigh as much as an adult, tend to both absorb and metabolize medicine more quickly than adults. Even if data are available on older children it is unwise to assume what happens in that age group will be replicated in a younger age group. The metabolic system in children, the way they rid their body of toxic substances and their excretion system, changes as they mature. An example of the age problem is illustrated by the speed with which a popular tranquilizing drug, diazepam, is absorbed and made available to the body. There was a threefold difference for infants compared to older children.

In spite of the efficacy and dosage uncertainty in children, it would be wrong to deny them a possibly effective drug. However, it must be recognized that there is a much greater risk of an untoward result when unproven agents are given to children. Intensive monitoring of the child is called for in that situation.

Minorities

It is sad, but probably not unexpected, that prejudice against minorities is also present in clinical research. Minorities, in general, and African-Americans in particular, have low clinical trial participation rates. There are multiple reasons for the oversight. Often physicians do not bother to discuss the availability of trials with minority patients, information about trials is frequently missing in their communities and it's unusual for the trial to take place near the areas where minority populations live.

Under-representation of Blacks and Hispanics exists even in HIV studies and raises questions about the applicability of the clinical research on AIDS to these patient groups. Ethnic and racial differences exist in the way patients respond to medicines. For example, Asians react differently than Caucasians to some drugs and this difference may also affect a study's outcome when there is a skewed racial distribution. Secondary illnesses are also more likely in some ethnic groups than others. Hypertension is an example where it is more common in African Americans than in Caucasians. Although the reason for this is not clear (it could be genetic or environmental), a trial excluding patients with hypertension will reduce a dispro-portionate number of Blacks.

In some instances a minority population may make up the entire patient data base, but that doesn't mean the researchers had the best interest of the subjects in mind when they conceived the trial. One of the most frequently cited examples of unethical research involved a study that was done exclusively in African Americans. The research project, known as the Tuskegee Trial, lasted from 1932 to 1972 and involved some 400 poor Black men with untreated syphilis. The men were fol-lowed, and compared with around 200 Black men free of the disease, to determine the natural history of syphilis. From a research perspective, medical people wanted to understand syphilis better. Since, at the time the study began, there was very little information on the course of the disease, the research organizers felt the study would serve a useful purpose. There was, at the inception of the study, only one syphilis treatment available and its efficacy was questionable.

Tuskegee was a rural community in Alabama with a high prevalence of syphilis. The U.S. Public Health agency, which set up and conducted the trial, believed it would be a good area to study syphilis. The disturbing and inappropriate features of this trial can be summarized as follows:

1. The participants with syphilis were never told they had the disease. In fact the experimental and control group were offered free burials, not as a gesture to somehow repay their heirs for the subject's participation, but because this was a way to perform an autopsy and determine the destruction caused by the disease.
2. At one point the subjects were given spinal cord taps (a potentially dangerous and painful procedure) to determine the disease status. However, the subjects were told that the rationale for the taps was because they had "bad blood".
3. Penicillin, discovered and used during World War II, was found to be highly effective for the treatment of syphilis. It became available for general use shortly

after the war ended. However, the Tuskegee subjects were never offered the drug because it would obviously interfere with the purpose of the trial – to study the natural course of the disease.
4. In 1969 the governmental health agency convened a group of experts to decide whether to continue or terminate the Tuskegee study. They voted to continue.
5. The local medical society in Tuskegee County agreed not to treat subjects with antibiotics for any disease because such an act would cause confounding of the syphilis trial.

The media exposed the badly designed and executed Tuskegee trial in 1969. A legitimately outraged Congress held hearings on the trial shortly thereafter and subsequently the heartless study was finally terminated. This case illustrates that a clinical investigator's goal should not be to obtain an answer to a research question if it means that subjects will be treated as the means to an end. There must not be a callous disregard for the subject's welfare for the sake of research goals.

National Differences

Almost everyone recognizes the disparity in health between rich and poor nations. The large discrepancy in infant mortality or life expectancy clearly distinguishes the developed and developing countries. However, few are aware of the inequities when it comes to medical research in such populations. Medical research concentrates its resources, not on where there's the greatest need, but where the return on investment is greatest. For instance, infectious diseases such as tuberculosis and malaria plague many poor countries, but the diseases are largely contained in the developed world. Hence, research sponsors in the industrialized world tend to use their resources to concentrate on the illnesses (e.g. heart disease and cancer) that are most common in the well-off nations they represent. Yet, when studies are eventually planned for the poorer nations, even more troubling issues of ethics and exploitation are raised.

Typically, researchers in developing countries cannot conduct their own research and must create partnerships with organizations in more developed countries. The idea that everyone should give informed consent before participating in medical research is very difficult to execute in some poor countries. Because of illiteracy it may be unrealistic to convey the detailed consent information expected in a prosperous nation. Thus, participants from third world countries enter research projects without understanding their rights or their risks.

The question of when placebo control is appropriate has also been an issue in research carried out in disadvantaged third world populations. In the U.S., the drug zidovudine had been found effective in treating AIDS and subsequent research also showed that when zidovudine was given to pregnant women, it significantly reduced the rate of transmission of the AIDS virus to the baby. Since zidovudine, an effective treatment, was available, the use of placebo controls in new studies involving pregnant women would appear to be unethical. However, despite this, studies were designed by trial planners in the U.S. that would take place in developing countries and included a placebo group for HIV-infected pregnant women. Opponents argued that this amounted to a double standard: the use of a placebo group was unquestionably unethical in the developed countries, but in poor countries, somehow this ethical standard no longer applied. The studies involved over 12,000 women in seven countries and it was estimated that more than 1,000 infants would contract the AIDS virus. Proponents of the trial contented that the study, as designed, was the only way to get a quick reliable result and the women were not deprived of therapy since they wouldn't receive zidovudine in the first place.

The World Medical Association responded to this dispute by sending out its strongest message to pharmaceutical companies and research organizations around the world. The Association had the power to revise the Declaration of Helsinki, which is the worldwide source for ethical clinical research, and it was altered in order to protect people in poorer countries from being exposed to unnecessary risks in a clinical study. The revised document called for the testing of any new treatment to include a "best current method" as one of the treatment options. Furthermore, in the presence of a drug known to be effective in the disease being studied, a placebo control group was not to be used.

> Research should not be carried out in countries in development just because it is cheaper and the laws are more lax. The same ethical rules should apply wherever research is being conducted. (A. Milton in B. Christie, British Medical Journal)

Reforming the System

Fortunately, U.S. government with the FDA taking a leadership role, instituted a number of ways to obtain better clinical trial representation of the overlooked populations. For instance, during the clinical trial-testing phase for each drug, the study sponsor must submit the number of women enrolled in clinical trials to the FDA on an annual basis. An even stronger requirement occurs at the time a sponsor seeks marketing approval for their drug. In this instance they must prepare an analysis of the drug's effectiveness and safety in women. The FDA has the option of refusing the approval application if the report is omitted.

A similar requirement applies to elderly people and minorities. The agency also established guidelines encouraging drug manufacturers to include more elderly patients in their studies. They recommended that protocols eliminate an upper age limit and that older people with health problems be allowed to participate if they were able. Although the FDA has no minority-specific programs to increase trial enrollments, it tries to make sure these individuals get information on how to get into clinical trials and has an 800 number just for that purpose. They also established a special office to give information to minority groups and minority physicians information about which pharmaceutical companies are doing clinical trials.

The greatest effort and most success has come in increasing the information on drug effects in children. The 1997 FDA Modernization Act made the greatest impact by giving companies a positive incentive to conduct studies in children. If they did studies requested by the FDA, they received an additional six months of market exclusivity. Pharmaceutical companies have produced well over 100 drugs that have taken advantage of this provision and the FDA estimates that about 80 percent of its requests for child-centered studies will be conducted. In addition, the FDA was granted the authority by Congress to require pediatric studies if they felt the drug would be used in a substantial number of children.

There is a continuing need to emphasize diversity in clinical trials. The medical research community should work with the FDA and Congress to come up with both positive (e.g. tax incentives) and negative (conditional drug approvals) innovations in order to obtain that diversity. Advocacy groups for under-represented populations should be encouraged to join the movement to be sure their constituents are not overlooked. There also needs to be attention directed at what should be measured in clinical trials that can shed light on how different groups respond to new treatments. For example, what test would be best to find physiological or genetic differences among different patient groups? There are many unanswered questions in medical research and finding strategies that will extract the maximum information from clinical trials need to be explored.

Chapter 12
Seven Deadly Flaws – The Clinical Trials' Achilles' Heel

Abstract Wrong results from clinical trials occur because of (1) mistakes by researchers in the planning and execution of clinical trials, (2) the complex and inexact nature of information researchers require and (3) factors that are beyond the control of the researcher. This chapter examines the last element and identifies seven fatal flaws that are inherent in the methodology of clinical trial:

The unknown population
The imperfect sample
The unequal treatment groups
The uncontrolled experimental setting
The breakdown of blinding
The impractical result
The insufficient sample size

These seven elements may or may not contaminate a trial and even if they do, they may not cause a significant distortion of the results. However, it's virtually impossible to know if their presence or their effect occurred, and as a result, researchers can never be certain that their study came up with all the right answers.

Keywords Experimental control · population · sample · sampling error · small sample size

The clinical trial is the backbone of medical progress. It is responsible for many of the important advances in treating dreaded diseases such as cancer. Survival rates for breast, uterine, prostate and bladder cancer all improved because of clinical trials. Clinical trials showed that breast cancer could be treated just as effectively with limited surgery as with major surgery, sparing patients unnecessary suffering and disfigurement. Clinical trials debunked the myth that a synthetic estrogen was useful to prevent miscarriages when in fact it caused more harm than good in women trying to maintain a pregnancy. Clinical trials showed that vaccines could prevent a wide variety of dreadful diseases – smallpox, diphtheria, tuberculosis, etc. Clinical trials identified effective drugs to treat debilitating illnesses like rheumatoid arthritis and multiple sclerosis. I can go on and on extolling the extraordinary successes of the clinical trial. There is no doubt that clinical trials can provide a valid answer to an important medical question. However, it can also end up with erroneous findings and the reason this is so needs to be articulated.

The (randomized controlled trial) is a very beautiful technique, of wide applicability, but as with everything else there are snags. (A. Cochrane in R. Kunz and A. Oxman, *British Medical Journal*)

In 2005 a prominent medical researcher declared that most clinical research findings are false in an article published by *PLoS Medicine*. That dour position is not universally accepted and I do not believe that's it's necessarily true. Nonetheless, there is no question that it is extraordinarily difficult, if not impossible, to know for sure if a clinical trial has come up with the right answer.

I am aware that issues raised in this chapter may not be unique to the clinical trial. Poor planning, sampling, etc. plague other research techniques as well and may be even more destructive in those settings. However, the clinical trial is the gold standard. It is the major research technique to advance medical science, and there needs to be a forthright discussion of its vulnerabilities.

As you would expect, surveys such as the one published in the *Journal of International Medical Research* show that medical researchers themselves believe that clinical trials are by far the best way to advance medical science. Practitioners also realize that without clinical trials they would have to practice medicine in an atmosphere of gross uncertainty. Even the public at large believes that clinical research is a great value. If it weren't for clinical trials, we'd be in big trouble. Ineffective and harmful products would be on pharmacy shelves across this nation.

Scientists who believe in the clinical trial also realize that improperly designed trials are all too common and researchers should be held accountable when this happens. In fact, failure to properly design, execute and publish a study should be and is considered by some to be a breach of ethics – the researchers should have known better.

Some of the incorrect findings generated from clinical trials are the result of inferior performance by investigators. Sloppy research leaves many clinical studies open to criticism. An assessment in 1982 appeared in the journal, *Methods of Information in Medicine*, and claimed that the majority of medical studies published over a 35 year period were uncontrolled or poorly controlled. Only about one in four was judged a decent study at that time. Sins of omission and commission were plentiful – trials failed to adequately control factors that could distort the findings, and outcomes of interest to patients were often overlooked. Incompetent planning led to an insufficient number of patients and resulted in unreliable results. Although there has been considerable improvement in the quality of studies since the 1982 critique, there remain many deficiencies in medical research today.

Again, there is no question about the many accomplishments earned by the clinical trial, but claiming it as the "gold standard" leaves the wrong impression. It is not infallible – far from it. Elements, beyond the control of even the extraordinary investigator can sabotage a study. Even if researchers do the best they can, they may still end up with the wrong answer. There are insurmountable obstacles facing investigators that keep them from getting at the truth. Should they bear guilt for things beyond their control? Not really, but too few discuss the limitations of their research methods. The truth is that researchers need a bit of luck to avoid all the pitfalls plaguing clinical trial research.

As we saw in preceding chapters, the most potent clinical trial is the randomized blinded controlled trial (RABCOT). It has all the desired qualities; a treatment and a control group, random assignment of treatments and double blinding. You can't do better than that. However, even though it's the best we have, it is far from perfect. There are seven inherent problems with a RABCOT that can corrupt the designed study and there's little investigators can do about them except hope that none of them infect their studies.

Some of the seven threats that menace clinical trials were touched on earlier, but all of them now need to be consolidated into a single list. The flaws are embedded in the heart and soul of the clinical trial and although the conscientious researcher can reduce the risk of a flaw, he or she can't provide complete immunity. The seven flaws are:

- The unknown population
- The imperfect sample
- The unequal treatment groups
- The uncontrolled experimental setting
- The breakdown of blinding
- The impractical result
- The insufficient sample size

The Unknown Population

The theory that grounds clinical trial research is based on the following paradigm.

1. Define the population.
2. Draw a representative sample from the population.
3. Do a research study on the sample.
4. Infer your results from the sample back to the population.

Note, it all begins with a precise definition of the population. The goal of research is to make statements about a population based on study results from a sample. It is important to know that population because it is suppose to be the source from which the sample is to be drawn. The whole idea of inferential research (using a sample to represent the entire population) depends upon an accurate identification of the population.

That's the theoretical model. In medical research that means that out there – somewhere – are all the people who a new drug is intended to help. In statistical jargon, that group of people is the "population". For example, a population could have been all the sailors who were at risk of getting scurvy. A population could be all bald-headed men. A population could be all the people who get a cold. Now it's clear we cannot treat all those people – and, of course, statistical theory doesn't require that we do that. But we are suppose to take a sample from the population that we want to help. Now we add to the challenge. Statistical practice requires that we take the sample in such a way that all individuals in the population have an equal chance of being selected. Note that in order to do that we must identify all the people in the population.

Here's the troubling part: in medical research we don't and can't adequately identify the population of interest. We don't know and have no way of knowing all the bald headed people in the world or for that matter, in the United States. Take the illnesses for which we want cures – cancer, heart disease, AIDS, Alzheimer's disease, etc. We cannot identify the entire population for these diseases. We can't even come close. In addition to the sheer size of a population, the definitions of diseases are not all that specific and people with a disease are often undiagnosed.

Contrast this situation with a poll you want to take to see whom might win the forthcoming election in your town. Only registered voters vote and a list of registered voters exists and can be readily obtained. The list of registered voters is the population. It is clearly the group you want to make inferences about. You can, with relative ease, identify people on those lists and produce a sample. Now you might not get them all to participate in your poll, but at least you have a legitimate sample from that population. Medical research is messier. In medical research, it can't work that way because of the unknown population.

But let's be realistic. Theory is one thing and practice is another. You're never going to identify all the people in the world, in the U.S. or in Los Angeles with a given disease. If you could identify many of them, and then assume that the ones you missed were similar to the ones you identified, you'd be in very good shape. However, even that's next to impossible to do and, as explained below, in medical research, the investigators must settle for less.

Remember the research model requires us to take a sample of individuals (i.e. patients) from the population, but that's not how it's done in medical research. We don't start by picking patients – the process begins by finding researchers and we're now heading down the wrong path. The patients that researchers have access to are a unique group of individuals. They are not representative of all patients that have the disease of interest (the population). A trial that begins with selecting researchers can easily end up with a set of atypical patients when we contrast that set to the set called for – the population. The results of such a trial cannot tell us for sure, how a treatment will work in the general pool of patients who have the disease.

Usually the researchers selected are the ones who are most interested in treating the targeted disease. He or she may apply for a grant to do a study and add other researchers who share an interest in the disease and who may well have access to patients. Sometimes a governmental agency may decide to sponsor research for a disease and it solicits researchers at important medical facilities to apply to be the experimenters; these individuals may have a convenient but specialized group of patients. Private parties such as pharmaceutical companies may also contact individual physicians or medical centers and ask those with available patients to participate in a medical study. There are many ways to recruit investigators, but note how all the possibilities violate the process of selecting patients from the population of those with the disease. Granted the subjects used in such medical trials come from some part of the desired population, namely the part containing all patients willing to participate in clinical studies and are under the care of researchers who perform clinical trials.

There is clearly a problem here – the limited population derived from physician recruitment is obviously different from the theoretical population we should be concerned about. However, how serious is this discrepancy? It all depends on how different the limited population used in the clinical trial is from the true population of interest. If the two populations are very similar, the results of a clinical trial could be very relevant and trustworthy. But without making a studied comparison, we do not know if that level of comparability between the populations is present or not. The comparability may be adequate for some trials, but again without deliberate study, researchers do not know what trials are OK and which ones are unrepresentative. Any trial may have this problem and that means the results from any trial may not apply to the true population of interest.

Amazingly, this qualification is rarely noted and researchers make broad generalizations just as if the legitimate population had been accessed. Researches publish their results for a drug with a great deal of fanfare, but only infrequently are we forewarned that those results may apply only to the type of patient treated at the research centers used in the study rather than the general assortment of patients in the population.

The Imperfect Sample

The second inherent flaw that afflicts clinical trials also has to do with the patients selected for the study. To become a participant in a clinical trial you first must volunteer for the study. You can't be a participant in a trial until you give your written consent. The problem that arises is whether the volunteers are the same kind of people as those who want no part of a RABCOT. Those who won't sign up for a clinical trial may be less desperate than those eager to find a treatment that may help them. Those who forsake a clinical trial will tend to be healthier as well. On the other hand, volunteers also are more likely to be risk takers – after all in a RABCOT, they take the chance that they will receive the control treatment rather than the more promising experimental treatment. The population of interest has both kinds of patients, those who volunteer and those who won't volunteer, and there is evidence that the two groups have different personal and health characteristics.

If, the differences between volunteers and non-volunteers have an effect on the outcomes measured in a clinical trial, then there is clearly a problem because the results apply only to the volunteers. Under this scenario, the clinical trial results are not relevant to people who would not choose to participate in a clinical trial.

Unfortunately, we are stuck with this potential dilemma because ethical standards demand that only individuals who volunteer and give their consent can be used in a clinical trial. However, it should be emphasized that this is only a potential problem and if the volunteers and non-volunteers have the same response to the treatments employed in a clinical trial then the results would apply to both groups. Unfortunately, it's not possible to known whether the responses by volunteers and non-volunteers are similar or different.

Unequal Treatment Groups

The best kind of medical study has a number of important attributes. It needs to include a control group and the make-up of the control group needs to closely match the treatment group. Typically, the control group receives a placebo, the experimental group receives an active medication and the results from the two groups are compared. So far so good, but any group differences are valid only if a critical condition is met: at the start of a clinical trial – the two groups should be equivalent in terms of the critical variables that affect the trial's end points. For example, we certainly wouldn't want to find that almost all of the sickest patients ended up in the same treatment group. The treatment given to that group could be at a terrible disadvantage.

In an earlier chapter, it was noted that randomization was the method used to try to create treatment group equality. However, it was also pointed out that randomization does not and cannot guarantee an equal distribution of critical factors among the treatment groups.

A rather simple example of what can go wrong might help to illustrate this issue. Imagine we have a study in which we compare two treatments using 12 subjects. Six of the subjects are males and six are females. We want to have six subjects on each treatment. Now we'll slip in a critical piece of information unknown to the research team – compared to males, females respond better to both of the two treatments we are testing. Because of this, any disproportionate gender distribution could muddle up the findings. This inconvenient truth is why randomization may not give us what we want – treatment group equivalence in terms of gender.

Here are the incriminating statistics. If a random sample is drawn from a group that has an equal number of males and females, there is a very good chance that there won't be a 50/50 gender split. There is even a chance that all the females will be in one group and all the males in the other. The probability of this latter event is small – on average only one sample out of every 64 will end up with that kind of distribution. A small risk, but it's not zero. The chance you'll get an even split is larger, but it is still far from certain with the chance being about 30 percent. If we have doubts about getting equality with one factor (gender) what can we expect when we have to worry about two or more factors (age, race, etc.). Clearly, the possibility of an unbalanced distribution rises as the number of important factors increases. In general, it is truly a matter of luck if the distribution of all critical factors is similarly present in all treatment groups.

Statistical theory gives us some protection when it comes to factors that confound the results, but it is hardly sufficient. First of all, the theory tells us that the larger the sample the more likely there will be group equivalence. So, if the study is large enough, the process of randomization will usually distribute the confounding factors fairly equally between the treatment groups. But there is no certainty that this will be so because the greater the number of factors, the greater the likelihood that the randomization will not provide treatment group equivalence.

The solution seems clear. Researchers can easily examine the data to see how any critical factor is distributed among the treatment groups. They can then try to adjust the data by sophisticated statistical methods in order to reduce any distortions caused by an offending factor. But, this solution is not possible if we don't know what variable to look for. The truth is medical science is constantly finding new factors that can affect the progress of a disease or the action of a therapy. Prior to their discovery, there is no way to know if study results were skewed because of their presence.

The Human Genome project is discovering all sorts of connections between our genetic makeup and a propensity to develop a disease or respond to a treatment for a disease. For example, in December 2004 the *New York Times* reported that scientists had made a discovery that surprised even them. They discovered a genetic variation that could predispose people to depression. The presence or absence of this gene could explain why some people respond to a certain antidepressant and others don't.

Obviously, failure to account for the disproportionate presence of this gene among treatment groups could distort results from an antidepressant study. Previous research findings from antidepressant trials could be at risk as well. Perhaps there was an unbalanced distribution of subjects with this gene that caused a positive or negative result, which was mistakenly attributed to one of the drugs employed in the trial. How many past medical research studies results are inaccurate because of the failure to account for unknown genetic differences among the treatment groups?

Uncontrolled Experimental Setting

There are other ways in which medical trials fail to get the right answer. In a clinical trial all experimental conditions except for the treatments being administered, are to be the same for the groups being tested. This condition simply cannot be met. You cannot restrict human beings so they behave the same way and have identical environmental exposures. There is enormous variation in terms of how men and women choose to live, what they eat, how much they exercise, the amount of stress they endure, etc. Human beings live in a broad array of environments that bring unique pressures and demands on them. The variety of settings and experiences people have can and do cause treatment group inequality. That inequality in turn can introduce considerable bias in any clinical study.

Efforts to control bias in research studies go back for at least three centuries, but only in the past 100 years has bias control been emphasized. Still, in spite of that recognition, and as hard as it may be to understand or justify the lack of detection, many researchers continue to take inadequate steps to control biases. Add in the problems that an investigator can't control, such as subjects not giving truthful information or forgetting to take their medications, and it's no wonder that misleading results remain a problem to this day.

Breakdown of Blinding

The failure to keep hidden which subject is getting which drug can poison judgments as well as assessments, and represents the fifth threat that can undermine a clinical trial. Good experimental practice requires that subjects be handled in the same fashion so that the effect of inconsistent patient treatment does not jeopardize the results. Knowing what they are taking also must be hidden from subjects so they don't let that knowledge bias their responses.

Blinds, however, can be broken by the patient and sometimes the research staff. Even if the exposure is unintentional, the study results are still compromised. Knowing or even suspecting what treatment a subject is receiving can result in inaccurate observations and evaluations. The degradation of a trial because blinding failed is a real possibility and successful blinding should never be taken for granted.

Impractical Result

The sixth flaw is definitely ironic because many of the factors that make the RABCOT so appealing turn out to contribute to its disadvantages. Take all the elements that researchers use to control the research environment: not allowing the "wrong" concomitant agents, using only the patients that are most likely to respond to treatment, making sure the subjects take the treatments as directed, etc. When we get a positive result (i.e., the experimental treatment is found to be more effective than the control treatment), it can apply to an almost unrealistic situation because of all the restrictions placed on a clinical trial. How do we know if the garden variety of patient will do as well as the highly selective ones used in a RABCOT? Note the many differences between real life and the rarified setting of a research trial. Do patients who forget to take their medications fare as well as subjects constantly prodded to take their trial medications faithfully? Do patients who see their doctors once a year do as well as subjects who are seen weekly? Do patients who eat poorly and rarely exercise do as well as subjects who are on a strict diet and exercise program? The typical RABCOT has an idealized setting and the "good" result may not be conferred upon a more "natural" situation.

Insufficient Sample Size

The final flaw is yet another blow to our high expectation for medical research accuracy – the concern over the number of subjects in a clinical trial. It stands to reason that the more observations you make, the greater the assurance of an accurate overall assessment. Take too few observations and you may miss finding something important. Concerns about the number of observations (i.e. number of subjects) are especially relevant to clinical trials.

A later chapter will show how the number of subjects for a clinical trial can be determined, but that calculation may require information that a researcher does not possess and it applies to one variable measured in a trial. However, a typical clinical trial involves scores of tests for a broad assortment of variables and for these assessments, the sample size selected for the main variable may be too small or too large.

At present, many wrong, or at least unreliable answers are generated because trials are too small. For example, a 1978 review appeared in the *New England Journal of Medicine*, and reported that among 71 clinical trials, half of them could have missed a 50 percent therapeutic improvement because of the small number of subjects studied. Another review, published over 25 years later in *JAMA*, noted that having too few subjects in clinical trials was still widespread. Clearly, trials have to be large enough to be sure they're coming up with correct answers.

A large treatment difference may be impressive, but if based on a small sample, it may not mean very much. Having a sufficient number of subjects is especially difficult when doing research that involves major outcomes such as life or death. A vast sample size is also necessary to identify a rare but perilous side effect. In these situation, researchers usually need an enormously large number of patients (5,000 or more) and time to complete (five years or more) such trials. If studies are not large enough it is likely that the answer generated may be due to chance. But even large sample sizes may not overcome all the threats that keep researchers from coming up with the right answer from a clinical trial.

Even outcomes of mega-trials (there are large trials containing 1,000 or more subjects) can give inconsistent results. A review article in the *Journal of Clinical Epidemiology* described 289 pairs of mega-trials, in which each pair contained the same treatment and type of subject. For example, the two trials would be identified that had the same kind of subjects (e.g. patients with elevated cholesterol) and the identical test treatments (e.g. the same active medication and control treatment). The outcomes (i.e. was the active treatment better than, equal to or worse than the control treatments) were then compared. Finally, a judgment was reached on whether there was consistency (e.g. both trials found the active treatment better) or inconsistency (e.g., one trial showed no treatment difference but the other trial concluded that there was a significant difference between the treatments). In spite of the enormous number of subjects in these trials, the results of 79 out of the 289 pairs (27 percent) produced inconsistent results. Using a different database to locate pairs of trials produced a similar finding. What do we conclude? Even when different trials research the same question, and the problem of small sample size is eliminated, there are plenty of other factors – sometimes known and sometimes unknown – that lead to inconsistent trial conclusions.

As I conclude this chapter it is important to point out that the reason clinical trials end up with incorrect findings come from three main sources. The wrong result occurs because of (1) mistakes by researchers in the planning and execution of clinical trials, (2) the complex and inexact nature of information researchers require and (3) factors that are beyond the control of the researcher. This chapter focused on the seven elements which investigators do not control. These factors may or may not contaminate a trial and even if they do, they may not cause a significant distortion of the results. Nevertheless, they are truly serious threats to the integrity of any study. They stand as reminders that as good as the clinical trial is, it may not be good enough. When selecting a group of subjects for a study there is a risk that the proper set of patients will not be chosen. Furthermore, as much as we think we know about the drug we're testing, the disease we're treating and the measurements we're making – that knowledge is incomplete. No matter how hard we try to control the subjects and the study setting so that we don't get a distortion in the findings, it can never be sufficient and elements that can bias the trial emerge. Our attempts to make a trial efficient turn on us and we are left with too little information, which leads to tentative rather than clear-cut conclusions. And in our effort to have a very efficient trial, we can end up with results that are not relevant or useful for the practicing physician.

> *The controlled trial has been placed on too high a pedestal and needs to be brought back to earth.* (Editorial, *British Medical Journal*)

Somehow in spite of all these threats from all these places, good results do surface and each of us owe the many research teams that conduct medical investigations a vote of appreciation for their fortitude, perseverance and perhaps a bit of divine intervention in their search for the right answers.

Part III
Tools of the Trade

Chapter 13
Statistics – Was the Finding Significant?

Abstract To appreciate how medical research works it is necessary to understand the vital role played by statistical analysis. How one can determine if a person is truly a psychic is used to introduce the concept of statistical significance – the criterion that determines whether an experimenter can claim he or she has found a treatment difference. The explanation relies on simple coin tosses and the creation of a testing standard to determine if a person claiming psychic powers should be believed. The role of the confidence interval, which is essentially the "margin of error" that is faithfully included in political poll results, is incorporated into the explanation as well. The need to establish a null hypotheses and appreciation for the types of errors that come from statistical analyses are also covered. In addition, the chapter presents issues that must be addressed to judge whether any treatment differences found are truly meaningful. Included are (1) the assumptions researcher must make to determine the number of subjects they need for a trial and (2) the role of clinical relevance.

Keywords Clinical relevance · sample size · statistical significance · Type 1 Error · Type 2 Error

> *Since World War II, the organization and conduct of clinical experiments have been radically transformed by medicine's encounter with the discipline of statistics.* (H. Marks, *The progress of experiment*)

We cannot appreciate how medical research works without understanding the vital role played by statistics. The data generated in a clinical trial are analyzed using statistical methods and the decision on whether there's a credible treatment difference is based on a statistical probability. Fortunately, the subject of statistics is not really as overwhelming as most people think. I'll begin by examining what happens when we flip a coin.

Suppose you meet a person, who claims to be a psychic and you are asked to verify if the person's claim is true. The most logical step is to have the person claiming psychic powers to correctly predict events. A simple test could involve correctly identifying the outcome for a series of coin tosses. A single coin flip wouldn't be a sufficient test – there is a 50/50 chance a person can correctly guess a single coin toss. So we need to do more than one flip. But how many should we do? We probably want to do enough flips so we're pretty certain that the psychic's predictions aren't due to good luck from guessing.

If we did two flips there are four possible outcomes. Here's how they would turn out:

Note that of the four possible outcomes there is one in which a correct guess occurs on both flips (outcome 1). The psychic could also get both flips wrong (outcome 4). In between these extremes is getting the first flip right and the second one wrong (outcome 2) or visa versa (outcome 3). There are no other possibilities (Table 13.1).

Table 13.1 Coin toss outcomes

Outcome	First flip	Second flip
1	Correct guess	Correct guess
2	Correct guess	Incorrect guess
3	Incorrect guess	Correct guess
4	Incorrect guess	Incorrect guess

Since among the four possible outcomes, only one outcome produces two correct guesses we can say that there is a 25 percent chance (i.e. one out of four) of two correct predictions by guessing. That doesn't seem too hard to achieve so let's try three flips. Now by chance alone there is one chance in eight (or 12.5 percent) that all predictions would be accurate. Maybe we should go to four flips where the likelihood of getting all flips correct would be 1 chance in 16 (or 6.25 percent). Let's see what's the chance of correctly predicting all the outcomes from flipping a coin five times – it's one chance in 32 (or 3.1 percent).

Probability

It's easier to work with probabilities so we'll convert the last outcome – one chance in 32 to a probability. The probability is .031 (we just divide 1 by 32). We could also express this result as a percent – i.e. 3.1 percent. Incidentally one chance in 16 has an occurrence probability of .062 (1/16) and one chance in 64 would be a .016 probability (1/64). The corresponding percentages would be 6.2 and 1.6 percent. Table below summarizes the results we have gotten so far and adds a few more.

Table 13.2 Proportion and probability for correct coin tosses

Number of coins tossed	Proportion of times all guesses are correct	Probability of getting all guesses correct
1	1/2	.500
2	1/4	.250
3	1/8	.125
4	1/16	.062
5	1/32	.031
6	1/64	.016
7	1/128	.008
8	1/256	.004
9	1/512	.002
10	1/1,024	.001

As shown in the last column the probability of a correct guess drops by half for each additional toss. With one toss the probability is .500, but it falls by half to .250 with two tosses. Due to rounding, the probabilities don't appear to follow the reduction by a half rule exactly (e.g. half of .125 is .0625 not .062), but rounding holds down the umber of digits that must be shown and makes the table more manageable.

I could continue adding coin toss results to the table and recording new proportions and probabilities, but I'd never get to the point where there is no chance of getting all guesses correct (i.e. a .0000 probability). We'd get close – after 10 tosses there is only one chance in a thousand (probability = .001) that a person could correctly guess the outcome of all the tosses. However, there is always going to be just the smallest probability that a person can make correct predications by guessing for even the longest set of tosses.

If there were no restrictions on time and the testing didn't cost anything we could just do more and more testing so we'd become more and more certain of being correct when and if we declare that the person really has psychic powers. But we have to stop somewhere – at some point we have to say that's enough testing. Furthermore, psychics don't have to be infallible – they're entitled to some misses. We can't demand that there can never be a wrong choice – that would not be fair. If we set too high a standard too many true psychics would be incorrectly identified as fakes. As a result, at some point we have to decide that that's enough testing and come to a decision if the person is a psychic or not. We need to appreciate the fact that the chance of all correct guesses drops each time we require an additional test. Thus the question becomes – at what level of probability are we willing to say this person is or is not a psychic. There is also the time and cost of doing more tests that wouldn't amount to anything in this example, but in other situations that issue can be a big concern. That leaves us with the momentous question – how many tests should we require. How about using four tosses – there is only one chance in 16 (a .062 probability) that all of the four tosses would turn our correct simply by guessing? Is the probability of .062 good enough? Or maybe we should use six tosses – there is only one chance in 64 (a .016 probability) that all those tosses could be correct by guessing. But remember the greater the number of tests, the greater the chance that a true psychic will miss a correct answer and be declared a fake.

If researchers conduct a study and find an impressive treatment difference they'd like to be reasonable sure that the difference they found was not due to chance. Probability plays a vital role in this decision because it determines the likelihood that the difference the researchers obtained was a chance occurrence. In the psychic example, probability levels were calculated for sets of correct guesses the psychic could make that were purely due to chance. However, we never set a probability value to accept or reject the decision that the person was a true psychic. In medical research, there is a generally accepted level to determine if observed treatment difference are due to chance. The standard used in medical research is a probability of .05 (1 chance in 20).

Researchers use the expression "p value" to refer to the probability value they calculate. For instance in a research report they could write, "All statistical tests were done with a p value of .05." It is understood that a p value of .05 means that there is a five percent probability that the result observed might be due to chance. They may also report just the p value they calculated and not refer to the .05 probability standard. For instance, they may simply write, "The treatment difference was associated with a p value of .02." In this case by mentioning the actual p value they mean there was a two percent chance that the result they obtained was due to chance. The larger the p value, the greater the likelihood that the outcome could have occurred by chance. The smaller the p value, the greater the likelihood that the outcome is due to a true treatment difference.

If the .05 probability level is achieved the term "statistically significant" is used when referring to the treatment differences. The researchers will state that the difference they found is statistically significant and that means they have found sufficient statistical evidence to believe that there is a true difference between the treatments.

It is most important to point out that using a probability level of .05 means that five percent of the time the conclusion that there is a treatment difference will to be wrong. Five percent of the time, they're going to say there is a statistically significant difference when one doesn't exist. Five percent of the time, they're going to come to the wrong conclusion. This mistake has nothing to do with the quality of the study's design or execution. It arises from a mathematical decision on how to control chance as a cause for a treatment difference.

Those who are used to getting a definitive answer from a mathematical calculation will be disappointed to hear that there are no such guarantees when it comes to the statistical tests used by researchers. In performing statistical tests, the chance of an outcome can not be assured with 100 percent certainty nor absolutely denied with 100 percent certainty unless the entire population is tested. In other words, the statistical test cannot end up with a p value = 1.0 nor a p value = 0.0. The probability of an outcome is somewhere between those two extremes. So at the end of a trial, no matter how convincing the evidence for or against a drug's effectiveness may be, a researcher can never come to an absolute unconditional conclusion.

The rules of the testing procedure employed for medical research always leaves open the possibility that the conclusion the authors reach is wrong. Here is but one more argument on why a single medical research study can never guarantee the right answer – the statistical methodology employed doesn't permit it. Technically, the rules of the game do not allow a definitive finding without any possibility of error. However, don't blow this concern out of proportion. The possibility of a mistake can get very small – one in five hundred or one in a thousand or one in a million. People would be foolish not to come to a confident decision about a treatment difference in those situations where the p value is exceptionally small. The treatment difference is beyond any reasonable doubt when the probability level is minute. To remain unconvinced when the possibility of an error is infinitely small would be foolhardy. Still, demanding absolute certainty is a luxury you can not get with statistical testing.

There is much to be said for using the probability standard. We certainly don't want to say a drug is effective if its perceived benefits are due to chance. A fixed value for the probability standard also keeps all studies meeting a common criterion. We wouldn't want researchers setting their own level – many might be too generous and a flood of inferior drugs would be the result. Without the .05 probability standard numerous results that occur by chance could be accepted as fact and we would be lot worse off than we are now. But that said, we must also realize that using a probability standard is essential, but not sufficient. There are other factors that influence the interpretation of a statistical finding.

The Null Hypothesis

Good research methods require the planners of a clinical study to declare a hypothesis for their project. They must formulate what is known as the null hypothesis. A null hypothesis is a statement that postulates that there is no difference between the study treatments. In most cases, it is not likely that researchers really believe the null hypothesis. Usually they are doing the clinical study in hopes that the experimental treatment is better than the comparison treatment. As a result, the null hypothesis is really just a straw man – a proposition set up with the intention of disproving it.

As we just saw, in the world of probability testing, nothing is ever proven absolutely one way or the other. Statistical tests do not give simple "yes" or "no" answers. Instead the statistical analysis determines the likelihood or probability that the result is consistent with the hypothesis that there is no difference between the treatments. Nonetheless, the failure to reject the null hypothesis doesn't mean that there is absolutely no difference between treatments. To the nonprofessional it may appear that failing to reject the null hypothesis means it should be accepted. That's perfectly logical, but in clinical research practice, failing to reject the "no difference" outcome does not always equal accepting it. There is almost always some kind of treatment difference, but it could be so small that it failed to result in a p-value of .05 or less. Consequently, clinical researchers often interpret a finding of no statistical significance to mean there was insufficient evidence to show that there was a difference. Given the structure for statistical testing this is a reasonable conclusion to reach.

Cautious interpretation is also required when comparing two active drugs. A comparison of two drugs (e.g. a new one versus the current standard) is often referred to as an equivalence or comparative trial. The real purpose of such a study is often to see if the new drug is as good as the drug that is the current treatment standard. In other words, an acceptable goal of the study sponsors is to be able to claim their drug is equivalent to currently used treatment. In this case the real objective is to come to a "no difference" conclusion – if the experimental drug is just as good as the current market leader, that's good enough. There may be advantages of the new drug (e.g. fewer side effects or a more convenient dosage schedule) that make equal efficacy a satisfactory outcome.

Because of the tendency to misinterpret the absence of statistical significance, reports on equivalence studies can be confusing. One investigation, which appeared in the *British Medical Journal*, looked into studies comparing two active drugs (e.g. a test drug against standard therapy) and found that an inappropriate claim of no difference appeared in 20 percent of these kinds of studies without any qualification about clinical or statistical significance. These incorrect assertions were probably due to careless wording rather than a mistaken belief that no effect or difference had been shown. However, readers of the articles – the practicing physicians who do not engage in research – may accept the "no difference" inference as fact and shape their medical decisions based on this erroneous conclusion.

The Type 1 and 2 Errors

Earlier we examined the risk of finding a difference that is not real because it is due to chance. As previously noted the .05 probability standard is set up to control this kind of error. If an investigator concludes that there is a difference, but in fact there really isn't one, that kind of mistake is called a Type 1 Error.

There is another risk that can lead a researcher to come to the wrong conclusion. Researchers can conclude that there is no difference when, in fact, a difference really exists. Statisticians aren't too imaginative and they call this kind of mistake a Type 2 Error. Note that the Type 2 Error is the opposite of the Type 1 Error. One mistake is to conclude that there is a difference when that judgment is wrong (a Type 1 Error). The other mistake is to conclude that there is no difference when there is one (a Type 2 Error). Sometimes the Type 1 and Type 2 Errors can be better understood by showing their relationships in a table that is shown below (Table 13.3).

Table 13.3 Relationship between a Type 1 and Type 2 error

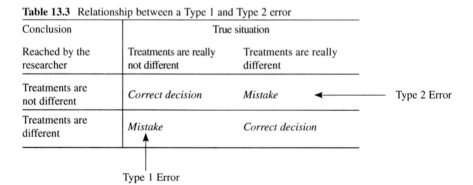

In the diagram, the left-hand column represents what the researcher concludes from a study based on the p-value. There are two possible conclusions – the treatments are not different (row 2) or they are different (row 3). The right two columns represent the actual truth. The treatments are really not different (column 2) or they are different (column 3). In the interior are the four cells that indicate if the researcher's conclusion is correct or not and the information is italicized. If, in fact, the treatments are not different and the judgment reached by the researcher is also that they are not different then, as indicated in the first cell, the researcher's decision is correct. If on the other hand the researcher concludes that the treatments are different, when in truth they are not different, then that is an error on the part of the researcher. As noted in the diagram that mistake is called a Type 1 Error. This mistake is controlled by the probability standard. It is set at .05 so the risk of claiming there is a treatment difference when it is not true can not exceed five percent.

For the cells on the far right, the true situation is that the two treatments are in fact different. However, if the researchers conclude they are not different then that is a mistake. That kind of a mistake is called the Type 2 Error. In the last cell which is in the right hand corner, both the true situation and the researcher's conclusion are that treatment differences exist and, as a result, the researcher has made a correct decision.

In most research trials the two types of error are not considered equally bad. The more serious blunder is the Type 1 Error. The reason for this can be appreciated by assuming the results of a study will be used to decide whether a drug will be approved for marketing or not. In this circumstance, to conclude a drug is effective when it is not, is considered the more egregious error. Allowing patients to take an ineffective drug is clearly unacceptable, especially if efficacious drugs on the market could be used instead. The other alternative, Type 2 Error, means a useful drug will not be available to patients – that's not good, but it's considered less serious than the Type 1 Error since there may be an ample number of alternative treatments available for patients. There is one important exception and that has to do with equivalence trials. If you remember in an equivalence trial the goal is to show equality not superiority. In this case it's important to focus on the Type 2 Error – incorrectly claiming no treatment difference when one really exists.

Sample Size

It's important to appreciate the connection between sample size (i.e. the number of subjects participating in a trial) and statistical testing. A failure to have enough subjects can lead to a serious error – an important treatment difference will not be declared statistically significant. But too many subjects always raises a problem – an excess number of participants can allow a declaration of statistical significance when there is only a trivial treatment difference.

There is a formula that statisticians use to determine the number of subjects needed for a trial. Most people hate formulas and I won't present one, but I must talk about the three elements in the formula – (1) the size of the treatment difference researchers expect, (2) the variance of the primary measurement researchers plan to use and (3) the amount of assurance researcher want that they will find the difference they specified in item 1. It may help to give a brief explanation of the second element, variance. Variance refers to the consistency of the response for the primary measurement by the subjects. There is low variability when all subjects have a similar response to a treatment. If subjects are inconsistent in their treatment response then variability is high.

The three elements that determine sample size affect the required number of subjects needed differently. Sample size is increased when:

1. A small treatment difference is expected.
2. A large variance occurs with the primary assessment.
3. A large amount of assurance is desired.

So if researchers want to (1) find a small treatment difference, (2) plan on using a measurement that is very erratic and (3) want to be real sure that they find a treatment difference they will need lots of subjects. Researchers obviously want to use as few subjects as possible so they like just the opposite set of circumstances – large treatment differences, a measurement with a low level of variation and a willingness to accept a low assurance level.

The sample size formula assumes the size of the treatment difference and variance of the primary measurement are known, but they are often not known. If researchers already knew what the treatment difference was, there would be little purpose in conducting the trial. However, researchers can approximate what is a likely treatment difference based on prior results. The expected variance can also be estimated from the results of past studies. To enhance the likelihood of low variance, researchers like to conduct studies with subjects who are alike. The homogeneity among subjects in respect to age, gender, degrees of the illness, etc. provides greater consistency in response than if the subjects are very different in respect to these factors. Substituting estimated values for the expected treatment difference and the variance usually result in the calculation of a reasonably accurate sample size, but it is important to point out if the estimates are incorrect then the calculated sample size will be off. For instance, if researchers overestimate the size of the treatment difference or underestimate the amount of variance, their trial will have too few subjects and they risk having a Type 2 Error (i.e. they will fail to show a treatment effect when there is really is one).

The third element in the sample size formula, the assurance level, requires a decision on the part of the researchers on how certain they want to be of finding a statistically significant difference. Do they want to be 75 percent certain that the trial will find the expected treatment difference or, if that's not good enough, perhaps they should be 99 percent certain. It would seem reasonable to pick a high degree of certainty, but that choice comes with a high cost – it will inflate the sample size. A larger sample size means more cost and more time to complete the trial. Typically, an assurance value of 90 or 95 percent is chosen, but if these choices end up with too large of a sample size, the study may proceed anyway with a smaller number of subjects and a greater risk of a Type 2 Error. Unfortunately, many published reports of clinical trials fail to describe how the sample size was chosen. When this information is eliminated there is no way to appreciate the chance of a Type 1 or Type 2 Error and we have yet one more reason to be suspicious of the result from a clinical trial.

One more comment related to the sample size question is appropriate. The sample size calculation is usually based on the primary effectiveness variable in a trial. There are many other variables assessed and corresponding p-values determined. For these other variables, the sample size determined for the primary variable may be grossly inappropriate. Nevertheless, the study is run as planned even though for most variables there will be too many, or more likely too few subjects, and in the latter case the Type 1 and 2 Errors will be much worse than that for the primary variable. In fact, clinical trials are very poor at finding conclusive evidence that a rare side effect is related to a medical treatment. The side effect could be lethal, but if it's rare, a trial with 10,000 or even 20,000 subjects may not be able declare that it is an effect of the treatment at the usually level used for a statistically significant finding. The sample size calculation, based on the principle efficacy assessment, is invariably insufficient when it comes to unusual but serious side effects. The Type 2 Error for these types of adverse effects will be extremely high because there are not enough subjects. Therefore, any given clinical study should not be relied on to fully determine the safety profile of a drug.

Clinical Relevance

A corollary requirement to judge whether the means of two treatments are truly different needs to be considered. Is the difference meaningful? When researchers conclude that statistical significance exist this means that there is a low probability that the findings occurred by chance. However researchers also need to answer the question: does the difference that was associated with the statistical significance have any practical value?

We have practical significance when a researcher looks at a treatment difference and says, "if this is the true difference then I would certainly prefer one treatment over the other." In the medical research area the terms "clinically significant" or "clinical relevance" are often used when a difference is judged to be important medically. There are no statistical tests to help physicians and consumers of research determine clinical significance. It usually requires clinical expertise to interpret research results, and decide whether the treatment difference has any clinical relevance. For example, researchers might design a study to evaluate a weight-loss drug that is taken for three months. If subjects in the experimental group lost an average of 23 pounds and subjects in the non-intervention group lost an average of 21 pounds, the 2 pound difference could turn out to be statistically significant. But this slight weight difference could have little clinical significance. Researchers must consider clinical relevance before coming to final conclusion about the success of the treatment. Unfortunately, there is evidence that far too many researchers have failed to do this in the past. A 1994 study published in *JAMA* examined slightly over 200 studies in which there had been a negative result (i.e. the experimental treatment was not shown to be effective for primary outcome variable). The selected articles had been published in major journals over a 20 year period and less than 20 percent made any statement related to the clinical significance of the observed differences. Another disturbing finding was that less than one in three indicated that there had been a sample size calculation to determine the number of subjects to be used for the trial in the first place.

The Type 2 Error has an important role when it comes to the issue of clinical significance. If there is a clinically important difference, the fact there is no statistical significance doesn't mean the treatment failed. We need to ask, how likely was it, given the size and design of the trial, that a clinically important effect was missed? The kind of response we'd want in this case would note that a difference of X would have been found Y percent of the time. Note that X is the clinically significant difference and Y is a percent based on the Type 2 Error. For example, take a study evaluating drugs to treat obesity where 5 pounds is deemed the clinically important difference. The authors could state that a difference of 5 pounds would have been found 50 percent of the time. This hypothetical statement means that an important difference (5 pounds) would have been missed half the time. Because of the likelihood that an important treatment difference could have easily been missed, the drug shouldn't be discounted until more research is performed.

It bears repeating: researchers always need to be cautious about the interpretation of a clinical trial that fails to find a statistically significant difference. In those situations, it would be helpful to know what kind of a difference could have reasonably been found. Inclusion of a statement such as the one given above that specifies the chance of finding an important treatment difference is particularly helpful when interpreting the results of a trial. It is invaluable to know how capable a trial was at finding a clinically important effect, and a study report that omits that information should be considered incomplete.

The Confidence Interval

Because of dissatisfaction with the use of the .05 probability standard, many researchers have turned to an alternative way to express the statistical quality of a research finding – it's called the confidence interval. A confidence interval is a range of values that tries to define the true difference between treatments. Since we use samples, we never know the real treatment difference for sure. However, based on the difference observed in a trial, we can develop an estimate of the true population difference. Nevertheless, there is uncertainty associated with that estimate. The confidence interval attempts to quantify the uncertainty associated with the observed treatment difference. Consider it as a range of plausible values. A short confidence interval implies an accurate assessment – the plausible values fall within a narrow range. A wide interval implies poor precision – the plausible values cover a broad range of values.

The usual convention is to calculate a 95 percent confidence interval. A 95 percent confidence interval should include the true value for the treatment difference

95 percent of the time. This means that five percent of the time the actual mean for the complete population would be outside the 95 percent confidence interval range. A choice of a 95 percent confidence interval is arbitrary, but as we will see in a moment, it is in synch with the .05 probability standard.

Let's again use a weight loss example that compares a drug against a placebo. Assume the confidence interval for a study gives a range of 5–15 pounds. This means that the true treatment difference is most likely greater than 5, but it is most unlikely that it exceeds 15 pounds. The center of the interval (in this case 10 pounds) corresponds to the observed mean of the treatment difference. The interval could therefore also be described as 10 plus or minus 5, but it is customary to present it using the two extreme values – i.e. 5 – 15.

Although statisticians hate this explanation, the researcher could say that he or she is 95 percent certain that the true treatment difference lies somewhere between 5 and 15 pounds. Of course, either the interval contains the population mean or it doesn't. As a result statisticians point out that there can't be a 95 per-cent probability that the interval contains the population mean because the inter-val either contains it (and the probability = 1.0) or it doesn't (and the probability = 0.0). Actually when a 95 percent confidence interval is calculated it corre-sponds to a process in which the calculated interval includes the true population mean 95 percent of the time. Thus, the criticism by statisticians is justified, but for practical purposes it seems like an unnecessary complaint to the simpler explanation. Perhaps a compromise is to say a 95 percent confidence interval gives a range of values within which there is 95 percent certainty that the popula-tion value occurs.

In our example of a 95 percent confidence interval falling between 5 and 15, we would have strong evidence that there is a treatment difference. There appears to be at least a difference of 5 pounds and it could be as great as 15. At either extreme the treatments is better than the placebo – it is only a matter of degree. However, what if the 95 percent confidence interval were −2 to + 8. The length of the interval is the same (10), but more importantly it now includes 0. A value of 0 is the point at which the treatments being compared show no difference at all. A value of −2 indicates that the treatment is inferior to placebo, but a value of + 8 supports the opposite conclusion that the treatment is better than placebo. In this circumstance the results are inconclusive. There is insufficient evidence to claim one treatment is better than the other.

The margin of error. There's a confidence interval that you are exposed to many times, but you're probably unaware of it. The exposure becomes very intense every four years and has a noticeable drop following the first Tuesday in November. What I'm referring to is the presidential election. We tend to be inundated with polls predicting the winning candidate. In reporting poll results it is now customary to cite a margin of error. Candidate X was preferred by 54 percent of the people with a 5 point margin of error. If you perform a little math the information translates to a range of 49–59 percent. The 5 point margin of error is simply subtracted (54 – 5 = 49) and added (54 + 5 = 59) to the mean value. The 49–59 range is in fact a con-fidence interval and although the newspapers never report this, it is almost certain that it is a 95 percent confidence interval. In this example, since the range overlaps 50 percent, pollsters report that the survey is inconclusive – the election is too close to call.

This situation is akin to a clinical trial in which patients receive two treatments and decide which one is better (i.e. preferred). If the sample size was the same as used in the political poll and 54 percent of the subjects preferred one of the treatments then the 95 confidence interval would match that from the political poll – i.e. 49 – 59. In this case there would be no statistical significance since the range included the no difference point of 50 percent.

In reality the use of the .05 significance standard or the 95 percent confidence interval will lead to the same answer regarding the presence of absence of statistical significance. They are just different ways of expressing the same level of certainty regarding an observed difference. They are not different ways to determine statistical significance. As a result the negative criticism of the .05 probability standard that it is an arbitrary standard also applies to the confidence interval. Still, there is an advantage in the use of the 95 percent confidence interval because it does a better job of illustrating the nature of the treatment difference.

With the .05 probability standard you usually only get the mean treatment difference – a single number that is declared statistically significant or not statistically significant. By specifying a range of values the confidence interval has definite advantages over the single value used with the .05 probability standard method. Let us assume a study has a sample size of 100 and another researcher investigating the same problem with the same measurement uses a sample size of 25. Both calculate a mean for the treatment differences and it is the same value. Also assume each study ended up with the same conclusion regarding the statistical significance. At this juncture there would be no way to differentiate the two studies even though one has four times as many subjects. However, if each researcher reported a confidence interval, the study with the larger sample size will have a shorter interval and be the more appealing result. The confidence interval gives more information because at its center we have the mean treatment difference, but there are also the lower and upper limits. They add information and provide a more comprehensive and meaningful way to understand trial results.

A good rule of thumb to follow when the confidence interval method of presentation is used is to take the lower value and decide what you would do if that were true. For instance, you could decide that one drug was better than the other one or perhaps the differences were not clinically important. Next take the upper value and do the same thing. If you would come to the same conclusion whether you used the lower value or the upper number then the trial has been successful since it produced one conclusion. There is only a small risk that the true difference isn't in the zone you looked at and led you to make the same judgment. If you would decide one way based on the lower number and reach a different decision based on the upper number, then the study has failed to provide a consistent result.

Statistics are a critical part of the clinical research world. However people who do not have statistical training, but are affected by the results from clinical research (e.g. health care providers and media reporters), can easily misunderstand clinical trial results. An understanding of concepts such as statistical significance, clinical significance and margin of error are vital to the interpretation of medical research findings.

Statistical analysis and evaluation to prove significance is the hallmark of modern medical science. The requirement for statistical significance is, however, not necessarily coupled to enthusiasm, understanding, or appreciation of practicing clinicians. (J. Rothstein, *Physical Therapeutic*)

Chapter 14
Analysis Issues – A Lot of Choices

Abstract In the statistical analysis of data from a clinical trial, one would expect the same set of data to lead to the same result. However analysts have many choices – what statistical test to use, what type of data to analyze, whether the underlying mathematical assumptions of the tests they use were met, etc. Depending on those decisions, different conclusions about a treatment's efficacy and safety could be supported. Furthermore, today the recommended research practice for analyzing a study is the intention-to-treat approach whereby all subjects the researcher intended to treat are included in the analysis, even if they didn't meet the protocol requirements or left the trial prematurely. This approach can cause a bias, but the alternative that allows researcher to decide who should be dropped and who should remain in an analysis can also introduce bias. The importance of statistical decisions is reflected in an astonishing report claiming that over half of all medical research findings are false. Too few subjects, small differences between treatments, the number of tests preformed and the incorrect interpretation of probabilities were used to support that premise.

Keywords Intent-to-treat analysis · multiple testing · statistical assumptions · statistical methods · statistical tests

In the analysis of data from a clinical trial, one would expect the same set of data would lead to the same result. However, an analysis involves many choices such as what statistical test to use to analyze the data. Depending on the analysis decisions, different conclusions about a treatment's efficacy and safety could be supported. As a result, there is no assurance that the same data set for a clinical trial will end up with the same conclusions. In this chapter, I explore the many choices research teams have when it comes to analyzing and interpreting the data from a clinical trial.

Huge sums of money are spent annually on research that is seriously flawed through the use of inappropriate designs, unrepresentative samples, small samples, incorrect methods of analysis, and faulty interpretation. (D. Altman, *British Medical Journal*)

Choosing the Statistical Test

There is a wide variety of tests available and the best ones are those that that give the analyst the most information and the greatest efficiency. Efficiency is defined as the ability of a statistical procedure to come up with the smallest number of required observations to find a treatment difference, if one exists. For instance, the statistical test that required the smallest number of cases to reach the .05 probability level would be considered the most efficient test. Unfortunately, the most efficient tests require a lot of assumptions and, as will be explained in a moment, it's at least difficult if not impossible to be totally sure that all the assumptions are met. On the other hand, the tests that require few assumptions are limited in what they can do. They are less efficient and give researchers less valuable information. The choices leave the statistician between the proverbial rock and a hard place.

One of the first questions that needs to be addressed when planning the statistical analysis is what class of tests is appropriate. There is one set of tests for variables that are considered numeric. A numeric measurement includes quantitative variables such as weight or a blood pressure reading. However, measurements can also be classified as categorical or ordered. In the categorical class, the measurement result can only be placed in a response category. The categories may be a patient's race (e.g., White, Asian, etc.) or whether the patient had to be hospitalized (e.g., a "yes" category and a "no" category). A categorical measurement is clearly different than a numerical measurement such as a blood pressure value since the outcome cannot be expressed as a quantitative value. A variable that belongs to an ordered scale of measurement falls in between the categorical and numeric scales. Like a categorical scale, an ordered scale has discrete categories, but they can be placed in a hierarchy. An example is pain that can be rated as none, mild, moderate and severe. Statistical texts refer to the measurement scales by alternative names, but those terms are not as descriptive (e.g. a categorical scale is called a nominal scale).

There is a group of statistical tests set aside for each measurement scale – one set for numeric variables, a different set for ordered variables and a third set for categorical variables. Within each class of tests there are also alternative statistical procedures offered. Consequently, analysts choose the test, within a class, that they considered most appropriate. The choice of a test is up to the analyst. Analysts have preferences and may not pick the same test to analyze the data collected in a study, which leads to the possibility that different statistical conclusions will be reached for the same data set.

There is also a related problem. Although it may appear that a given variable will distinctly fit into one of the three classification groups, that is not necessarily the case. Take temperature which can clearly be considered a numeric variable. However, temperature can also be considered an ordered scale by assigning temperatures over 101 degrees to a class called "high fever"; 99–101 degrees to a class called "fever" and those below 99 degrees to the "normal" class. Temperature can also be treated as a categorical variable by just recording "fever-present" or "fever-absent". The way an analyst classifies a variable is important since the ability to find a statistically significant difference can be influenced by the class chosen. Statistical significance is more readily declared when a variable is considered numeric and less likely if it is judged to be in the categorical class. Therefore, much could depend on whether temperature is recorded as a numeric, ordered or categorical variable. The chance of finding a statistically significant difference would be more likely if temperature was judged a numeric variable and least likely if it were determined to be a categorical variable. It's evident that different choices by an analyst can lead to different judgments about the effects of a treatment.

Selecting the data to be analyzed represents another decision facing the researcher and statistician. I'll use a hypothetical example to illustrate this situation. Assume the trial used 50 patients with hypertension who were randomized to receive either an authentic or a sham acupuncture treatment. The primary outcome was based on blood pressure readings that were taken before and after treatment. There are three choices for selecting the data to be analyzed:

1. Compare the post treatment scores only.
2. Compare the differences between the post treatment and baseline scores.
3. Compare the post treatment scores while adjusting for the baseline scores.

A different statistical test would be appropriate depending on which of the three data sets is used. Significantly, each choice could lead to a different result.

Another concern is the fact that statistical tests are based on mathematical models and those models require assumption about the data used in an analysis. As might be expected, the "best" tests are also the most complicated ones and it's not just the math that is more tedious. The group of tests considered the most powerful also has the most demanding set of underlying assumptions. If the assumptions for the test are not met then the results using that test are obviously corrupted. This situation gets even messier because the decisions on whether the assumptions are met do not have clear standards. For the most powerful and sophisticated tests, the assumptions are very stringent and satisfying the assumptions for these tests becomes even more problematic because there may be no way to adequately test them. In the end, a statistician has a lot of latitude in making decisions about whether test assumptions are met. Different decisions equate to dissimilar test choices and that means there is the possibility of inconsistent statistical decisions about a treatment result.

One last example of statistical methodology options involves combining treatments into broader groupings and then analyzing the data based on the newly created groups. The grouping of treatments is not a bad step if it is done in a logical and fair manner. It may be valuable to compare different classes of drugs rather than individual drugs to see if one class is better than another. By combining the results, the sample sizes are increased and that can increase the sensitivity of an analysis. But it is important that the merger of individual drugs into a class be done rationally. In the next example this was not the case.

Sometimes an improper analysis decision surfaces when a study is looked at closely. A report in *JAMA*, by two researchers at Copenhagen University, illustrates this possibility. In the process of preparing a meta analysis, the researchers noted that the investigators for one of the trials they planned to use had combined the results for two drugs. They also recognized that one of those drugs was known not to be useful for the indication under investigation. In addition, almost 80 percent of the patients taking the other drug took it orally rather than intravenously. The oral form was known to be much less effective. The results for the two drugs were merged and then compared to a third drug. Not surprisingly, the third drug showed superiority over the two-drug combination. In this dreadful case, the fact that the third drug turned out to have better results, and therefore declared superior, was a totally deceptive answer.

It seems obvious that this was a case of intentional manipulation of the options available to the analyst in order to show a drug's superiority. The researchers weren't particularly clever, but it is also disconcerting that the medical journal that published the original trial may have played a complicitory role when it accepted the study for publication. At a minimum, the journal was clearly inept in performing a reasonable review of the submitted study. Once medical research gets published, even bad research, the medical community and the general public are the ones who eventually lose out.

Taking a more cynical view, it is also possible that faced with a negative result (when a positive finding was hoped for), a statistician may try different types of statistical tests, reclassify data and cases, or change the outcome variable until the desired positive result can be described as statistically significant. An article in *PLoS Clinical Trials* noted that there is evidence that this kind of behavior is probably a greater problem than most people think it is.

The potential problems discussed above can be mitigated by requiring a statistical analysis section in the protocol that specifies, in advance, what statistical test(s) and data sets will be used to analyze the data. If there are valid reasons to alter the analysis plan, a full explanation for the change should be provided in the final study report. The CONSORT guidelines, developed by an august body of leading medical researchers, include standards for reporting the statistical analysis methods for clinical trials. That section begins by providing an example that clearly supports the belief that the analysis of clinical trials be based on a pre-established analysis plan.

The intent-to-treat approach. A critical decision in any study has to do with the inclusion and exclusion of subjects from the analysis. Today many researchers believe the recommended research practice for analyzing a study should be based on the "intention to treat" (ITT) approach. This means that all subjects the researcher intended to treat and were allocated to a randomized treatment group should be included in the analysis. This includes subjects with the following characteristics:

1. Subjects who did not take any \study medication or they did not receive an adequate course of treatment
2. Subjects who dropped out of the study before it's completion
3. Subjects who were admitted by mistake and were actually unqualified for the study
4. Subjects who did not follow the protocol, missed important assessments and took unapproved drugs that could interfere with the assessment of the study drugs

There are a number of reasons given to accept this standard. If subjects are excluded for any reason, their removal changes the make up of the treatment groups and jeopardizes the goal of having equivalent groups. It is also argued that including subjects in the analysis, even though they never took the drug or were on an inadequate dose, is like real life and they should be included to demonstrate what will happen when the drug is in general use. As a matter of fact, ITT advocates believe slightly deviant behavior, here and there, is good because there's always some level of it in real world. The ITT supporters also favor including misclassified subjects who never should have been in the trial. Perhaps they were too old or had the wrong diagnosis. The argument in this case is that if false inclusions occur in the controlled environment of a trial, it seems inevitably that misclassification will also occur in routine clinical practice and therefore the subjects' experiences should count.

It's not clear when the intent-to-treat approach became the preferred method, but a 1997 study in the *British Medical Journal* found that only two percent of the clinical trials reported in the medical literature explicitly stated that all randomly assigned subjects were analyzed according to their original treatment assignment. A much larger number noted that ITT analysis was used, but the investigators provided insufficient data to support the claim. Clearly, there were also other investigations that eliminated subjects from their analysis if they felt the subject did not have a fair course of treatment.

The ITT procedure is often viewed as a conservative approach since it tends to make it more difficult to find statistically significant treatment differences. A rather bizarre example illustrates this position. Assume none of the subjects included in a trial have the correct disease. As a consequence, the value of an effective drug for the disease cannot be demonstrated. As a matter of fact, no treatment can demonstrate superiority or inferiority when the wrong subjects are treated. The process of excluding subjects also has drawbacks since those very difficult decisions can become arbitrary and favor one treatment over the other. Neither situation is desirable, but note that the two approaches test different research questions. An analysis that eliminates subjects for cause provides a result for patients who follow the protocol rules, but the intention-to-treat analysis gives a result that applies to both compliant and nom-compliant patients. The current trend favors the use of the ITT method as the primary analysis for a clinical trial and major journals such as *JAMA* instruct authors to include an ITT analysis in the reports they submit for publication.

A related concern is what should be done if the decision is made to retain a subject in the analysis, but the follow-up results for the subject are so incomplete that there is no meaningful evaluation of a treatment effect? For example, the subject drops out before any meaningful outcome measurements are taken. Researchers faced with inadequate outcome data are left with a few unwelcomed choices. They can eliminate the subject from the analysis, forsaking the ITT goal and live with any bias that this decision may cause. They can also try to estimate what the final outcome would have been (e.g. by using the last outcome assessment they had no matter when it occurred or employing a mathematical model to predict the final result). Choosing one of these options rather than another can have an impact on the results for a study. One subject may not matter very much, but if there are a number of subjects the effect could be important.

Multiple Testing

The .05 probability standard discussed previously applies when there is a single statistical test. In other words, with just one statistical test, there is only a five percent chance of concluding a drug is effective when it really isn't. However, in a clinical trial many statistical tests are performed, never is there only one test. In a typical trial, many variables can be used to determine the safety and efficacy of a drug and a statistical test performed for each variable. In addition, some of these variables may be assessed more than once during the trial. In doesn't take long before analysts have performed a large number of statistical tests.

Two other situations lead to even more tests. They are interim analyses and subgroup analyses. Interim analyses of the primary variable(s) occur when a clinical trial runs over a relatively long period of time. During such a trial, it is important for researchers to monitor the results so the trial can be terminated prematurely if patients are at risk because one of the treatments is unexpectantly very ineffective or unsafe. Analyzing the data at periodic intervals during a trial is therefore reasonable and necessary.

Another reason for multiple testing is related to subgroup analyses. In a study, it is often interesting to know how certain demographic groups did in a trial. Were the results similar for whites and non-whites or did one gender do better than the other? The overall results that include all study participants can be misleading if they do not apply to important subgroups. Essentially, what is being looked for is a differential effect. If the subgroup were gender, researchers would like to know if males and females had a similar result. Knowing how a treatment works in subgroups can be especially valuable to the practicing physician. If the drug has minimal efficacy in females, and was found effective because of a very positive effect in males, that information may temper a physician's decision as to use of the drug in women.

The statistical implications of multiple testing are not insignificant. When multiple testing takes place, statisticians worry about what is known as the experiment-wise error rate. The experiment-wise error rate considers the possibility of a statistically significant result, given all the analyses performed. When there is only one statistical test, the probability standard is also the experiment-wide error rate. They both are .05 and that means there is a .05 chance that the experiment will result in a conclusion that there is a statistically significant difference when one does not exist. However, if there are two or more tests, the probability that one or the other or both will be declared statistically significant is greater than .05 (.095 to be exact). Instead of there being a five percent risk of a false positive result in a study with a single statistical test, there is now almost a 10 percent risk of at least one false positive result when there are two statistical tests performed in that study. Obviously, the more tests conducted, the greater the risk of having a false positive finding associated with one of the analyses conducted. A failure to compensate for multiple comparisons can have important consequences; a new experimental drug may be declared superior to an existing drugs, when it is, in fact, only equivalent.

Fortunately, for analysts that want to control the false positive error rate associated with making multiple statistical tests in a study, there are mathematical techniques that can do that. However, there is no guarantee that each of the methods used to control multiple testing, will give the same answer concerning statistical significance. The various methods should produce similar results, but if a treatment difference is at the marginal level of statistical significance, it could be altered one way of the other depending on the technique used.

There are other important issues regarding multiple testing that need to be mentioned. Multiple statistical tests are performed in the analysis of all clinical trials, but some variables tested are more important than others. For example, the primary efficacy variable is usually the single most important variable. The statistical test for this variable is the premiere test – and as such, it is tested at the .05 probability as if it were the only test. However, planners may recognize there is another statistical comparison of major interest. For instance, they feel they must do a subgroup test for gender because prior research indicated that males and females were likely to respond differently to the experimental treatment. Consequently, the subgroup test is conducted using one of the methods to adjust the result for multiple testing so that the .05 experiment wise error rate is retained.

All the other variables are considered secondary and it would be unrealistic to do those statistical tests using one of the available multiple testing methods. As a result, when interpreting the results from tests on secondary variables, it just has to be understood that some false positive results will occur among the analyses performed. On average, without a multiple test adjustment, there will be about one false positive result for every 20 statistical tests performed.

That still leaves the question about unplanned analyses. For example, what if a subgroup analysis wasn't anticipated, but at the conclusion of the study there are clearly major differences between some groups. If the females fared poorly and the males did extremely well, that situation cannot be ignored and nothing done about it. Clearly, the finding needs to be examined and a statistical test conducted to determine the chance that the result was due to chance. But if that test turns out highly significant, even after adjusting for multiple testing, the interpretation is very tricky because the gender difference was not anticipated. There are a great many potential subgroups in a clinical trial (gender, race, age, etc.) and some, by chance alone, can show a large difference. No matter how strong the subgroup test turns out, researchers must be skeptical and not proclaim that they've uncovered a major gender difference. This kind of after-the-fact revelation is equivalent to betting on a horse after the race is over. Interesting subgroups identified after a study is completed deserve to be reported and possible reasons for the difference explored, but (and this is the main point), the finding needs confirmation based on the results from a second independent trial.

Here is an example, that was reported in a 1991 article in *JAMA*, that supports the need to confirm unanticipated subgroup analyses with a second trial. After completing a study, subgroup analyses showed that benefit was confined to heart attack patients (1) under the age of 65 (2) treated within six hours of the onset of symptoms and (3) who had heart damage in a unique location. However, new trials and a review of findings from older completed trials failed to support this conclusion. In fact, benefit took place irrespective of (1) age of patient, (2) time from the onset of symptoms or (3) of site of heart damage.

It should also be pointed out when interim analyses or subgroup testing is anticipated, that intention should be specified in the protocol. Accommodating the extra test(s) results in an upward adjustment to the sample size, however, the credibility of the study is enhanced and it is well worth the cost of the additional subjects.

Statistics and Medical Research

The extraordinary role statistics plays in medical research is evident when we recall the astonishing report that claimed over half of all medical research findings were false. The individual who caused the fuss over the quality of medical findings, J. Ioannidis, was Professor and Chairman of the Department of Hygiene and Epidemiology at a medical school in Greece. A prolific contributor of medical research articles, he also held an Adjunct Professor position at Tufts University School of Medicine. His major argument for the high percentage of incorrect medical findings had to do with statistical issues such as small studies, small differences between treatments, the number of tests preformed and the use of p values as a way of demonstrating conclusive research findings. However, he also pointed out that other factors such as difficulties with outcome definitions, loose trial designs as well as conflicts of interest on the part of investigators also contributed to spurious results, but it was the statistical problems that most concerned him.

The medical community met Ioannidis' claim that most published research findings were false with deafening silence. In the six months following his article, there were three short responses, published by same journal that published the Ioannidis essay. Although they each found his contention provocative, they basically offered helpful suggestions regarding the statistical issues he raised while accepting his basic premise. The low level of criticism or support is in contrast to the fact the article apparently was of high interest with over 100,000 downloads from the publisher's Web site. The article even made it into the popular press with a *Boston Globe* editorial referring to it as a "cult classic". Perhaps the lack of criticism was due to the emphasis on statistical issues. The editors of the journal that published Ioannidis' original article noted that parts of his position were based on assumptions that even they did not fully understand.

There was a little more reaction in 2007 as three other articles appeared, but only one by Goodman and Greenland challenged Ioannidis on his conclusions. The other two essentially accepted his suppositions and expanded on its ramifications. The contrary article agreed that there were more false claims in medical research than many would believe were present, but they challenged the over 50 percent figure.

They felt that the over estimate by Ioannidis could be traced to a flawed mathematical model he used to "prove" his point.

The material in this chapter shows the important role statistics play in medical research and the recurring theme is that there are many opportunities for error when it comes to analyzing the data from a clinical trial. The type of measurement to be tested, the data set to use, satisfying the assumptions of a statistical test all can vary based on who the analyst is. There are also problems related to multiple testing that are not easily solved and can lead to inconsistent statistical conclusions depending on how analysts address the problems.

Is it any wonder, given all the choices that must be considered when it comes to the statistical analysis, that the same data may end up with a different result. This pessimistic statement in no way reflects on the quality or intelligence of the researchers and analysts involved. They are almost assuredly dedicated and well-educated professionals. However, the environment in which they must operate precludes their ability to guarantee their analysis has provided the only true result.

Chapter 15
Meta Analysis – An Alternative to Large Trials

Abstract A large series of studies on the same treatment and for the same indication often include trials that lean one way while others go in the opposite direction and a few are just neutral. A relatively new statistical technique, the meta analysis, is seen as a hopeful method that can take a large body of studies and provide an overall assessment of a treatment effect. The technique, admired because of its ability to take many small trials and blend them into a consensus finding has its detractors as well. There are methodological issues such as accounting for unpublished studies, or the inclusion of published results that are of poor quality. The absence of individual patient data can also be a deterrent to a sound analysis. Examples of meta analyses cases illustrate where the method has provided useful revelations as well as questionable conclusions. In the end, however, because there is an incomplete understanding of the technique, caution is called for when interpreting the results from a meta analysis. There is clearly a need for meta analysts to educate the health care professions about the strengths and weaknesses of this promising technique.

Keywords Meta analysis · publication bias · research quality · review article · systematic review

> *Meta analysis cannot make a silk purse out of a sow's ear.* (S. Simon, *Statistical Evidence in Medical Trials*)

Because of the inherent difficulties surrounding medical research, there may be many trials investigating the value of same experimental treatment in the same condition, but they fail to end up with a common finding. Still all that research creates a very large body of data and shouldn't there be some way to obtain an overall assessment of the treatment? A meta analysis may be the answer.

Meta analysis is a procedure that combines the results from many studies that research the same question. It is a complex method, but when competent professionals perform a meta analysis it has the potential to provide unusually valuable findings. This analytical approach is seen as an attractive alternative to doing large, expensive, and logistically difficult clinical trials. Supporters of meta analysis are optimistic that results from completed trials can provide the necessary number of patients and the pooled data will lead to the detection of important findings about treatments that were lost in the conflicting results from individual studies.

Although the first meta-analysis was performed in 1904, its first use in medical research took place almost 50 years later. Even by 1987, less than 100 meta analyses had been performed by medical researchers. Then the technique caught on and in 1996 there were over 800 meta analyses recorded for the medical field. The slow start was in part due to the fact that the initial meta analysis was shrouded in controversy. And meta analysis remains a controversial issue to this day. Opponents refer to it as "meta-silliness" while proponents prefer the term "Newtonian".

It's no wonder meta analysis is popular among its proponents. The meta analysis uses result from completed trials so researchers don't have to recruit and examinee subjects, worry about dropouts nor wait years to get an answer from their research project. The raw data already exists – the analyst only has to execute the meta analysis process, but unfortunately, that's not a fail-safe endeavor.

To do a meta analysis, the studies that investigated the treatment and indication of interest, need to be identified and this involves a thorough literature search. An analyst wants to find all relevant studies, however, that's not as easy as it may seem because not all clinical studies get published. If a research project produced a positive result, that was also statistically significant, then that trial will almost certainly be published. On the other hand, studies that were equivocal and failed to satisfy the .05 probability standard may never be published. Omitting this latter set of studies could easily bias a meta analysis. If only positive studies are used, an overestimate of a drug's effectiveness is the likely result. In fact, the authors of a *British Medical Journal* article on selecting studies for a meta-analysis cautioned that published trials tend to demonstrate a greater benefit of treatment than unpublished trials.

However, even if a study with a negative result does get published, it may not be easy to find. Positive studies are more likely to be published in widely read journals that are almost certain to be written in English. Studies with negative results, on the other hand, have a greater chance of publication in non-English journals. Analysts must carefully examine the non-English literature to be sure no study is overlooked. It is also possible for the same clinical trial to be published more than once and the duplication must be recognized so only one version of the study is included in the database. Finding a duplication can be challenging because the study title may change and the authors very often will be in a different order and names may be added or deleted from one report to the next. Even the number of subjects used can vary so the duplication may not be easy to spot. There can be good reasons for multiple publications. The original study data may be reworked to fit the special interest of a journal – concentrating on a subset of the original group of subjects with an illness that is the journal's focus.

An article in the *New York Times* reported on an investigation that looked at 84 studies that had been performed on a drug for the same indication. It initially appeared that there were almost 12,000 patients involved in those trials. However, after taking a closer look, it was discovered that some of the studies collected had been published twice. After sorting out the confusion, it was discovered that there were really only 70 studies, in less than 9,000 patients. More importantly, it was discovered that the duplicated data would have led to a 23 percent overestimate of the drug's effectiveness.

After identifying studies for the analysis, an analyst may decide to eliminate those of poor quality. After all, including poorly planned and executed trials could have a deleterious effect on any kind of analysis. However, analysts again face a difficult decision when it comes to identifying studies to be selected for a meta analysis. There are no standard rules to guide decisions about what studies should be included and which ones should be excluded and, as a result, the study selection process could introduce unwanted bias into the proposed meta analysis. Because of this concern, some authorities believe it might be better to escape the study selection step altogether and just include all trials.

For analysts who believe study selection is necessary, a research team establishes its own criteria for study selection. Some analyst may simply confine the database to RABCOTs that use the ITT principle. However, an attempt to have only one type of study included in a meta analysis can eliminate other research such as a carefully designed and executed cohort trial that contains valid and useful information. Other researchers may select criteria that they believe would be appropriate such as requiring studies to be randomized, double blinded and published in a reputable medical journal. Analysts are free to select additional criteria such as a strict definition for an acceptable drug regimen that had to be followed, or the minimum length of time the subjects had to be treated. As a result, each meta analysis researching the same question can easily end up with a different set of trial data and that means the findings may differ.

It should be noted that there is a unique advantage in retaining all kinds of studies in a meta analysis. Some of the characteristics that differentiate the studies can be treated as variables in the analysis. In other words, the researchers may include studies that were randomized and those that were not to see if that factor (i.e. randomization) influenced the results of the trials. Other factors about the studies, providing the data are available, may also be examined in a meta analysis. For example, did the results show a different outcome based on gender or age? The researcher is clearly testing subgroups, which as we know is a problem, but it is often nullified in a meta analysis because of the large sample size generated by so many trials.

Another challenge analyst's face in a meta analysis is the need to combine the outcome effect from each selected studies to get at the overall effect. If all studies use the same outcome measurement the studies can be pooled without difficulty. But working with many different studies can pose a major problem when the studies use different endpoints. For example, take a look at studies investigating the value of a new appetite suppressant against placebo. Some researches could use weight change as the outcome variable, which seems to make sense. However, another set of researchers may prefer to measure calories of food eaten and a third group use a 10 point rating scale based on an evaluation the subjects made on how hungry they felt. Now we have results based on pounds, calories and a number from 1 to 10. Clearly, these data can't be combined to get a meaningful average.

In the event that the available studies have different measurements, the meta analysis relies on the concept of effect size for standardizing the results. An easy method to achieve this is to find the percent change from the baseline period (just before treatment started) and the end of therapy. For instance, if the study using pounds showed an average weight of 160 pounds at baseline and a weight of 140 pounds at the end of treatment the difference is 20 pounds. There is therefore a 12.5 percent reduction (divide the 20-pound loss by the starting weight of 160 and multiply the result by 100). In the study measuring calories if the caloric consumption began at 4,000 calories a day and ended at 3,200 calories a day the percent change would be 20. Finally if the rating on one's physical condition improved from a value of 6 to a value 5 the percent change would be 17. Now all the outcomes are measured in respect to the same measurement (i.e. percent change) and can be successfully combined and analyzed.

As noted earlier, because of the larger sample size generated in a meta analysis, researchers can often legitimately examine outcomes for subgroups. However, some meta analyses may have to work with summary data from the published report rather than individual patient data. Combining data across studies may be impossible unless all of the studies provide data on the same subgroup. For example, a subgroup for "elderly" subjects may include different sets of subjects depending on how the various studies defined elderly.

This dilemma could be overcome by gathering individual data for all subjects in all trials. Unfortunately, gaining access to the results for each subject in a large number of trials is not easy to do. Researchers may have confidentiality agreements that forbid such submissions or they may simply be reluctant to have their data scrutinized by a third party. Until there are ways to facilitate the sharing of clinical trial data, the meta analysts is left to rely on summary information.

Because meta analysis is a relatively new technique, as far as clinical research goes, many physicians are unable to neither appreciate its strengths nor recognize its weaknesses. Meta analysis can be a powerful tool for medical research providing attention is paid to the selection of studies, the consistency of the outcome measurements, and other factors that could lead to a biased result. A 1997 article in the *British Medical Journal* on the potential and promise of meta analysis included an intriguing story illustrating the value of this methodology. The story begins with an influential editorial stating that there was no clear evidence that beta-blockers improved long-term survival after a heart attack despite almost 20 years of clinical trials. Then a meta analysis came out showing that a considerable beneficial affect, both clinically important and with a high level of statistical significance, was present for beta-blockers. What's ironic is that the studies included in the positive meta analysis were completed years before the editorial was written that questioned the benefits of beta-blockers. In addition, subsequent clinical trials involving over 13,000 subjects confirmed the value of beta-blockers. In the same year (1997), an analysis published in the *New England Journal of Medicine* put the meta trial is a less favorable light. The results of 12 large randomized, controlled trials (involving 1,000 patients or more) were compared to the results of meta-analyses published earlier on the same topics. The outcomes of the RABCOTs were not consistent with those of the meta analyses 35 percent of the time. Since results from a large RABCOT were considered the best evidence on the efficacy of a medical treatment, the assumption was that the meta analysis finding was wrong.

There were other results that suggested the findings from a meta analysis were off the mark. A 1995 *British Medical Journal* reviewed the rise and fall of magnesium treatment in which a meta analysis played a major role. The article noted that, based on a meta analysis, it was concluded that magnesium treatment represented an effective, safe, simple and inexpensive intervention for patients with a heart attack. It was recommended that magnesium should be introduced into clinical practice without further delay. However, a few years later a large clinical trial reported negative results for magnesium treatment based on heart attack survival. This was a setback not only for magnesium, but it was a rebuke to meta analysis as well.

When there is a great deal of information about a treatment, journals usually publish a review by an expert that synthesizes the information from many clinical studies and formulates an overall evaluation of the treatment. Clinicians rely on the reviews to give then a comprehensive summary of the available information about the treatment. Essentially these reviews and a meta analysis are examining the same information and since the practicing physician tends to accept the expert reviews as a fair and reliable assessment of the treatment, they easily could treat a meta analysis in a similar fashion. Whether meta analyses are given a great deal of weight in how these physicians prescribe drugs is not known, but they not be influenced very much. An example to support this possibility appeared in a *British Medical Journal* article titled "Meta-analysis – Potentials and Promise." The article offered a telling story of how physicians appear to use meta analyses. The focus of the article was on dissolving blood clots in order to reduce the mortality rate for those who suffered a heart attack and noted that the use of thrombolytic agents increased only after publication of two large RABCOTs in the late 1980s. The same lowering of the death rate had already been shown in two earlier meta analyses that used a number of small studies as the database. But it took the publication of the first RABCOT to establish that dissolving blood clots was an appropriate treatment for patients who had suffered a heart attack. It's entirely possible that meta analyses are now having a greater impact on the practice of medicine as clinicians become more familiar with the methodology.

In conclusion, due to the difficulties inherent in clinical trial research, inconsistent findings are unavoidable. The meta analysis offers some hope that a reasonable consensus decision can be reached when there is a large body of inconsistent research finings However, because there is an incomplete understanding of the technique, caution is called for when interpreting the results from a meta analysis. There is clearly a need for meta analysts to educate the health care professions about the strengths and weaknesses of this promising technique.

Part IV
The Real World

Chapter 16
Research Results That Clashed – What's the Right Answer?

Abstract This chapter uses a series of case studies to illustrate that inconsistent research findings are all too common. The first case deals with the use of mammography to screen for breast cancer and how the appearance of a negative study, after a run of studies that supported the use of mammography, caused the medical community to rethink the value of mammography. Eventually after a consensus was reached that mammography could detect early cancer and save lives, doubts lingered because of the harm caused by false positive results. The second case follows the disastrous plight of the contraceptive device, Dalkon Shield. Reports claiming the Shield caused a pelvic inflammatory disease became so pervasive that the product had to be withdrawn, but the number of lawsuits drove the company into bankruptcy. However, it appears likely that its downfall may have been due to shoddy research and overzealous regulators. The final example involves aspirin use to prevent a heart attack. Using the same kind of subject (doctors) and similar designs, contrasting results between major U.S. and U.K. trials occurred. Although additional research supported the US findings of a positive effect, the FDA never approved this use of aspirin.

Keywords Aspirin · cost benefit analysis · intra uterine devise · mammography · outcome measurement

There is probably no disease in women that is more feared than breast cancer and rightly so – the statistics are alarming – one in eight women will develop the disease. Mammography can find the cancer early and thereby improve the chances of survival. But, not everyone believes that this is the right way to go. This chapter and the next use case studies, such as the quixotic path mammography has taken, to describe controversial major health issues that emerged because of inconsistent research findings. A second case, a bit dated and many readers may not be familiar with it, but it is nevertheless invaluable because it shows how contradiction in study results can have a devastating effect on a medical product. The last case looks at aspirin, the all time favorite remedy for our ailments, but controversial research let to a dispute on whether it could actually save lives. These three cases have a common theme – patients, doctors and health authorities can be left bewildered and confused as researchers struggle to find the right medical answer.

Mammography – Should I or Shouldn't I?

Many women you know have either had breast cancer or have been faced with that possibility – friends, neighbors, relatives as well as young mothers, career women and senior citizens. Articles about breast cancer, touting a new discovery or questioning an old one, appear regularly in the newspaper or on TV. Yet, in truth, there are other conditions that possess a greater threat to a woman's health. The chance of developing heart disease is actually much higher than that of breast cancer. Other forms of cancer such as lung or pancreatic cancer, are equally devastating and harder to cure than breast cancer, but it's breast cancer that produces the most terror. Maybe that's because almost everyone knows someone who's had it. Or, despite the greater rate of heart disease in all women, it may be because breast cancer is the leading cause of death among women under age 55. Or perhaps the fear is related to the possible disfigurement from breast cancer surgery.

A mammogram is nothing more than a low-dose x-ray that examines breast tissue. It uses about the same amount of radiation as an x-ray of your teeth. It is a screening device that helps women find cancers that are too small to be found during self-examination of the breast. Early detection is vitally important since a successful outcome is vastly improved by starting treatment as soon as possible.

Mammography, as a screening device, has its proponents as well as opponents. In use since the 1960s, there still remains a lack of consensus on the benefits of mammograms. Contradictory results from clinical trials and concern with the accuracy of the test cast doubt on its value for fighting breast cancer. As a result, thousands of women are confused because they cannot get a clear answer about the value of the procedure. The research reported in medical journals, newspapers and magazines leaves many health providers baffled as well. One can read forceful arguments that "prove" harm or benefit from the procedure. What has made this issue such a bewildering muddle?

The first experimental study to show that mammography could reduce breast cancer mortality was done in the U.S. in 1964. The study, utilizing the records of the Health Insurance Plan of Greater New York, involved 62,000 women – an enormous number for research in that era. The women, aged 40–64, were randomized to receive mammography examinations or not. After only a few years the findings were impressive – significantly fewer breast cancer deaths occurred in the mammography group.

There appeared to be some consistency among the different research methods used to evaluate medical innovations. Case reports, exploratory studies and experimental studies all found mammography effective. The exploratory studies generally found it more effective than the experimental studies, but what mattered most was that both approaches demonstrated efficacy.

By the 1980s, mammography came to be widely accepted because of the belief that it could detect early cancer and save a woman's life. Early detection of breast cancer meant the disease could be discovered before it spread. Treatment that was less damaging and more effective could be used as a result of early detection. There were some unresolved issues about its value in younger women and the frequency of tests for older women, but that did not influence the majority of women who marched off to medical labs to get their annual mammogram.

The good news continued. In 1993, results from five research centers in Sweden were reported in *Lancet* and they showed a positive effect for women who had had a mammography compared to those who did not. Although the results among the centers were mixed, after the data from the centers were pooled, the authors found that mammography clearly lowered the breast cancer mortality rate by almost 30 percent. Additional experimental studies done in Canada and Scotland also resulted in positive findings, supporting the value of mammography. In 1995, American researchers used a meta analysis to evaluate mammography and published their findings in *JAMA*. In this case, the data set contained the experimental studies mentioned above and four other exploratory studies. As most observers would have expected, the analysis led to a positive assessment of mammography. What could be better – there was an overall positive result based on data from an array of different countries – Sweden, Scotland, Canada and the U.S. The value of mammography looked secure.

And then the trouble began. An exploratory study conducted in Sweden came out in 1999, published by the *British Medical Journal*, with a most surprising result. It found no decrease in breast cancer deaths among women who had used mammography as a screening procedure, contradicting the earlier findings from Sweden. This discordant result peaked the interest of researchers in Denmark who went back and looked closely at the positive Swedish mammography trials discussed earlier. The Danish researchers' review prompted a 2000 article in *Lancet* that questioned whether screening with mammography was justifiable. The Danish team found that three of the five Swedish trials were of poor quality and felt that the positive results concerning the efficacy of mammography from these trials had to be ignored. Of the two "acceptable" studies, one showed a slight decrease in breast cancer mortality with mammography; but the other showed an increase in the number of deaths. Combined, the two studies showed no advantage for mammography. These extraordinary revelations placed the presumed unquestionable value of mammography in doubt.

The results shocked the medical world and received wide media attention. *CBS Evening News* used the turn of events as their lead story. The findings were featured in the *Washington Post* and *Time* magazine. Confusion reigned among adult women and the physicians who cared for them – should they continue to have annual mammograms or not?

The shadow of doubt was also raised over another of the positive studies. The analysis of the 1964 U.S. trial, showing that mammography was effective, used the number of deaths due to breast cancer as the key outcome. The Danish researchers disagreed and felt that the most important indicator of success had to be all deaths, not just deaths due to breast cancer. Using the number of deaths from all causes had a profound effect – the positive finding for mammography all but evaporated. To find a positive effect, only breast cancer deaths could be considered.

What should be the appropriate outcome measure for a cancer trial is an ongoing debate. Many researchers favor the all death standard because it can measure direct as well as tangential effects of a procedure. But others prefer to use the disease-specific deaths because it's more straightforward. Most of the time the two choices lead to the same conclusion. This time, however, they didn't and the lack of agreement added fuel to the controversy stirred up by the Danish investigators.

As you can imagine, the lead researchers of the five Swedish studies responded firmly. They defended their findings as appropriate and their methodology as sound. In 2002, they also published a follow-up report on the Swedish trials in *Lancet* based on a longer observation time. It showed that their "positive results" for fewer breast cancer deaths held up.

Most scientific controversy is aired in the medical literature by sending "Letters to the editor" of prominent journals. In this controversy, supporters of both sides entered the fray. Scientists have their unique way to vent their frustration and anger and there were plenty of nasty exchanges in the mammography controversy. The Swedish researchers were accused of withholding information by not reporting critical information about imbalances among the treatment groups used in their trials. They were charged with concealing information by their failure to include in their report that adjustments for age were made in the analysis. An effort to denigrate the Swedish research through these charges was clearly evident.

On the other hand, the Danish researchers also came under attack by the pro-mammography forces. They were accused of making accusations without supporting evidence and including irrelevant arguments riddled with misrepresentations, inconsistencies and errors. Other failings included applying made-up criteria to suit their personal objectives and conducting a flawed analysis.

There was, of course, no resolution in this bitter debate. The battleground stretched to another arena – cost-benefit analysis. The opponents to mammography relied on cost-benefit analysis to justify their position. They believed that mammography was not warranted because its liabilities exceeded its benefits. Yes, it can save a life, but it can also contribute to the loss of a life because of a false negative report that fails to detect a cancerous breast. Furthermore, a false positive diagnostic error causes psychological distress and unneeded medical procedures including a biopsy and even breast removal.

The truth is there are always false negative and false positive results with any screening test. Consequently, women should not take too much comfort in a negative result – the test may have failed to identify the cancer. And now the stakes are raised – the belief in a "no cancer" report may keep a woman from noticing or reacting to other signs and symptoms that indicate cancer is present. By the time the correct diagnosis is made, the women's chance for recovery may be severely reduced.

However, the more common error of mammography, as is true for many screening tests, is the false positive. A false positive occurs when the test is positive (i.e. the finding indicates that cancer is present), but the test is wrong (i.e. there is no cancer). A mass is detected, but it turns out not to be malignant. A perfectly well woman, who ends up with a positive mammogram, is presented with a considerable dilemma that she should never have to face. At one extreme she can do nothing and risk dying from the disease. At the other extreme, she can pursue a vigorously treatment program that can lead to significant costs, unnecessary pain and surgery which was not necessary. A middle ground position, in the face of a positive test, is to do more investigation to determine whether or not cancer is truly present, but that takes time and when it comes to cancer delaying treatment can be fatal.

The quandary women face is complicated by the unreliability of mammography, but it's next to impossible to find an accurate figure for the percentage of false negative and false positive tests. Age, weight, skill of the radiologist, hormone use, time between mammograms, breast density are just some of the elements that affect accuracy. As a result, the absence of accurate percentages for false negative and false positive results only add to the puzzle. Estimates range between 5 and 15 percent for false negatives and 10 to over 50 percent for false positives.

Even the benefit side of mammography may not be as good as it first appears. The major benefit of mammography is limiting the number of breast cancer deaths. But those "saved" tend to be older women. Thus, the number of years of life restored is relatively small and this causes the benefit from mammography to be smaller than one would expect.

Those who challenge the value of mammography argue that the limited financial resources of health care systems should be channeled into more cost effective channels. One option is to spend more on public education about the disease, especially aimed at high-risk groups such as women with a family history of breast cancer. Another choice is investing in the development of more accurate screening tests.

Still, based on what public health authorities have recommended and what many patient's physicians recommend, mammography won out over the groups who claimed there was a negative cost-benefit balance. In the end, although the Danish findings created quite a stir, they had little impact on U.S. health policy. Mammography continued to be advised by the National Cancer Institute and the American Cancer Society recommended yearly mammography starting at age 40 to be continued as long as a woman was in good health. Clinicians continued to believe annual mammograms were useful as well. This is aptly illustrated by a survey of gynecologists in Sweden, Denmark and the U.K. that was conducted a few months after the Danish researchers published their report challenging mammography. The mammography controversy was most intense and well publicized in these countries. Nevertheless, the survey showed that over 90 percent of the gynecologists had not changed their favorable attitude toward mammography screening in spite of reading or hearing about the negative findings from the Danish research team.

The mammography case is intriguing because it illustrates just how crucial the choices researchers make in a research project can be. Trial design decisions researchers make seem perfectly reasonable to them, but when viewed by other researchers they can judged seriously flawed. Define an outcome one way and the procedure is a success – pick an alternative outcome and it's a failure. This case also shows even when science gets it right (i.e. mammography can and does detect early breast cancer) other considerations (e.g. cost benefit analysis) may intervene and place make the decision about valuable of the procedure in doubt.

> *There will come a time when all the study patients have been followed up, all the analyses have been done, all the expert groups have met, and all the editorials have been written, and we still won't be sure how much benefit and how much harm are caused by mammography.* (S. Goodman, *Annals of Internal Medicine*)

Dalkon Shield – Destruction of a Company

The mammography debate is not alone in producing controversial results and creating a confused public. The Dalkon Shield was an extremely popular contraceptive method in the 1970s. It was classified as an intrauterine device or IUD, because it was placed in the uterus of women who wanted to prevent a pregnancy. IUDs of one kind or another had been around since the early 1900s. Manufactured in many different shapes such as a squiggly S or the number 7, modern IUDs were usually made of plastic and inserted by a gynecologist. An IUD was very effective in preventing a pregnancy, relatively inexpensive, and could be removed easily when a woman no longer needed it.

The Dalkon Shield, developed in 1970 by a physician at Johns Hopkins University, was a particularly big hit. Beginning in January, 1971, it was marketed by the A.H. Robins Company and soon became the most popular IUD in the U.S. Based primarily on case reports, the Shield was found to be a safe and effective device – a boon to women. However, a problem with the device emerged. Reports claiming the Shield caused a condition known as pelvic inflammatory disease or PID started to roll in.

Bad news for Robbins, but there was even more dire news on its way. A startling case series, reporting 10 deaths in pregnant women using the Shield, appeared in a leading U.S. journal, the *American Journal of Obstetrics and Gynecology*. Although there were almost three million women using the Shield, the manufacturer was in deep trouble. During the 1970s other studies, many using the case-control methodology, also incriminated the Shield. One review published in the *Journal of Reproductive Medicine* even found that the Shield caused more than a four-fold increase in PID. The FDA reacted. In 1975 it advised Robbins to withdraw its product.

In the mid 1970s litigation against Robins took off. One case found Robins guilty and awarded the plaintiff $600,000 plus another $6.2 million in punitive charges. The plaintiff in the case had to have an abortion due to an infection in the uterus. Even though her infection wasn't in the pelvis, she won her case on the grounds that Robins failed to warn her, or her physician, about the potentially dangerous character of the Shield, thereby preventing her from making an informed decision on the use of the IUD. Now the floodgates were opened. Robins soon had over 1.5 million cases pending and it was estimated that they would cost the company around $3 billion. What could it do? The company filed for bankruptcy; the product was removed from the market.

In 1976 the National Institutes of Health (NIH) commenced the Women's Health Study (WHS), a retrospective review of IUD use. The WHS was an exploratory study of the case-control variety which focused on IUDs and the likelihood of contracting PID. Based on records from 16 hospitals, WHS published its results in 1981 in the journal *Obstetrics and Gynecology*. It was not good news for the IUD industry. The researchers reported that IUDs, in general, increased the risk of pelvic infections and it was especially high for the Shield. Although the Shield had already been removed from the market, this was still bad news for Robins because lawsuits were still wending their way through the legal system and the WHS obviously supported a belief that IUDs were harmful.

In the 1970s a rash of other studies had actually investigated the relationship between the Shield and PID. When there were significant results, they tended to incriminate the Shield. The WHS, and the mass of data that preceded it, seemed to prove the guilt of the Shield as well. By and large, there was no vital news during the rest of the 1980s. But, as we've seen in the world of medical research, the tide can turn and sure enough in 1991 researchers from the University of Washington published a report in the *Journal of Clinical Epidemiology* that re-examined the original data from the WHS case-control study. A bold move considering the WHS was an NIH sponsored trial.

The University of Washington group felt that some women had been eliminated from the study pool without satisfactory scientific rationale. They also suggested that adverse publicity about the Shield, at the time of the WHS trial, could have biased patient recall about their medical history. In addition, they raised a concern that doctors may have been more likely to diagnose PID infections in women who used the Dalkon Shield, after hearing about the problems with the product. The University of Washington researchers came to a momentous conclusion – the WHS trial was flawed in its design, conduct, analysis and interpretation of results.

The battle lines were drawn. The WHS researchers responded quickly and tersely, saying that the University of Washington re-analysis was replete with error, misrepresentation and overstatement. Clearly aroused, the WHS scientists conceded their study may not have been perfect, but claimed the Washington researchers misrepresented facts and rendered opinions that were not adequately supported. Raising the ante even more, they pointed out that their critics had served as expert witnesses for Robbins, clearly implying that they had a conflict of interest. Pretty harsh language for brethren of the same medical research fraternity.

In the next year (1992) even stronger support for the Shield showed up in the journal *Fertility and Sterility*, even though the Shield and Robins were no longer around. The authors worked at the Center for Research on Population Security (CRPS), a non-profit organization specializing in reproductive research, and they looked at all the IUD trials conducted to see their effect on PID. These researchers wanted to see if the type of research method (exploratory vs. experimental) influenced the final results. They determined that the incriminating evidence against the

Shield was almost all from the 18 exploratory trials included in their database. From the pooled 71 experimental studies, the researchers did not find any connection between the Shield and PID. They concluded that the indictment of the Shield was a mistake.

In that same year, T. Farley and associates reviewed the World Health Organization's IUD clinical trial database and came to a very interesting conclusion. Their work, published in *Lancet*, found that PID was a risk with IUD use, but only during the first 20 days of use. Thereafter the risk was low and not unusual. Equally important was their finding that PID among IUD users is strongly related to the insertion process. Combined with the other 1992 study, there was now impressive evidence that the Shield had indeed been safe and effective, providing (and this was their major contribution to the situation) it was inserted by a skilled and experienced physician.

However, just to confuse matters even more, back in 2000, epidemiologists at the UCLA School of Public Health, starting with essentially the same set of studies that had been in the 1992 CRPS analysis, came up with a contradictory conclusion. Their meta analysis found that there was a positive association between the Shield and PID. This striking and different conclusion may be traced to the reason for conducting the UCLA analysis. As noted earlier, the cumulative data set for the first analysis by CRPS included a range of studies. Some studies showed IUDs were harmful and others did not. There were also studies that provided no clear answer.

The 2000 analysis, however, was undertaken precisely to find the reason for the inconsistency in the 1992 results. Thus, the analysts restricted the type of study they would use in their meta analysis requiring studies that had to have information on a number of factors which might account for the inconsistency in results (e.g. whether a patient had a prior PID). Consequently, using these criteria, they ended up with a much smaller number of studies involving the Shield. In fact, there were only 12 studies out of the original 89 trials the CRPS assembled. Of these 12, there were 11 that used the exploratory research model – the type of methodology that condemned the Shield in the first place. Remember that the goal was not to determine whether the Shield was safe, but to try and find an explanation for the inconsistency in the 1992 results. The authors did find that the rate of PID in women using the Shield varied and depended on whether the women had or did not have a prior history of PID. They also noted that results varied based on the kind of comparison group used. Different answers were generated depending on whether the controls were women who had other IUDs, women who had not previously used contraception or women who used a contraception method other than IUDs.

What does all this mean? There appears to be a good chance that questionable research analyses led to the demise of a useful product. Today only about 1 percent of the women in the U.S. use an IUD, even though it has the highest satisfaction rate of any contraceptive method. Elsewhere in the world IUDs are the most popular form of contraception with more than 100 million users. It has been more than 25 years since the last Shield was inserted, but its troubling legacy keeps IUDs from gaining any popularity in the U.S.

This case illustrates how utterly confusing medical research can become – for patients, doctors and heath officials. Select a different type of research method, and the results change. Select a different kind of comparison group, and the results change. Select a different type of patient for the study, and the results change. In spite of the lack of clarity public health decisions must be made – and those choices have momentous repercussions. What's the truth about the Dalkon shield and PID? The best one can say is "it depends".

Aspirin – Does It Save Lives?

Almost everyone has taken aspirin – it's the most widely used drug in the 20th century. And it's been around for a long time. Willow bark which is a primitive form of aspirin was prescribed for pain by Hypocrites back in the 5th century BC. But, as far as medical research is concerned, it's just another compound over which research findings and tempers have clashed.

Although it never went through the rigorous clinical testing that new agents go through now, aspirin's ability to reduce pain is well known and universally accepted. However, aspirin's popularity is also due to other uses besides pain relief. One of the most significant is its ability to affect the way blood clots. When an artery is narrowed by heart disease, a blood clot can block the artery and cause a heart attack. When you take aspirin, blood is less likely to clot and block an artery.

Medical research had demonstrated that for people who had a heart attack, a daily aspirin dosage would help prevent a second heart attack. However, the next logical question was: could it prevent people from having a heart attack in the first place? Because of aspirin's side effects – it causes stomach ulcers, bleeding in the gastrointestinal track and even brain hemorrhages – the benefits had to be large in order to offset its risks. Research studies were needed.

In the 1970s the needed research results began to appear, but they lacked consistency. A case-control study by the Boston Collaborative Drug Surveillance Program raised the possibility of a significant benefit from aspirin to prevent a heart attack. However, the findings from a cohort study that appeared in the *British Medical Journal* were less upbeat about the value of aspirin. Using all heart related deaths as the outcome variable, there was little difference between people who never used, seldom used or often used aspirin. Note that the outcome variable the cohort trialists used was death from any heart-related event. As a result, they counted deaths from causes such as a blood clot or an obstructed artery in addition to death due to a heart attack. This contrasted with the case-control researchers who had concentrated on nonfatal heart attacks. In the following years, two more publications on this subject appeared. There was another case-control trial published in *Circulation* and an update from the Boston Collaborative investigators. The case-control trial again used the broad outcome of death from multiple heart-related causes, and the authors concluded that the results failed to show a preventive role for aspirin. However, the Boston Collaborative group had completed a second case control trial and it too supported a positive effect from aspirin. Given the inconsistent results, and the shortcomings of the exploratory methodology, the issue on the value of aspirin to avoid an initial heart attack looked to the controlled clinical trial for resolution.

In the 1980s two major experimental trials, one in the U.S. and the other in the U.K., set out to provide a more definitive answer regarding the value of aspirin to ward off an initial heart attack. The U.S. trial was organized by the Harvard University Medical School and designed to investigate whether aspirin could pre-vent cardiovascular deaths in people without a prior history of heart problems. Researchers at Oxford University planned the U.K. trial to do the same thing. The two trials both used only male physicians as subjects.

The trial in the U.S., the Physician Health Study (PHS) and the U.K. study dubbed the British Doctors Study (BDS), were similar in many ways. They both used placebo as the control treatment, randomized the subjects and observed subjects for about the same amount of time (approximately five years). However, although the researchers collaborated with each other, they pretty much designed their studies independently. The PHS trial was blinded, the BDS was not. The PHS gave the aspirin every other day; the BDS gave a higher dose of aspirin on a daily basis. The U.S. study enrolled over 20,000 doctors equally divided between the aspirin and placebo treatments. The British study used only about 5,000 participants and for every two doctors assigned to aspirin treatment, one was given placebo.

In spite of the design differences, a compatible result was anticipated. But that's not what happened! The major end-point, fewer heart attacks, showed up only in the U.S. study. Indeed, the reduction of heart attacks in the U.S. trial was sizeable. Compared to placebo, there was close to 50 percent reduction in heart attacks for those taking aspirin every other day. Conversely, the U.K. study found on their aspirin regimen almost no reduction in heart attacks. There was clearly a differ-ence in the aspirin dosage used in the two studies, but it was the study with the higher aspirin dose that failed to show a positive effect from aspirin. More side effects on aspirin would make sense, but not less effectiveness. Since the U.K. study was so much smaller then the U.S. study, their results were less precise, but this factor could not account for the wide discrepancy in heart attack rates between the two trials.

Other important end points produced disappointing results, but they, at least, were relatively consistent between the two trials. There was an insignificant increase in strokes for aspirin-users in both trials. Both studies also showed no dif-ference between aspirin and placebo in terms of deaths due to heart disease. So here we have two trials, both using the "gold standard" research method, and for their primary outcome they end up with conflicting findings.

What is interesting is that in this same time frame, a relatively large cohort study (over 10,000 participants) was also underway in the U.S. conducted by researchers at the University of Southern California School of Medicine. It dif-fered from the U.S. experimental trial in important ways. The cohort study used participants (males and females) from a retirement home in California and they were considerably older (on average by about 20 years) than the doctors participating in the clinical trials. The findings from the cohort trial, published in the *British Medical Journal*, appeared in 1989, a year after those of the two experimental studies. In respect to the major end point (i.e. heart attacks) the cohort study had results more consistent with the U.S. study. The magnitude of the aspirin benefit was less, but it was still sizeable with about a 30 percent reduction in heart attacks among aspirin users. Again there was an increase in strokes on aspirin and no important difference in term of the number dying from all heart-related events. However, there were some unique findings in the cohort trial – an increased risk of kidney cancer in the aspirin group as well as an increased risk of heart disease (i.e. disorders such as arrhythmias and angina that indicate that the heart was not functioning normally).

It took another 10 years before new clinical studies were completed on this issue. Three RABCOT trials, the Thrombosis Prevention Trial, Hypertension Optimal Treatment Study and the Primary Prevention Project employed low-dose aspirin, averaging less than 100 mg of aspirin per day. A total of over 10,000 subjects (mostly males) served as subjects. Each of these studies confirmed the value of aspirin to prevent non-fatal heat attacks. Adding these results to those studies already completed supported a conclusion that aspirin did indeed reduce the risk of non-fatal heart attacks, but its effect on stroke and all other heart related deaths remained unclear. All in all quite an impressive results.

In spite of all these trials and all these subjects the FDA never approved the use of aspirin to prevent an initial heart attack. Did the FDA fumble the ball? No – they too have their own experts, and that group provided the rationale to withhold approving aspirin for this new indication. The FDA's advisory committee, also a group of highly respected medical experts, looked at the same data, but came to a very different conclusion. There would be no recommendation to use aspirin to prevent a heart attack. Several things troubled them: the low representation of women in the studies, the failure to lower overall death rates and the fact that aspirin causes life-threading adverse reactions. For patients with a low heart attack risk, the chance of experiencing one of aspirin's serious side effects meant they faced an unsatisfactory benefit-risk ratio.

To better appreciate the FDA's position, look at the situation from their point of view. What's the risk if they don't permit the new indication for aspirin? Not approving the indication really just keeps the aspirin manufacturer from advertising their product as a way to avoid that first heart attack. It's not like people can't get the drug without a prescription. Aspirin is readily available – you can even buy it at grocery stores and gas stations. Hopefully the FDA action also may encourage doctors and patients to talk over the subject and decide what is best for the patient. Still this case reinforces the pattern we see in medical research – inconsistency in findings, interpretations and conclusions. Too often the result is a perplexed public and medical community.

That doesn't mean the medical community as a whole agrees with the FDA. There are prestigious groups that take a different position. Medical associations as well as a U.S. Preventive Services Task Force, a special panel sponsored by the government but consisting of independent research experts as well, ended up creating guidelines for the use of aspirin to prevent heart attacks. The recommendations supported the use of low-dose aspirin for otherwise healthy men and women providing they had a higher than normal risk for a heart related event. Thus, those who had risk factors for heart attacks such as obesity, high blood pressure or tobacco use were advised to use a low-dose of aspirin to ward off heart related problems.

This case study also illustrates that there can be conflict between two experimental trials using the same kind of patients and comparing the same two agents. A satisfactory explanation for the conflicting findings between the U.S. and U.K. aspirin trials has still not surfaced. Except for the unexplainable failed trial using physicians in the U.K., the other studies had similar findings favoring aspirin. Did some condition related to heart attacks that we are not aware of affect the U.K. trial? There are so many possibilities beyond the researchers' control that could have produced the unique U.K. outcome. Who knows, maybe U.K. doctors working in a national health system have less stress than their counterparts in the U.S. who work in a pressure-packed free enterprise system. The lower level of stress may keep heart attacks at bay.

One more comment must be made. Note that the expert group recommending aspirin included women as well as men in their recommendation, even though only a small minority of the subjects were female. As noted previously, the extrapolation of medical research results, when the studies contain a small proportion of women is a dangerous, but frequent practice. Unfortunately for the experts in this case, it appears that they got it wrong. An experimental trial of close to 40,000 women, published in 2005, revealed that aspirin therapy to prevent first heart attacks did not have the same benefit for women as it did for men. For too many years, after conducting clinical trials on male subjects, researchers have assumed that the same result applied to women. But at last, more and more researchers have realized that differences in women's biochemistry, hormone profiles, and body structure make a big difference in the way they react to drug therapies.

Chapter 17
Hormone Replacement Therapy –
The Silver Bullet That Misfired

Abstract Hormone replacement therapy (HRT) had gained a positive image due to results from the Nurses Health Study, and other cohort trials, but randomized clinical trials wiped out many of its presumed benefits. In 1998 the results of a large clinical trial challenged a crucial claim that HRT protected the heart. Then a second study, sponsored by National Institutes of Health (NIH), found that HRT not only didn't reduce the risk of heart disease – it increased it! The NIH trial covering 16,600 postmenopausal women also found other damaging evidence such as increased risk of stoke and breast cancer. Even some of HRT's heralded advantages such as an improved quality of life were not supported. An explanation on why the nurses cohort study apparently got it wrong is traced to the nurses taking hormones who turned out to be healthier, better educated, from a higher socioeconomic class and with better health care access compared to the nurses not taking hormones. Key differences between the cohort studies and the clinical trials are also examined to see if the differences between them could account for some of the conflicting results as well.

Keywords Heart attack risk · heart and estrogen/progestin replacement study · hormone replacement therapy · nurses health study · women's health imitative study

If there were a list of landmark cases in medical science, the trials and tribulations of hormone replacement therapy (HRT) could well head the list. The history of HRT research is a story of the rise and fall of a celebrated pharmaceutical product and illustrates the enormous difficulty medical research faces. As the 21st century began, almost everyone was singing the praises of hormone replacement therapy (HRT) in large part because of the findings from the Nurses Health Study (NHS), that large and prestigious trial that we read about in the chapter on cohort trials. Middle-aged women swore by products containing estrogen – it was their miracle drug. At last, the depressing symptoms of menopause could be relieved. Most women dreaded menopause, the time when menstruation ceased and there was a large reduction in the production of female hormones; most notably estrogen. Many women experience a variety of difficulties related to the decrease in hormones such as hot flashes. Sleep disorders caused by night sweats and the dreary days that followed, took the place of a more peaceful existence. It made sense to replace natural occurring hormones by taking pills containing estrogen, the most versatile female hormone. Taking hormone replacement therapy was thought to be the best way for a woman to get through this difficult time in her life.

It all started in 1942 when Premarin, a pill containing estrogen, was approved for marketing to American women. Premarin promised to control symptoms associated with menopause – in particular the hot flashes and vaginal bleeding women experienced. In the 1950s and 1960s the Premarin legend grew. Estrogen seemed capable of bestowing all sorts of miraculous benefits to women. The book, *Feminine Forever* published in 1968 and still in print, made estrogen therapy sound like a second fountain of youth. The book celebrated estrogen for multiple reasons. It could prevent the dreaded aging process and much more. HRT eliminated the menacing menopausal symptoms and women would not have to face the mood swings associated with their middle-years. Because of estrogen's positive effects of skin and hair they could also avoid becoming dull and unattractive. A fantastic opportunity to live a better life – what women in her right mind would want to be left out?

The accolades for estrogen continued to roll in. Not only could it make a woman look and feel better, it could prevent bone deterioration and reduce the risk of a heart attack or stroke. The dreaded problem of mental deterioration could also be postponed because hormones could enhance a woman's memory. In particular, dementia, the loss of memory and language could be defeated. To end up with Alzheimer's disease, the best known form of dementia, was an unbearable thought. Even more good news followed – there were claims that estrogen provided protection against breast and uterine cancer.

Given this glowing profile it is no wonder that Premarin became one of the most prescribed therapies in the U.S. It didn't seem to matter that the evidence to support all the positive claims came from exploratory research methods rather than clinical trials. For most people at the time, medical research was medical research – the form of the research was unimportant. It was easy and felt good for doctors and their patients alike to have a positive outlook when it came to estrogen therapy.

The first hint of trouble appeared in the 1970s. That's when a report, by the Coronary Drug Project Research Group based at the University of Maryland, reported that estrogen provided no heart benefit in men. But that study was in men and not women. Still the result was unexpected. Furthermore, the men taking estrogen had more blood clots and cancer, prompting the researchers to halt their trial prematurely. They reasoned that if the trial were continued, men who were assigned to the estrogen treatment group would be vulnerable to an avoidable health risks, and that was unacceptable.

In the mid 1980s, however, there was major news about the effect of female hormones on heart disease. The news regarding hormonal effects on the heart was mixed, but the good news seemed more believable than the bad news. The well-regarded Framingham Heart Study (FHS), described earlier, published findings in 1985 in which they reported that in their cohort of women, those who took hormones had more heart disease related deaths and a higher risk for stroke than women not using hormones. However, that bad news was pretty well wiped out by a report from the NHS that appeared in the same journal, the *New England Journal of Medicine*, at the same time as the FHS report. This research project following nurses, had about 100 times more women in the trial than Framingham. The NHS did not just find no difference, it reported that the rates of heart disease in women were much lower for women on estrogen. It was easy to accept this latter result since most other exploratory studies during this time-period had found good effects by hormones on heart disease as well.

Armed with these favorable results, in 1990, the manufacturer of Premarin, the most used form of estrogen, asked the FDA to approve their product for heart disease prevention. Their request was denied. It was one of the few times the FDA did not accept an advisory committee recommendation – the FDA advisory board had approved the change (with only a single dissenting vote). As far as the FDA was concerned, the evidence wasn't strong enough. Where were the experimental studies to support the claim?

Then the biggest story of all came out in 1996 when the NHS researchers in a follow-up report claimed that HRT decreased the risk of heart disease by a whopping 40 percent. In the same year, a case-control study reported in *Obstetrics & Gynecology* noted that long-term hormone use lowered overall mortality rate in postmenopausal women and the reduction was mainly due to less heart disease.

Heart disease wasn't the only game in town, however. The effect of hormones on other diseases and problems had slowly dribbled in and raised important issues for women. What, for example, did the drug's risk-benefit profile look like? There was no clear answer. On the down side, women had to worry about cancer and a potential problem when it came to strokes. On the up side were new promising uses of hormones to prevent hip fractures and potentially other conditions such as dementia.

For some researchers and members of the medical community, the propensity for hormones to stimulate uterine and breast cancer meant that a link between estrogen and cancer always loomed on the horizon. Back in 1976 a *New England Journal of Medicine* article had reported that female hormone therapy was linked to breast cancer. As the 1980s begin, there is a break in the bad news. It was discovered that by adding a second hormone (progesterone) to the usual estrogen therapy, the higher risk of uterine cancer could be overcome. With the combination of estrogen and progestin, the synthetic form of progesterone used in many hormone medications, a women's risk was no higher than the normal risk.

Then the dam seemed to burst. A 1989 article in the *American Journal of Obstetrics and Gynecology*, indicated that women taking estrogen could have up to a 10 times greater chance of developing uterine cancer than women who didn't take estrogen. The news more than offset a 1983 governmental case-controlled study by the Centers for Disease Control that had found no increase in breast cancer for women who had used oral contraceptives at sometime in their lives. The women ranged in age between 20 and 54 so the news, although positive, did not completely exonerate estrogen use in postmenopausal women.

By the end of the 1980s the picture became even more confusing. The estrogen-progestin combination that had been found to safeguard women from uterine cancer was also found to potentially have a serious adverse effect. Studies published in the *New England Journal of Medicine* showed that the combination appeared to markedly increase the risk of breast cancer. However, a few years later, data from the NHS provided a way out. A 1995 article, by the NHS epidemiologists headed by G. Colditz, noted that both estrogen alone and the estrogen-progesterone combination increased the risk of breast cancer, but the increase was seen only in women who took HRT for five or more years. A review of articles published in the 1990s noted the widespread inconsistency in results among exploratory trials when it came to estrogen use and breast cancer. In their 1999 *JAMA* article on this topic Bush and Whiteman concluded that any risk must be small or must occur in a very limited population. If this were not so, a greater risk would have been detected by now.

In the end women faced a dilemma – take HRT and receive its likely benefits (including the lower heart disease risk), but run the risk of breast cancer. Women and their physicians were left to answer this question, but based on HRT sales during this time, it appeared that most preferred the benefit of hormones over the cancer risk.

A warning signal had been raised on the connection between strokes and hormone treatment as early as the mid 1980s, but after years of research the situation was still confused and unclear. A review in *Cephalalgia* showed that the set of completed exploratory stroke studies had come up with all sorts of incompatible results. You couldn't tell if hormones increased, decreased or had no effect on the risk of a stroke. It seemed that the link between HRT and stroke would never be settled. Whenever there was a step forward, it was followed by one backward. For instance, in 1993s paper in the *Archives of Internal Medicine* by a group of researchers in the National Center for Health Statistics, described the outcome for women who did not have a history of stroke. Followed for an average of 12 years, the women who were on hormones experienced a large reduction in the risk of a fatal stroke. However, this time the NHS put up the red flag. In an *Annals of Internal Medicine* publication by F. Grodstein and other NHS colleagues found a weak relationship between postmenopausal hormone use and the risk of stroke. Compared to women, who never used hormones, the women taking the highest HRT doses appeared to have a slightly higher number of strokes.

There was much more consistency when it came to hormone benefits. Almost all exploratory studies came up with positive findings for HRT use in the reduction of hip fractures. With osteoporosis being a common threat to older people this was especially good news. Also on the bright side were additional reports that hormone therapy in postmenopausal women staved off dementia. However, the results were still inconclusive for there were prospective cohort studies reporting no benefit.

By now a reader is probably dazed trying to keep track of all the results from HRT treatment. You're in good company – doctors, patients and the public at large were also overwhelmed. Based on my premise that you shouldn't believe the results from any single research project, the litany of "answers" serves as an ideal illustration to support that argument.

The plethora of incompatible results and FDA's reticence to act amid all the confusion, it was left to the practicing physician to make sense out of this puzzle. On the positive side, long-term hormone use to ease the symptoms of menopause remained an uncontested benefit. It appeared reasonable to add preventing osteoporosis to its advantages. Other uses, such as forestalling dementia, also held out hope even though there was too little information to be sure. The uterine cancer scare seemed to be checked by adding a second hormone to estrogen. You could go either way with stroke. However, the risk of breast cancer couldn't be overlooked. That left one important effect to be factored in – heart disease. The jury was still out, but heart disease was a major illness that could lead to thousands of deaths in postmenopausal women. Could the hope of less heart disease trump the nagging concern over the possibility of breast cancer? In this debate, as any statistician would have gladly pointed out, a reduction in heart disease of almost half would overwhelm any anticipated increase in the risk for breast cancer. For instance, in 1994 there were a little over 200,000 deaths from heart disease compared with about 30,000 deaths from breast cancer in women older than 55 years. The potential benefits of HRT had an enormous public health impact. The medical community listened. Based on a 1995 survey of physicians, more than half said they would prescribe estrogen for the prevention of heart disease.

As the end of the 20th century approached, the scorecard for hormone treatment was clearly on the favorable side. However this record was based almost exclusively on exploratory trials. Even well into the 1990s, few clinical trials had been conducted and those that were performed tended to be too small to be helpful. However, in 1997 an effort was made to pool the available RABCOTS and see what the accumulated results showed. The authors, who published their results in the *British Medical Journal*, had to make do with variations in the reporting of the selected studies, their small size and limited duration of treatment. The goal of the research was confined to seeing what effect HRT had in terms of heart disease and cancer. Based on 22 trials and over 4,000 subjects on HRT or control treatments the authors found a great deal of variation from one study to the next. However, contrary to what the exploratory trials found, the authors were able to conclude that the pooled data could not support the notion that HRT prevented heart-related events. For cancers, the numbers of reported events was too low to arrive at a reasonable conclusion.

Major Clinical Trials

The FDA's rejection of the heart-protection claim made it clear, positive results from the exploratory studies weren't enough. They could not and did not establish causality. Well-designed clinical trials, which were less subject to bias than exploratory studies were not only needed, they were essential to help establish the truth about HRT.

In the mid 1990s, two research teams launched large experimental studies to evaluate hormones in postmenopausal women. The first study was the Heart and Estrogen/Progestin Trial (HERS) paid for by the maker of Prempro (the top selling HRT drug that combined estrogen with progestin into a single pill). They would sponsor an experimental trial to satisfy the FDA. Close to 3,000 women with heart disease participated. The goal was to see if hormone treatment could reduce the risk of a second heart attack. It was a randomized, double-blinded, placebo controlled RABCOT. It was a multi-center trial using 20 clinical centers. The subjects had a maximum age of 89 and a mean age of about 67. There was, on average, a little over four years of observation per subject.

The second major experimental trial was the Women's Health Initiative (WHI). It was a massive undertaking, sponsored by the influential National Institutes of Health, that set out to assess the incidence on major diseases associated with the use of Prempro. It was also a RABCOT, using placebo as the control treatment, and took place at 40 clinical centers across the U.S. Over 16,000 postmenopausal women between the ages of 50 and 79 enrolled. The average time the women were treated was just over five years. These women were unlike those in the HERS trial because they did not have heart disease when they entered the trial and it is important to keep this fact in mind as you read the results from the two research projects.

Before the two RABCOT trials reshaped the positive profile for HRT, the exploratory study researchers defended their findings and they commanded a great deal of respect in the research community. The NHS researchers conceded that experimental studies provided stronger evidence of cause and effect relationships. However, they also pointed out that there were limitations with experimental studies that were not found in exploratory studies. In particular the experimental studies could not, in general, determine long-term effects, whether these effects be positive or negative. It was up to exploratory studies to find the more long-term consequences. They also emphasized the more unnatural environment of experimental studies versus the "real world" setting for cohort trials. Nevertheless, they rightly believed that only when the evidence from a number of different kinds of studies had been completed could one come to a firm conclusion about a cause and effect relationship. They were particularly supportive of the experimental WHI study, which was underway when they were making their views known.

In 1998 the HERS investigators published their initial report in *JAMA* and a follow-up report (HERS II) four years later in the same journal. The results did not bode well for the Prempro faithful. The researchers found that women who had heart disease and took estrogen plus progestin had more than a 50 percent increase in the number of heart disease events during the first year of treatment. However, by the fourth year of treatment there were fewer episodes reported for the women taking the hormones compared to those on a placebo. In other words, in the first year the women were in trouble, but by the fourth year the danger had disappeared and they even seemed to be a little better off. The experimental HERS study also had more bad news, however. It found that hormone therapy could cause blood clots in postmenopausal women taking hormones. The possibility that hormones could affect blood clotting had initially been seen in studies of oral contraceptives, but was not supported by early exploratory studies of postmenopausal estrogens.

The HERS study noted that their women showed a doubling of the risk for embolism, a potentially dangerous free floating blood clot.

When the new century began the pluses and minuses of hormone treatment continued to be reported. The researchers of the NHS study found their earlier reports in 1995 were substantiated in a 2000 follow-up analysis that they published in *Annals of Internal Medicine*. They also noted, however, that the breast cancer risk was still there, but remember, it didn't appear until after five years of hormone use. In contrast, the HERS trial had mainly challenged the positive effect of HRT on the heart, but according to their study, the higher heart disease risk didn't seem to last long and it occurred in a unique group of women: those who already had heart disease. By and large, the believers in HRT continued to believe. On balance, HRT was still a good bet, but due to the HERS results, doctors and their postmenopausal patients had a bit more to worry about when it came to their continued use of hormone treatment.

The findings from the experimental HERS trial were troubling, but the patients were somewhat unique because of their heart disease history and, in general, the medical community felt that they could get reasonably reliable answers from well-done exploratory studies such as the NHS in spite of the handicaps associated with this method or research. After all, exploratory studies had a decent track record and besides, experimental studies could come to incorrect conclusions as well. For many it was more sensible to rely on good prospective cohort studies when experimental studies did not exist or the trials applied to a specialized patient population. The alternative was to ignore the benefits hormone therapy promised – an unacceptable choice for many physicians and their patients. As noted previously, the dominating NHS that had found so many worthwhile benefits, was clearly a carefully executed study. It was huge in terms of participants. It was methodologically sound and used a contemporary control group observed over a long period of time. It was based at Harvard and the subjects (nurses) were health advocates and thus responsible providers of information.

The favorable profile for HRT however, was torn asunder when the second experimental study, the Women's Health Initiative or WHI, announced it results in 2002. The hormone combination not only increased the risk of breast cancer, there was also a stunning reversal when it came to heart disease. HRT didn't decrease heart disease – it increased it! The researchers were so convinced of their result that they felt they could not ethically continue the trial and subject women on hormone treatment to the higher heart attack and breast cancer risks. Consequently, the Prempro portion of the WHI came to a premature close.

Other results from the WHI trial indicated that hormones also increased the risk of stroke and blood clots, but it did confirm the advantage of hormone for protecting against fractures. Furthermore, the HERS trial, which raised the possibility that hormones might reduce heart disease in women who already had heart disease, reported in 2002 that their 1998 finding about less heart disease after four years of use was not sustained after an additional three years of follow-up. The three-year extension allowed all subjects some form of hormone treatment so it was not blinded. Nevertheless, the researchers concluded that there was no significant decrease in heart disease and recommended that hormones not be used to prevent heart problems in women who had a heart condition.

Besides the heart disease issue, a second critically important difference from the experimental study results and the exploratory trials having to do with breast cancer surfaced. A studious review in the *Annals of Internal Medicine*, examined exploratory studies on the breast cancer question and located almost 40 studies done from 1970 to 1990. Most studies found no difference at all, but there were four that reported a significant decrease and seven that found a significant breast cancer increase from hormone use.

A second review, published in *Obstetrics & Gynecology* in 2001, looked at all studies conducted between 1975 and 2000 that examined the breast cancer and hormone use relationship. Once again, the analysts found there was little consistency in terms of developing breast cancer from the use of HRT. However, when it came to deaths from breast cancer, the incidence was higher among hormone users compared with nonusers. The analysts concluded that, although an increased risk of getting breast cancer with long-term use of hormones could not be ruled out, the likelihood of such a result had to be small. This relatively benign finding for hormones turned out to be in direct conflict with the WHI result that showed an approximate 25 percent increase in the development of breast cancer for women taking hormones. Since the WHI was a RABCOT, its results carried the day making the few epidemiologists who had conducted case-control studies and found a high risk of breast cancer from hormone use before the WHI study published its results, look like visionaries.

Actually the WHI consisted of several parts or sub-trials, but the Prempro portion of the project that focused on heart disease was the main trial and the first to publish findings. A second part of the project looked at the effect of estrogen alone versus placebo in women who had had a hysterectomy. Since the hysterectomy removed the uterus there was no need to worry about uterine cancer and progesterone was not required. Over 10,000 women participated in this double-blind trial of estrogen alone versus placebo, but it too ended early because of the harm done by estrogen. In this study, published in *JAMA* the year after the first WHI report, estrogen was found to increase the risk of stroke and appeared to be no better than placebo in respect to heart disease. In both the main trial and this trial, about the only good news for HRT advocates was that hormone treatment reduced bone fractures, but that advantage had not been in dispute.

Finally another area was examined by the WHI and published by the *New England Journal of Medicine* in 2003. In spite of all the negative results associated with hormonal therapy for postmenopausal women, there were still many believers in the drugs. Many women and their doctors said that the hormonal drugs had quality of life benefits. By that they meant they relieved symptoms such as hot flashes and night sweats. In addition, hormones made them feel more energetic, made sex more pleasurable and improved their memory. The women who took hormones simply believed in the product. They were convinced they were doing much better because of their daily intake of hormones.

Then the medical findings from the WHI quality of life trial destroyed that myth. Even the researchers who did this phase of the study were surprised by the results.

The women on hormones, compared to those on placebo, did no better in terms of vitality, mental health, depressive symptoms or sexual satisfaction. There was just a touch of good news, but it was not that impressive: women had less problem sleeping. The difference, however, was marginal. Physical activity was just barely better and there was a minimal improvement in respect to pain. Hot flashes were alleviated by three out of every four women on Prempro, but if they were on placebo, two out of four women reported improvement as well. Not much of a difference considering all the positive anecdotal reports by those who swore by hormonal therapy.

Wyeth Pharmaceuticals, the drug company making Prempro, raised questions about the findings. They said the study subjects were not typical hormone users because they did not have the severe symptoms of menopause. They added that their quality of life was already so high that it was unlikely to improve while in the study. Few minds were changed by these arguments.

The early reports, that hormone therapy in postmenopausal women staved off dementia, had come up with a risk reduction that went as high as 30 percent. However, the results were mixed and there were cohort studies reporting no benefit. As you might guess, the hope that women could protect themselves from dementia was dashed in the 2003 report from the WHI researchers. Not only was there no benefit, there was actually an increased risk of dementia in hormone users over the age of 65.

The final example of WHI's disastrous attack on HRT had to with stroke. The exploratory trials had been all over the place with some showing a decreased risk, others showing no effect and yet a number coming up with an increased risk. Would the experimental studies clear up the confusion? The WHI researchers reported that hormone treatment caused an increase in strokes by a striking 41 percent. But that monumental difference didn't totally eliminate the state of confusion. The HERS trial found there was an insignificant relationship between hormone use and strokes. There may be a simple explanation for the difference was confined to women who had had heart disease and the WHI study used only women without such a history.

The picture gets a big more foggy or clear, depending on your point of view, after the exploratory study results for stroke enter into the picture. The fashionable NHS study found a 45 percent higher risk for stroke among women taking estrogen combined with progestin compared to those who had never taken hormone therapy. This was unusually similar to the 41 percent higher risk found in the experimental WHI trial, but that left HERS as the odd man out. Any questions about a connection between stroke and HRT were pretty well settled by a 2005 meta analysis published by the *British Medical Journal*. Based on 28 trials and almost 40,000 subjects, the authors found close to a 30 percent increase in strokes for women using HRT.

The Conflicting Results

What caused this mass of confusion about the role of hormone treatment in post-menopausal women? The WHI ruled the day and its supremacy was barely threatened. Among the WHI findings, the one that was the most sensational had to do with heart disease. It should be clear that there were doubts about the advantages of hormonal therapy for postmenopausal women when only exploratory studies were available. Not all exploratory study results found hormones helpful in controlling heart disease, but most did. An analysis in *Preventive Medicine* of about 30 exploratory trials had half the studies finding a significant reduction and only one with a significant increase in heart disease. How could so many studies be wrong? Especially since the RABCOT WHI study found that there was not just no difference – there was an increase of heart disease of almost 30 percent for the subjects receiving Prempro!

What may have caused the NHS, the premiere exploratory study, to come up with an incorrect answer as it related to heart disease. Why did their results strongly suggest that HRT would prevent heart disease? To begin, there were obvious problems with the NHS's selection of subjects which epidemiologists recognized long before the WHI results appeared. In fact, the NHS researchers often qualified their results by noting that nurses were more health conscious, they had better medical care and enjoyed a life style that was far above that of most women. But they and others were reticent to say that this kind of subject selection bias could have a significant effect on the study results, especially on the claim of heart disease protection. But after the WHI findings became known, there were numerous articles written that pointed out that the relatively healthy women used in the exploratory hormone studies were behind the misleading results that favored hormone users.

An important 2002 analysis, in the *Annals of Internal Medicine* by L. Humphrey at the Oregon Health & Science University and her associates, lent support to the belief that the life style factor had indeed confounded the results of the exploratory studies. Shortly after the WHI results became available, the researchers performed a meta analysis using a set of well-done exploratory studies that investigated hormone use and the incidence of heart disease. Variables, especially those known to be risk factors for heart disease such as age, smoking, high blood pressure and family history, were examined. Also included were the socioeconomic level and the educational level of the study participants. These last two variables were felt to be reasonably well correlated with a healthy life style.

It was found that failure to adjust study results based on the socioeconomic and educational factors resulted in an outcome that showed a heart benefit for hormone use. The exploratory studies that considered these factors did not find the heart benefit. Simply put – the studies that failed to take into account socioeconomic status and education tended to produce more favorable results. When these aspects were factored into an analysis, hormone use was not associated with a better effect on the heart.

However, remember the two RABCOT studies had raised a question about (HERS) or shown (WHI) a harmful heart effect from hormones. Accounting for socioeconomic level and education among the exploratory trials had only brought the heart effect to a neutral position. Therefore, inequality in socioeconomic level and educational status could not be the whole answer. And in fact, the women on hormones had other traits that could have influenced the exploratory study results.

Hormone users were more likely to have access to health care and if there were troubling signs of disease they could avail themselves of effective preventive treatments and never come down with the illness. They also may have engaged in more health-screening programs that caught very early problems and treated them before they turned into more serious condition.

Hormone users were very likely to have a greater level of health awareness as well. As a result, they may have been more likely to take other medications that protected their heart such as blood pressure drugs or cholesterol lowering agents. Many exploratory studies took place at a time when there were questions about the safety of hormones. Physicians could have prescribed HRT only to women who they judged as being in excellent health. It's also been observed that during the hey-day of exploratory studies the standard *Physicians' Desk Reference* suggested estrogen should not be prescribed to women with heart disease. This meant that physicians would have been reluctant to even start HRT in many women who had a risk for heart disease. This latter group of women could end up in the non-estrogen arm of a cohort trial, but they were at a high risk to develop heart disease. Under this scenario it would be predicable that the women not taking HRT drugs would end up with a higher number developing heart disease.

Researchers who worried about the biases possible in exploratory studies also expressed another concern about the relationship between hormone use and heart disease. Research at the Northwestern Medical School had shown that people who are conscientious in taking placebo medication in a medical study had fewer heart problems than the subjects on placebo who are less diligent. In fact, a 1997 report in *Archives of Internal Medicine* noted that negative heart related events were significantly lowered in the people who carefully adhere to the treatment schedule they were asked to follow. Now, assuming that women who took hormones, especially for long periods, had to be very good medication compilers, we have another possible difference between the hormone users and non-users that could contribute to the misleading positive results found in the exploratory trials.

An additional source of subject selection bias was also raised as a possible reason for the erroneous heart disease results. Many of the women in the exploratory studies were on hormones to prevent the symptoms of menopause, osteoporosis and bone fractures. These women tend to be thinner and to have lower levels of naturally produced estrogen compared to the non-hormone users. There was research that showed these factors protected women from developing heart disease. Thus, body-type bias would be yet another reason for the overstated heart protection claim.

The preceding discussion shows that there were a number of ways that the exploratory studies could come up with the wrong answer. Hormone users and non-users were different in important ways. The women taking hormones were healthier, better educated and from a higher socioeconomic class. They had better health care access, were more conscientious about taking their medication and had a more ideal body type. However, there were additional problems that could have contributed to the ill-advised heart prevention claim.

It's also possible that subjects in the NHS and other exploratory studies could have been assigned to the wrong treatment group when they enrolled in a cohort trial. If a study enrolled only current users of hormones then women, who had started hormone treatment but then discontinued it when they became ill, could have been assigned to the non-user group. Because of their poor health, they would be more prone to heart disease thereby inflating the incidence of heart disease problems in the non-user group.

The designers of the NHS also noted another classification problem. The NHS updated the information on their subjects every two years. If a woman started hormones, but then stopped HRT in the same two-year period she ended up in the non-HRT group. If in that same two years she had a heart related event it counted against the non-HRT users. That heart problem could have been caused by the HRT the woman took, and she therefore should have been counted as an HRT user with a heart event. But as it worked out, the wrong side took the hit.

There were, in addition, some elements from the NHS and other exploratory trials that troubled scientists. A dose-response relationship had not been found. In other words, as hormone dosage increased there was no sign of more protection. Furthermore, a longer duration of hormone use was not associated with a reduction in heart problems. In fact, there seemed to be less benefit with long-term use compared to short-term use. On the other hand, additional factors lent support to the positive effects hormones had on heart disease. The biology fit. Estrogen was known to lower LDL cholesterol, the bad kind of fat that was one of the causes of heart disease. It also raised the level of HDL, the good cholesterol, which was associated with a strong heart. In addition, estrogens altered other biological substances that tended to affect the heart in a negative way. When it came to HRT, there were no easy answers.

Divergent answers in the medical research on HRT could also be due to other reasons beyond those already presented. For example, there were key differences between the NHS and WHI in respect to the type of subjects studied and the way HRT was given. In particular, notable differences were present for (1) ages of the subjects, (2) length of time since menstruation began before beginning hormone treatment, (3) the type of HRT regimen and (4) the duration of treatment. The WHI subjects were much older, had started treatment much later and were treated with different hormone products for a shorter period of time.

Age

Women in the WHI were, on average, in their mid 60s (an age range of 50–79) when they started hormone treatment and, as a result, they were on average more than 10 years past menopause. On the other hand, the women in the NHS were between 30–55 years old when they began taking hormones. The age discrepancy raises the question of whether the heart benefit could have been realized in the WHI, if younger women had been enrolled and if they started taking hormones as soon as they were enrolled.

Commencement of Treatment

Note the time when HRT is initiated was also very different in the two trials. In the NHS study about 80 percent of the subjects started hormone use within two years after menopause. For the WHI women, menopause had begun many years and even decades before the hormone treatment began. Subsequent investigations consistently revealed that the timing of HRT initiation may indeed be critical in its impact on the heart. Wait too long and the window of opportunity is shut – hormones no longer could protect the heart. Were the WHI women, a decade or more into their menopause, unable to derive a heart benefit from HRT?

Incompatible HRT Regimens

In the experimental trials, Prempro was a specific type of HRT and subjects took it on a fixed-dosage schedule. In the exploratory studies a variety of hormone products were used and the dosage schedules were extremely variable. Most importantly the exploratory trials used estrogen alone or the combination of estrogen plus progestin. However, the prevailing treatment for the combination therapy included progestin for only 10–14 days out of every month. This differed markedly from the WHI trial which used a single pill, Prempro, on a daily basis and women thereby ended up taking progestin every day of a month. In addition only the oral route was tested in the WHI. Could different routes of administration (e.g. the estrogen patch) produce different results? It's also true that the fixed dosage schedule used in the WHI was relatively high, compared to the dosage given in the NHS and many other exploratory trials. It's easy to wonder how much of the harmful effects were due to the rigid WHI dosing schedule.

Duration of Treatment

There was also a major difference in the long-term exploratory studies and the experimental studies when it came to the duration of hormone use. In the NHS about 30 percent of the nurses used hormones for 10 to 20 years and in other exploratory trials that found a positive affect on the heart, the use exceeded 20 years. The follow-up in the WHI was at best about seven years. Could it take long-term use for hormones to protect the heart?

It is also relevant to point out that biases could have existed in the WHI as well. There was greater unblinding of the hormone treated subjects and there is speculation that this could have resulted in artificially higher detection rates for heart problems among the hormone users. The blind was prematurely broken for over 40 percent of the HRT users and less than 7 percent of the placebo users. The staff that broke the blind didn't necessarily make that information known to those making assessments about heart disease. However, the women themselves could have disclosed the information to research staff members. It is also noteworthy that a relatively high rate of discontinuation of hormone therapy would lower the level of exposure for the HRT group and that could cause an underestimate of heart problems.

The point here is that experimental trials and long term exploratory trials produced results that were based on very different kinds of subjects, treatment regimens and operating rules. The differences may have had little effect on causing the conflicting heart disease result, but the fact they exist is always troubling when there are conflicting findings. For my purpose they represent yet one more example of the unbelievable difficulty in getting a valid answer from any single medical research project, no matter how distinguished.

It's even been postulated that there may be no conflict between the WHI and the cohort study results – perhaps everyone was right. Here's the reasoning. The average duration of HRT treatment in the WHI was about five years. In comparison, the subjects in the cohort trials were treated, on average, for a much longer period of time. If it is assumed that the initial cardiovascular effect of HRT is negative, and it takes long term hormone use to reverse the process and provide a beneficial level of protection from heart problems, then the WHI had it right (a negative short-term effect) and so did the cohort studies (a positive long-term effect). Another theory can be advanced to support the contention that the results from WHI and the cohort studies were compatible. In the cohort studies estrogen without progesterone was the most common treatment. The WHI, on the other hand, combined the two drugs and patients took the combined products every day. If estrogen alone causes heart problems, but by adding progesterone that liability is converted to a beneficial effect, the findings from the two research approaches would make sense. This explanation loses some of its appeal because the cohort investigations that included the combined therapy, reported protection from heart ailments just as those only using estrogen. Then again, the combined treatment in the WHI trial was given every day, but in the cohort investigations the progesterone tended to be taken with long breaks (up to two weeks every month). If progesterone has to be given on a daily basis to offset the harmful impact from estrogen, then the theory that there is no incompatibility between the two types of projects holds up. Although these possible explanations may be far fetched, the unpredictability of medical research shouldn't totally rule them out.

Medical research is incredibly difficult even when the best researchers are involved. Unexpected and uncontrollable controllable factors can influence a result and no matter how careful they are, researchers might get the wrong answer. In the case of hormone replacement treatment, the belief is that the experimental studies got it pretty right and the exploratory studies had some wrong answers. But that is not clearly the end of the story. More research may will modify what we know now. Maybe there is more truth in the exploratory studies than we are willing to concede at this point in time. The goal of epidemiology is to learn why some people acquire a disease and others are spared. Note that in the review of why exploratory studies missed the boat on heart disease sensitive variables such as life style could not be studied because information on the variable was not collected. How many other variables that may play a role in the development of heart disease are there? How many can we afford to study? The hormone and heart disease issue shows that getting at the truth is a long term and frustrating process and no one study can guarantee that it has produced the right answer. It may be that for some women hormones increase heart disease, for others it decreases heart disease and for still others it has no effect. Sorry to say but until more research takes place on the effects of hormones on the heart we won't know for sure what's the clear-cut answer.

Just before I end this chapter a note on the repercussions from the perplexing results of the medical research performed on post menopausal hormone therapy seems in order. When the dust cleared, HRT was left with an unsatisfactory risk versus benefit comparison for many women and their doctors. It helped with menstrual symptoms and bone fractures, but on the negative side were heart and cancer risks that definitely trumped the benefits. At a minimum there was confusion – at the extreme there was outrage.

A leading women's group called the National Women's Health Network (NWHN) called the situation a case of corruption by the medical and scientific community. Their anger was aimed at all manufacturers of hormone products, but especially the major company, Wyeth Pharmaceuticals. The belief that hormones were good preventive medicine was a triumph of marketing over science, according to NWHN. They were particularly outraged that the manufacturers were allowed to skirt drug promotion restrictions and reap large sales from a flawed product. Hormones over the short term had been nowhere near as helpful as patients and their doctors were led to believe, and the long term dangers were life threatening. The NWHN in fact published a book detailing their concerns. In addition to women health advocates female physicians and scientists were authors of the book.

However Wyeth was not the only group criticized. The press, which will be examined in a subsequent chapter, was also a candidate for blame because of their failure to add appropriate qualifications to the results from exploratory trials. The epidemiologists who conduct exploratory trials were also singled out because of the dedicated belief they have in their methodology. By not being more reserved in promoting their results, physicians, patients and health authorities eagerly accepted them too easily. D. Sackett, a prominent clinical epidemiologist, writing in the *Canadian Medical Association Journal*, went even further when he blamed the "medical experts" who advocate preventive treatments that shape medical and public-health policy without ever being validated in RABCOTSs.

Putting aside who, if anyone, should be blamed for the early belief in HRT's "sensational" advantages, almost all medical authorities accepted the experimental study results and urged individual patients to consult with their physicians about the decision to continue or halt hormone treatment. However, the practicing physicians were placed in a quandary. What should they do? Their patients trusted them and it appears they let them down. And if they continue prescribing HRT, how much liability do they face?

Not surprisingly the sales of HRT products, including the market leader Prempro, plunged. Sales were cut in half in 2003 and yet there were still well over five million users. The FDA also reacted to the news. They required the manufacturers of estrogens to include a warning with their product that there was an increased risk for heart disease, heart attacks, strokes, and breast cancer. The warning also emphasized that these products were not approved for heart disease prevention and were not to be used as a first-line treatment for osteoporosis – one of the few condition for which estrogen was clearly efficacious.

Research involving ongoing hormone studies also presented their sponsors with a serious challenge – should they continue or stop. The National Institutes of Health asked each of its major therapeutic research areas to decide what it planned to do about any ongoing hormone studies and it also wanted to know the rationale for their decision. The decisions varied depending on the status of the research project. For example, we know the main heart study of the WHI had been stopped, but other areas of research were continued. The dementia portion of the WHI went on until it ended up concluding hormones caused more not less problems for menopausal women. Another NIH study testing the effect of hormones on lupus erythematosus, an arthritic type disease that often involves skin lesions and weakness, was halted.

The impact on patients required them to come to their individual decisions after conferring with their physician. A task force created by the U.S. Public Health Service came up with recommendations to guide physicians when making those decisions. The recommendation advised against the routine use of estrogen and progestin for the prevention of chronic condition noting that the benefits were unlikely to offset the harms. They urged physicians to engage in a shared decision-making approach with their patients about what to do when they enter menopause.

The HRT case study is a classic example of showing that no one can know for certain when a study has got it right or wrong. An interesting evaluation supporting this point of view appeared in 2005 and was based on major research articles published between 1990 and 2003 in prestigious journals. The analyst, J. Ioannidis writing in *JAMA*, looked to see if the conclusions from the original publication stood up when a subsequent clinical study was carried out. There were 34 original studies that had published positive findings and 19 did in fact have their results confirmed. But that left 15 or a scary 44 percent with inconsistent findings. In eight of those cases, the inconsistency was due to a more recent study showing that the first article had overestimated the effect of treatment. There was a good result, but not as good as what the initial study claimed. In the other seven, the new results contradicted the original findings. The latter statistic is sobering and supports the contention of this book that neither health care professionals nor the public can ever rely on the results of a single study.

There were only two case series trials and four cohort studies included in the original set of 34 studies, but none of those results held up in the second study. Perhaps this can be offered as additional evidence of the superiority of the clinical trial, but remember those trials were also far from perfect – almost a third of its new trials could not be reproduced in the follow-up research. And also do not assume the second study is right and the first one is wrong. Maybe it's the reverse. The analysis could only detect an inconsistency not what trial (if any) got the correct result.

It is clear there will be no more studies about hormones that are comparable to the WHI. The cost of the trial, estimated to be over $600 million, simply rules out new studies. Yet the WHI tested a specific HRT formulation and there are many hormone products that have not been tested. Without a comprehensive experimental trial, we will never obtain the quality and quantity of information that's needed for untested hormone products. However, this is not just a cost issue. The organizers stopped the WHI early because of the high heart attack and breast cancer risk. The benefits of HRT could not compensate for these disturbing adverse effects. Future researchers will need unusually strong evidence of new advantages for hormone treatment before subjecting healthy women to the dangers of hormone therapy. A major negative study dooms a treatment and offers its proponents little hope for redemption.

New HRT trials may be dead, but the WHI trial is a fantastic database. Shouldn't researchers tap that gold mine of information to learn more about hormones and their effects on women? Wouldn't it be possible to identify subgroups from the completed study and see if the original results stand up for the sets of patient identified? Did one age group do better than another? Does the degree of sexually activity make any difference? There are many subgroups analyses that offer tantalizing results. But, as mentioned previously, there are many problems with a subgroup analysis. Analysts may come up with intriguing results, but they should not pawn them off as definitive answers. They really represent hypotheses that need verification from other research endeavors.

In fact, in 2007 a WHI subgroup report appeared in *JAMA*. The authors had a legitimate interest. They wanted to know if the elevated heart disease and stroke rates with women on hormones was across all ages. What they found surprised them. Women in their 50s did not appear to have an increased risk of heart attack, but women who were in their 60s and 70s who still had hot flashes and night sweats had an increased risk of heart attacks, especially if they were taking hormones. They wisely warned that interest in an age analysis was not specified when the study was first designed, and the analyses should be viewed as providing exploratory rather than definitive answers. So far so good. However, by the time the results made it into the media, the following expressions, in a 2007 *New York Times* article, were attributed to the lead researcher concerning the study results: "clear as could be" or "And we know for sure that…".

This case study also illustrates that medical research is like trying to solve a jigsaw puzzle that has a number of missing pieces and extra pieces that aren't needed. Relationships and principles can be identified from the research, but some are right and some are wrong. We have to study the pieces we have, discarding some and imagining what others would look like. It takes time, patience and often a bit of luck to get a clear image of the complete puzzle. And it takes a lot of trial and error to reach that point – and sometimes we don't.

Chapter 18
Publishing – Getting the Word Out to Doctors

Abstract The lifeblood of scientific discovery is information. Unless research findings are published and reach the medical community, they are of little value. However, there are problems with the present method of publishing medical research results. Peer review, a process by which experimenters review each other's work in order to weed out poor research, may not catch important errors. The results from some clinical research trials with negative findings may not be published and that also represents a serous problem. Paxil, a drug that some believe leads to juvenile suicides is used to illustrate this issue. A major Paxil trial with a positive result was published and presented at medical meetings, but a similar trial with a negative result ended up with no publication. The case illustrates that a drug's safety and efficacy problems can be deliberately hidden from the medical profession and the public. There are therefore calls for a clinical trial registry, which would contain the results of all clinical research investigations whether or not published in a journal. In addition, an innovative plan by faculty members of the London School of Hygiene and Tropical Medicine is used to suggest a radically way to change the current publication system.

Keywords Clinical trial registry · medical journal · peer review · publication bias · unpublished studies

> *Most physicians are not formally taught how to critically evaluate published results of clinical trials.* (H. Rubins, *Controlled Clinical Trials*)

The lifeblood of scientific discovery is information. The findings from each research project serves as a base for new research in a continuous chain. Each clinical study contributes to an evolving body of evidence. To make the process work, research findings must be published and be easily available to the medical community. The sharing of ideas, successes and failures, helps researchers discover new knowledge that leads to better health for everyone. But, anyone familiar with medical research recognizes that there is a litany of challenges with the publication process.

After completing a clinical study, the researcher's attention turns to writing a report of the trial and getting it published in a medical journal. Not all medical journals are equal and the most important research findings usually end up in the top U.S. and U.K. journals. The best journals publish a wide variety of articles covering molecular research, clinical practice developments, political issues, and ethical behavior. There are also excellent journals for every kind of medical specialty, from allergy to urology. Thus, researchers have a choice of a broad array of journals where they can submit their research papers. Frequently a medical journal is produced by a medical society. For instance *JAMA*, a highly regarded journal, is the property of the American Medical Association, but journals may also be owned by for-profit originations. The well-respected journal *Nature*, for example, is owned by the publishing house Macmillan Ltd.

Peer Review

Medical journals serve as a key link in the information chain that runs from basic research on medical treatments to their broad use by millions of patients. Quite simply, they act as the gatekeepers for the veracity and usefulness of medical science news. Editors of journals naturally want to publish only well-executed studies that are accurate, relevant and presented with clarity. To achieve these goals, the editors rely heavily on what is called peer review to ensure the quality of the research they publish. Peer review can be defined simply as the process by which journal editors solicit evaluations of submitted articles from outside experts who remain anonymous to the authors. The role of journals as the filter for scientific work dates to the 17th century in Great Britain, though the modern process of "blind" peer review is much more recent. Until the mid -20th century, many papers were approved solely by a journal's editors rather than by independent reviewers, and for some journals this is still the case. The explosion of scientific productivity after World War II strained the review process, significantly extending the lag time between submission and publication. More personnel were needed and peer review was the answer.

In time, peer review not only speeded up the editing process, it also strengthened the ability to identify incorrect or inadequate work and improve the accuracy and clarity of medical reports. In theory, it provides a rational, fair and objective way to assess scientific reports. Peer review, then, should weed out serious methodological and content errors, but that assumes there is an ample supply of experts in multiple fields to review the article. It's true that the goals of peer review are appealing and the system has a long proud history, but the system has its critics and there has been little research to prove that peer reviews achieve the purposes for which they were established.

In general, medical journals enjoy a high degree of respect for their selection and vetting process. But as in any media enterprise, there are critics as well. One of those critics was J. Kassirer, an insider – the former editor of a top medical journal, who wrote a critical review of his fellow journalists in the journal *Annals of Internal Medicine*. He cataloged the following flaws, which represent a broad array of issues that he found in too many published studies.

1. The use of intermediate endpoints rather than meaningful clinical outcomes
2. Results rendered meaningless because of small numbers of subjects
3. Strong conclusions based on findings that barely reached statistical significance
4. The use of placebo controls instead of insisting on active drug controls
5. Conducting unplanned analyses of variables based on the study results
6. The rejection of exploratory studies that provided useful information
7. Permitting authors to describe the value of their work rather than getting them to help readers to understand the weaknesses as well as the strengths of their studies

Indeed, it's not surprising that, in spite of good intentions, there are frequent errors in published research articles that have gone undetectable by peer reviewers. Obviously, such errors had to exist before the peer review process began. From the publisher's perspective, it often may not be possible to detect the errors based on what reviewers have to work with – a manuscript written by the researchers. The journal editor and the assigned peer review team, for instance, almost never have the individual case reports, the protocol, the record of decisions made before, during and after the trial was conducted. They receive a finished product. But that product may well lack the details on how it was assembled and produced in the first place.

An example of a flawed trial that made it into print is covered in a report published in *Circulation* by an NIH researcher G. May and his colleagues. The drug involved was Anturane, a medication approved by the FDA to treat gout, but early studies showed it also was an effective anti-clotting agent and that property could keep some patients from having a heart attack. It therefore made sense to conduct a study investigating the ability of Anturane to prevent cardiovascular deaths. The results, published in a leading journal, claimed that after using Anturane there was a 74 percent reduction in sudden death in patients who had suffered a heart attack.

However, unlike a medical journal, the FDA receives the raw data for a trial and when the FDA reviewed the data from the Anturane trial, it recognized that mistakes had been made on the way causes of death were classified. After correcting for this error and reanalyzing the data, the FDA determined that Anturane had no effect in reducing the rate of sudden death in recent heart attack victims. As this sorry example shows, articles on flawed studies can appear in distinguished peer reviewed journals because not enough information is available to either the editor or the peer reviewers.

Other problems such as authorship integrity, plague medical communications as well. A number of articles in medical journals, claiming to be written by the researcher who conducted the trial, are actually written by professional ghostwriters experienced in technical writing. These writers, whose names never appear in the report, are employed by the sponsor to make the report more appealing to readers. The opposite problem occurs as well, the name of highly respected co-author may be added, but the person may have played no role in the study and didn't know that his or her name had been added. Journal papers have had to be retracted once this masquerade was discovered.

Journal articles can also leave out information without providing a rational explanation for the omission. For example, a 2005 critique of published studies found that not all outcomes in clinical trials are reported. In this telling review, published in the *British Medical Journal*, it was found that some outcomes measured in a trial were simply omitted in an article because of the authors' decision that it lacked clinical importance or it failed to be statistically significant. As a result, the medical literature can represent a selective and biased subset of study outcomes and readers need to be aware of this possibility. Here's an example that further illustrates the problem. An analysis of study protocols, and the corresponding published report by five noted research methodologists, came out in a 2004 paper in *JAMA*. It showed that the reporting of trial outcomes were seriously incomplete. About 50 percent of efficacy outcomes and 65 percent of harms were incompletely reported. Furthermore, over 60 percent of trial reports had at least one primary outcome that was added, changed, or removed from the protocol. Obviously, the consequence of these acts may well lead to a serious bias in the overall study result reported in a journal article.

To overcome this problem, it has been argued that protocols should accompany the submission of a research report to a journal. Requiring authors to submit the trial protocol along with their manuscript is in effect at some of the major medical journals today (e.g. *British Medical Journal* and *Annals of Internal Medicine*). With concurrent submission of the protocol, editors do not have to chase after authors when they run into a potential problem because the manuscript indicates that protocol deviations may have occurred.

Gratefully, editors of leading journals are not at all complacent about the content of study reports. An attempt to have high standards for what should be covered in a clinical trial article led to the creation of publication guidelines and represented a major accomplishment in elevating the reporting of medical research. A group of scientists and editors developed the CONSORT (*Con*solidated *S*tandards *of R*eporting *T*rials) guidelines to improve the quality of clinical trial reports and their publication. These standards include a checklist and flow diagram that authors can use when writing up their results. Many leading medical journals have adopted the CONSORT standards since they facilitate the preparation of a clear and informed description of a clinical research project. Nevertheless, as valuable as standards are, they cannot overcome all the many issues associated with the quality of medical publications.

Statistical Review

Previous chapters emphasized the vital role statistics plays in medical research. The report on a clinical trial benefits from the presence of statistical expertise in the preparation, execution and write-up of a study. Nonetheless, how often statisticians participate in a clinical study is not known. An estimate of their rate of participation comes from a survey, by D. Altman and associates, who contacted the authors of clinical papers appearing in two of the leading medical research journals (the *Annals of Internal Medicine* in the U.S., the *British Medical Journal* in the U.K.). They asked the authors if they received assistance from a person with statistical expertise and the nature of any such contribution. They found that there was no statistical input in over one quarter of the papers. And in some of the papers that claimed there was statistical input, the assistance did not come from a professional statistician or epidemiologist.

The absence of sound statistical advice during a trial makes it more likely that there will be statistical errors in the manuscript submitted to a journal for publication. Unfortunately, the chance that statistical errors will be caught at the editorial review stage is problematic because, in spite of their importance, less than one in three medical journals does a statistical review. A related issue is to ask how many statistical errors get through the editorial and peer review system. The one study that looked for such errors appeared in *The Economist* in 2004. The examination was confined to two highly valued journals, both published in the U.K. They found that 38 percent of the papers in one journal and 25 percent in the other journal contained one or more statistical mistakes. Most of the errors were not likely to lead to grossly erroneous conclusions, but there were key mistakes that caused non-statistically significant conclusions to be incorrectly presented as significant ones. The editor of one of the journals subjected to the statistical critique noted that attempts to avoid numerical problems were handled by their routinely asking for the raw data, but the data were seldom received. On the other hand, a deputy editor of one of the journals also wondered whether it would be a good use of reviewers' time to scrutinize countless numbers and perform tedious calculations.

There have even been calls in the publication field for mandatory sharing of data to be a safeguard against fraud and the mishandling of patient information. In spite of a certain appeal for this approach, it has its negative aspects as well. As noted in previous chapters, there are so many subjective decisions in data analysis that sharing the study data from a trial could open up a Pandora's Box. Re-analyses of trials would become popular sport and few original conclusions would escape a "new" analysis that could easily reverse the initial findings.

The large number of statistical mistakes found in medical articles again suggests that statistical expertise may be missing or underutilized in too many medical experiments. It's entirely possible that research teams, that do not include a qualified statistician, allow the medical researchers (who may have only a shaky grasp of proper statistical techniques) too much leeway. No one knows how many medical findings claiming statistical significance have been wrong; the result of poor statistical technique. Since it is often felt that a key factor in the acceptance of an article for publication is a statistically significant result, there are clearly incentives to stretch the data and the analysis in order to declare there was a statistically significant finding.

The concern over an impartial statistical analysis has also motivated *JAMA* to add the condition to all industry-sponsored studies. *JAMA* will not accept a study for publication, if the data analysis was conducted only by statisticians employed by the company sponsoring the research, unless there is an additional independent analysis performed at an academic institution such as a medical school.

Publish or Perish

Researchers obviously want their study results to appear in a medical journal – the more prestigious the journal the better off the researcher. Publications add to their stature among their peers and are a requirement to get additional funding to do more research. Higher stature and remuneration from their institution are additional motivations to publish a lot. These incentives can lead to their writing articles that gloss over problems and exaggerate what was found. Outright lying and faking results also takes place and the forged manuscript can sneak past journal editors as well as those doing a peer review.

How quickly one can publish also becomes an issue for clinical researchers. Being first brings much acclaim, being second is far less rewarding. However, the chances of getting a reasonably correct answer in a medical study can fall in the rush to publish. Quality control steps may be sacrificed, the search for alternative explanations minimized and ambiguous information ignored in order to beat the competition with a significant result. As a result, contradictory information from subsequent studies on the same topic is commonplace.

There are hundreds of medical journals looking for articles and an estimated two million new research articles are published worldwide each year. However, there are contrasting forces in play when it comes to publishing so many research articles. On the one hand, researchers are encouraged to undertake multiple projects and publish their findings thereby expanding the scientific knowledge base in their field. Yet, the net result can be information overload with few in the field of medicine able to keep up with the ever-increasing volume of information that never seems to end. It is therefore, disappointing to realize that some researchers are urged to milk a single study for as many papers as possible. The practice results in a more impressive curriculum vitae, but the redundancy can fool others into thinking there's been replication of a finding and, as noted earlier, it can have a negative impact on a crucial meta analysis.

Absence of Reports

In December, 2003 clinical researchers held a meeting in Puerto Rico and FDA reviewers met in Washington DC to resolve a problem. The same question was probed by each group – does the use of antidepressants in children lead to an increased risk of suicide? The meeting in Puerto Rico included many of the researchers who had conducted studies on three extremely popular antidepressants.

However, this group faced a formidable problem – they did not have access to all the data they needed to cone to an informed conclusion. Because of confidentiality concerns, the drug companies that sponsored the trials refused to provide the requested data.

The suicide issue was first noted by British regulators who had earlier asked drug companies in their country for some of the unpublished data from the antidepressant trials they had conducted. In this case, the data the British authorities asked for was turned over to them. A review of that data suggested that a bizarre event could occur – antidepressants may prompt young people to attempt suicide. The possibility of suicide was not apparent from the published studies. It was only revealed in the unpublished studies. One drug, Paxil, seemed to be the most obvious offender. When the news media got hold of the story, the manufacturer of the drug, GlaxoSmithKline, was asked about the results from all their studies. They replied that all the results of their clinical trials had gone to the FDA, as required by law.

Paxil was originally approved for the treatment of depression in adults, but after securing approval, GlaxoSmithKline sponsored five trials of the drug in adolescents suffering from depression. By researching the drug in young people, the company hoped to extend the drug's use to this age group. In the process, they would also be entitled to a five-year patent extension for the drug because they had sponsored research in young subjects. Unfortunately, for the manufacturer only one of the five trials produced a good result for the drug. The investigators of the favorable trial published their results, but there was no publication of the any of the four failed trials.

As it turned out, not only did the unpublished trials fail to show any benefit for the drug in ameliorating depression in adolescents, they suggested that it might increase the risk of suicide. The FDA, which had all the Paxil data, now went to work establishing a regulatory position on Paxil. After completing their review, including the concern over teenage suicides, the agency recommended that Paxil not be used in children and adolescents for the treatment of serious depression. The FDA determined that each anti-depressant manufacturer should also include a warning statement that recommended close observation of adult and pediatric patients treated with these agents for "possible worsening of depression or suicidality". Then things got even worse for GlaxoSmithKline – in 2004, the Attorney General of New York filed a lawsuit against the drug maker.

The NY lawsuit claimed that the manufacturer engaged in fraud by failing to tell doctors that some studies of Paxil showed that it did not work in adolescents and might even lead to suicide. Instead of warning doctors, the lawsuit claimed that the company promoted the use of Paxil in youngsters. The Attorney General argued that the company was making selective disclosures of information and did not give doctors all the evidence available. Relying on FDA rules, that allow the results they receive about clinical trials for new drugs or indications to be treated as confidential on the ground that it is proprietary company information, the company disputed the charge. Therefore, GlaxoSmithKline took the position that they had acted responsibly in conducting and distributing the data from their pediatric studies.

The criticism of the company focused on two particular studies, which were used to show the inconsistency in the company's behavior. Both studies were multicenter trials and were very similar except that one was conducted in the U.S. (study 329) and the other in countries outside the U.S. (study 377). Study 329, the positive trial that showed that Paxil was effective in adolescents with depression, was completed first. Its results were presented beginning in 1998 at several medical meetings. The study was published in 2001. In the case of Study 377, the one with negative findings, there was no publication – not even a press release. However, one of the investigators, a Canadian who conducted one of the segments that made up the multicenter trial, expressed a desire to report the findings from study 377. He felt that even though the results were negative, they could reveal trial design flaws and that revelation could help others design better antidepressant trials in adolescents. The Canadian researcher presented his study results at a scientific meeting, taking this action after the manufacturer told him that they did not intend to publish the results of the multicenter study.

Two and a half months after the lawsuit charging fraud was filed, GlaxoSmithKline settled. The terms of the settlement required the company to place negative data on the safety and effectiveness of its drugs in a registry that could be accessed at its web site. The company would also update the information as new data became available, and keep it available for at least 10 years. The Attorney General who brought the lawsuit noted that the settlement sent a signal to the other pharmaceutical manufacturers that there now was a new standard with regard to disclosure of clinical studies.

This case illustrates a major problem in medical research publication: results of negative clinical trials sponsored by drug manufacturers are not widely published. As a result, the medical profession can remain ignorant of safety and efficacy problems with a drug. Experts have long faulted the tendency in the industry to publish mainly positive clinical trials, arguing that this distorts the knowledge base of medicine. The term "publication bias" is used for this method of preferential selection. Research is more likely to be published if it has a positive finding supported by statistical significance. Reporting that (1) one drug is better than another, or (2) that one treatment produces fewer side effects than another, or (3) that one patient group has a better prognosis following treatment than another seems to be more interesting than research that finds no significant treatment differences.

In addition, it's worth repeating that the drive to reach a statically significant result is a quest industry and academic researchers can't resist. Thus, there is an incentive to tweak the data so that the all-important "statistically significant" label can be stamped on their findings. In fact, there are software packages for "data mining" that rumble through databases looking for every possible kind of relationship that has "statistical significance". That approach may be great for business organizations that collect masses of data and want to see what kind of relationships exist that may help their marketing approach. But for clinical research, data mining can be terribly misused. Clinical research studies are based on a single a priori hypothesis and data mining is an after-the-fact "discovery" which comes about after testing a vast number of possible relationships. Any remarkable result, positive or negative, is essentially accidental. In clinical trials to claim statistical significance for a relationship found through data mining is ridiculous. At best, data mining results can suggest hypotheses that need further study, but they should never sneak into a report as an "extraordinary" finding.

From a commercial standpoint, it's useful to examine the rationale by pharmaceutical companies to withhold full disclosure of clinical research. Certainly, they are the ones with a lot to lose from a negative study about one of their products. Drug companies, however, have other explanations as well. They say that because they pay for a trial, they own the data and that their concern about data confidentiality is not intended to suppress possibly negative trial findings, but to make sure that data is properly analyzed before it is released. However, when this rationale is applied to a medical school that has researched one of their drugs, it is not particularly convincing, Medical schools run many clinical trials for pharmaceutical companies and the quality of their research is highly regarded as is their competency to properly analyze data. Yet the results of their studies may never appear in print because of the control exerted by drug makers. The reason for the omission lies in the data disclosure clauses contained in the pharmaceutical company contracts that medical school researchers sign. Those contracts generally forbid them to publish data without the company's permission. It is generally believed that unless medical schools take tough stands on issues like confidentiality and publication rights, their ability to publish will continue to be restricted. Leading academic research centers with a lot of clout and can get around this issue and eliminate such clauses, especially when they are the only ones conducting a study. But medical school researchers have less ability to set terms for a multicenter trial that is run at many academic and private testing centers. They may be able to publish the results from their center, but that's only one piece in a large puzzle and can be misleading.

A Clinical Trial Registry

In response to growing criticism about unpublished research, the American Medical Association urged the federal government to set up a public registry of all trial results. The editors of some of the world's most prestigious medical journals joined the crusade and want to require drug companies to register their trials publicly as a prerequisite to publication. The World Health Organization became involved in the effort in 2004, calling for the registration of all clinical trials to increase the public trust in medical research. Leading drug companies such as Eli Lilly and Schering-Plough also supported the proposal to create a public database that would include the results of all drug trials. The announcement of the creation of the clinical trial registry was made on International Clinical Trials Day, 2006 – a day devoted to raising awareness about the methods and challenges of medical research.

While the announcement was met with general approval, there still remained the issue of whether the registration of trial data would be mandatory or voluntary. Proponents said a mandatory program would eliminate the harm done by concealing negative data and provide researchers, physicians and the public, information they need.

The trade association for pharmaceutical companies, however, took a more conservative stand and supported a voluntary program. Supporters of voluntary registration pointed out that mandatory registration could reveal information that manufacturers consider proprietary, such as the results of small or exploratory studies and that could expose their research strategies and progress to competitors.

Perhaps the major roadblock to a mandatory program was that it would require Congressional action and whether that would happen depended on the unpredictability of political action. The answer came in 2007 when Congress passed and President George Bush signed the FDA Revitalization Act. A provision in the new law required the registration of all but early exploratory clinical trials to be placed in a public database.

The importance of a drug registry played a leading role in one of biggest uproars over unsafe drugs that also occurred in 2007. In this brouhaha, the manufacturer was again GlaxoSmithKline and their drug, Avandia used to treat diabetics, came under attack in 2007 because of a meta analysis that reported an increased risk of heart attacks with the drug. The analysts from the highly regarded Cleveland Clinic published their findings in the *New England Journal of Medicine*. They used as their data source, trial results that were on the GlaxoSmithKline web site listing results from clinical trials with their drugs. The database used by the Cleveland Clinic analysts contained 42 studies and about 16,000 patients on Avandia plus an additional 12,000 patients who made up the control group. In their paper, the Cleveland Clinic author's noted that their approach had limitations because it had been necessary to rely on summary data rather than patient-specific information. They also acknowledged that there were weaknesses in a meta analysis, but in spite of these caveats, they still believed there was evidence of a potential serious risk of heart attacks with Avandia.

After the meta analysis by the Cleveland Clinic researchers appeared, there were Congressional hearings, accusations that the FDA had again failed to do its job, and charges that the manufacturer knew years ago of the heart attack risk, but did too little about it. GlaxoSmithKline reputed the charges and argued that it would be a big mistake if the FDA acted against Avandia prematurely. The company had a major trial going on that was looking into the heart related risks with Avandia and until those data were available, it would be unwise to remove the drug from the market. An interim analysis of the data from that study was performed, published in the *New England Journal of Medicine* and concluded that the findings were inconclusive. This was not unexpected since the trial was only about half completed. Nevertheless, critics of Avandia pointed out that the interim analysis showed the rate of heart attacks were higher on Avandia. However, they conceded that the rate was not as high as that found in the Cleveland Clinic analysis.

That was not the end of the story. In August, 2007 a paper in the *Annals of Internal Medicine* described a re-analysis of the data used in the Cleveland Clinic analysis and it should come as no surprise that the new analysis, which employed different meta analysis options, had come to a different conclusion. By choosing this alternative approach, the second group of analysts concluded that a greater heart attack risk with Avandia was uncertain and that neither an increased nor a decreased risk could be established.

In the end GlaxoSmithKline again escaped the axe. An FDA advisory committee recommended that Avandia remain on the market, but with stricter label warnings. In addition the company also had to institute an extensive educational effort regarding the proper use of Avandia and the committee also requested further studies because none of the ongoing clinical trials was likely to provide a clear answer concerning the absolute heart risk for the drug.

Amending the System

For many, the system for the publication of clinical trial results is broken. Problems with peer review, the need to publish clinical trial findings fast and frequently on the one hand and not to publish them at all on the other, are symptoms of a ailing system. However, it would be terrible unfair to place the blame for the current situation primarily on the editors of journals. They pretty well inherited a flawed process and, in fact, have been in the vanguard promoting change. Nevertheless, editors and editorial boards are inclined to make modifications incrementally and that will take a lot of time and may not be enough in the end. Consequently, extraordinary changes may be the answer. For example, an innovative plan has been developed by faculty members of the London School of Hygiene and Tropical Medicine that would radically change the current system.

They propose that trial organizers post on the web, a review of the existing evidence about an experimental treatment they plan to study including its effectiveness and research needs in the future. A new trial would be registered and its protocol would appear on the web site, as well as the names of the research team members and their roles. The protocol would need to specify any planned subgroup analyses, stopping rules etc. Any interested party could add their comments about the information (e.g. completeness of the evidence, reliability of the research methods, etc.).

The proposed statistical analysis would be explained and when data collection was over, the full dataset would be added to the site. Description of the methods to avoid data fabrication and falsification would also be included. In addition, when data collection was over, the entire dataset would be uploaded and the statistical analyses presented. There would be no investigator commentary permitted. However, at a designated time the research team would be expected to prepare an updated review of the evidence concerning the treatment.

The London proposal offers some appealing features such as the emphasis on the totality of the evidence about a treatment rather than a focus on a single trial. There are, in addition, deterrents to unreported protocol changes and unwarranted statistical manipulations. Furthermore, in this plan there would be better control over the issues of multiple reports and no reports.

However, the advantage of having a great deal of input also means lots of opportunities for biased opinions, masquerading as honest critiques, to get equal attention in an arena without referees. In an entrepreneurship society, other avenues to present medical research studies could result in more chaotic and unfair systems. Nevertheless, what is needed, in addition to better-quality medical research, are new ideas and proposals to increase the timeliness, thoroughness and accuracy of medical findings so in the end researchers, public health officials, practicing physicians and their patients have the right information so they can make more informed medical decisions.

Chapter 19
The Public Forum – Sharing the News with the Public

Abstract What the public learns about medical research usually comes from newspapers, television, magazines and the Internet. This requires a journalist to translate a medical report into a newsworthy story, but the media and medical research professions each have a distinct method of operation, different standards and certainly different goals so that the communication between these two bodies can lead to incomplete and misleading articles. The media largely gets its information from press releases prepared by the organization that sponsored the medical research study and that can cause a lack of objectivity. Another source of information is a scientific conference where researchers present new work to colleagues, but the papers presented are usually a work-in-progress and based on exploratory research without the safeguards of peer review or thorough analysis. The way data are presented can influence a person's interpretation of the significance of a story and too often only the more sensational statistics makes it into print. Direct-to-consumer advertising by the drug industry is also an issue and the strong differences of opinion that exist are reviewed.

Keywords Absolute difference · direct-to-consumer advertising · medical reporting · press release · scientific meeting · relative difference

> We've come to a point where, unless we can communicate to people outside of medicine, we can't achieve a lot of our goals. (D. Satcher, US Surgeon General)

The public has a voracious appetite for medical news. They're aroused by startling headlines such as "Study: No Heart Damage from Diet Drug," and "New Therapy Builds Bone Without Unpleasant Side Effects". Health stories are regularly found on page 1 of newspapers and appear as daily segments on prime-time television newscasts. The amount of medical news that fills the headlines seem to increase dramatically every year and in the process, it plays an increasingly vital role in society. However, the media and medical research each have a distinct method of operation, different standards and certainly different goals. To be sure, the interaction between these two institutions can be awkward and distressing. A good illustration of the conflict between the two fields is how the results of a clinical trial finding

R.R. Gauch, *It's Great! Oops, No It Isn't*,   185
© Springer Science+Business Media B.V. 2009

should be interpreted. The results of medical studies, which invariably use statistical testing, give results that are based on probabilities (not certainties). However, to appeal to the public, reporters are trained to use commanding headlines and unambiguous descriptions rather than qualified conditional statements and conclusions. In the media world, the best story is one that is black and white, clear-cut and simple, but these are attributes that medical research can't posses.

Press Releases

The public and many physicians often first learn about new medical research through the news media. In turn, the media largely gets its information from press releases. The title of a scientific article, not to mention the text, are usually far too complex for the common reader. As a case in point, how many people would be interested in reading the article "Inducible nitric oxide mediates systemic micro-vascular leak following acid aspiration and mechanical ventilation"? The value of a press release is that it simplifies the information and transforms it into information that is newsworthy. Press releases, however, are usually prepared by the very organization that sponsored a successfully completed study and, as would be expected, that can cause a problem in objectivity. Often the sponsor is a pharmaceutical company, but press releases are also written by medical journals and other sponsors such as medical schools and governmental agencies. Whatever the source, press releases it's been argued often exaggerate the significance of the research findings, fail to highlight important caveats and overlook conflicts of interest.

One investigation of medical journal press releases, by physicians at the Dartmouth Medical School, concluded that press releases did not routinely highlight study limitations. Furthermore, the article, published in *JAMA* in 2002, noted that study findings could be presented in a manner that elevates the perceived importance of the research results. This conclusion is ironic because the editorial staff, and the process used to review manuscripts prior to publication, are preoccupied with making sure the articles fairly represent study findings; no exaggeration tolerated. Editors try to ensure that the articles they publish acknowledge important limitations of a study. Still, over 100 releases from medical journals were examined in the above mentioned study and less than one quarter of the releases noted study limitations. Industry funding of the trials was noted in less than a quarter of the releases as well. Since many believe that the sponsor who provides the money for a trial can affect nearly every aspect of the research, the identity of the sponsor is important to understanding the context of the findings and should be included in any press release and resulting news article.

Scientific Meetings

A scientific conference is intended to provide a forum for researchers to present new work to colleagues. Conferences provide a platform for researchers to share information and learn about each other's projects through the presentation of research papers, long before the results will ever appear in print. Science reporters attend scientific meetings looking for noteworthy stories though the material presented may be preliminary and may not yet have gone through a true peer review process. Frequently, what is presented is a work in progress and many projects fail to live up to their early promise.

Despite this limitation, scientific meetings can be used as a public relations opportunity by researchers or sponsors to court the media present. Thus, premature or not, investigators who make presentations and their institutions may become headline news and receive priceless publicity. Unfortunately, press coverage at this early stage clearly presents very real risks, leaving the public with the false impression that the data are in fact fully verified, the methods valid, and the findings widely accepted.

No question, the general public has a strong desire to know about the latest developments in science and medicine, and a scientific meeting holds the promise of dramatic stories about new cures, discoveries, and breakthroughs. Without a doubt, the early results from a clinical trial that are presented at a scientific meeting can receive substantial attention in the news media. But premature dissemination of medical research in the media often brings findings to the public before the validity and importance of the work have been established in the scientific community. Adding to this concern, the abstracts receiving media attention may involve studies that have weak designs, are small, and based on animal or laboratory rather than human subjects. These distinctions may or may not be made clear in media articles touting the latest medical "breakthrough".

There are numerous examples of early promising results reported in the press as significant that ended on the trash heap of clinical research. One that illustrates that the problem can occur when too much credence is directed at a preliminary finding, is described by Schwartz and others in *JAMA*. A clinical study, reported on at a 1998 meeting of a major medical society, the American Society of Clinical Oncology contained sensational news. Stories appeared in many publications including a front-page report in the *New York Times*. The media described the trial as the first to show that screening reduced prostate cancer deaths. However, after the research was completed and analyzed, and the full set of results published, the trial was discredited for serious errors in methodology.

The reverse can happen as well – condemning a drug before all the facts are in. Concern about the drug naproxen, the active ingredient in the popular pain reliever Aleve, produced the following headlines:

"Aleve Ingredient Joins Painkillers Linked to Risks" the *Washington Post*;
"Another Painkiller Tied to Heart Attack Risk" the *Boston Globe*
and
"Study Links a Fourth Painkiller to an Increase in Heart Problems" the *New York Times*.

In this case the news media alerted the public to the "risk" before the risk was determined to be real. Reporters want stories that attract readers because the news is startling and useful. Scientists are, or at least they should be, more cautious. In the Aleve story, the two approaches collided. The researchers of the study that prompted the newspaper headlines had reported preliminary figures. They did not know whether these figures represented actual risks, or whether they were just the result of coincidence. In any study, there is a possibility that an outcome, such as a higher heart attack rate, occurs randomly. This is why scientists must first determine whether the results are statistically significant. In this instance that determination hadn't been made.

Media Coverage

Similarly, journalists who use articles published in medical journals as their source material may not recognize that the scientific report is based on exploratory research and that its limitations are inadequately described in the medical article. As already noted, case-control and cohort studies are not equipped to demonstrate that a treatment causes a specific outcome. They show there is an association, but media accounts are likely to confuse causation with association and thereby misinform the public. Due to deadline pressures, journalists are often constrained to fully evaluate the quality of evidence presented in a medical article or recognize the significance of a medical report. For instance, prior to the publication that brought down hormone treatment for postmenopausal women, there were too few stories directed at the general public about the negative effects of HRT. Had there been more comprehensive press coverage, maybe the shock that HRT was harmful could have been softened.

Journalists are keen to get their stories right and have a strong sense of responsibility about reporting medical research accurately. They can routinely translate medical jargon into readable news, but reporters are less able to report the credibility or importance of the research. They rely heavily on the journal peer review process and the opinions of medical experts they may contact to compensate for these shortcomings.

There are a number of outstanding reporters at major media organizations who do a responsible job of reporting medical news in a reasonably balanced fashion. However, they can only work with the material they are given and too often the information they receive directly from the researcher of the sponsoring organization may be biased. To obtain better objectivity, a journalist may turn to an independent source to comment on the material the journalist has gathered and incorporate those views into the story. A good plan, but their independent expert may have received financial aid from the sponsor or have a professional connection with the researchers that are unbeknownst to the journalist. Under those circumstances, even the best reporter may not get the truly independent opinion he or she sought.

It is also true that there is tension between writing responsibly and producing articles considered newsworthy. Faced with a strict word limit, journalists may find it impossible to include all the caveats and qualifying statements that need to be included in research reports. In the end the public can get an exceedingly optimistic impression of a medical finding. Conversely, if it's bad news they can come away with an overly pessimistic concept of the situation. An apt illustration comes from a 2000 paper that appeared in the *New England Journal of Medicine*. The ABC, NBC, and CBS television networks included a broadcast about a conference in which the results of a RABCOT study for a drug to counter osteoporosis were presented. All three stories gave only the relative reduction in risk, stating that the new drug could reduce the incidence of hip fractures by 50 percent. One commentator described these results as "almost miraculous." None of the stories cited actual event rates in treated patients (1 percent) and untreated patients (2 percent). Only one network mentioned gastrointestinal distress as a potential adverse effect from drug usage and no story disclosed that the study investigator being interviewed had received funding for the study from the drug manufacturer.

I should re-emphasize that when reading news stories it is essential to know who sponsored a study. It's not surprising that some research has indicated that studies sponsored by industry are more likely to have a positive outcome in favor of the experimental drug, which is the sponsor's drug. Certainly, more and more research is funded by private industry, nevertheless, just because a pharmaceutical company sponsored a study, it doesn't mean the study is biased. For example, in the hormone replacement episode, the maker of the drug (Wyeth) sponsored the critical trial that showed that their drug was associated with more rather than fewer deaths.

The 2000 *New England Journal of Medicine* investigation cited above also uncovered other extraordinary findings. The authors sought to determine how well the benefits and risks of medications were covered in the news media and they to do that studied news stories about three medications used for the prevention of common maladies such as cardiovascular disease. They examined whether benefits were stated in a meaningful manner and potential harms were identified. They also noted whether the cost of the treatment, and any connections between the researchers and industry, were included in news stories. The authors collected data on over 200 newspaper and television stories and discovered that more than 50 percent of the stories did not include information about potential harms. They found that 70 percent of stories made no mention of cost and a majority of the stories citing a study group or an expert with a link to the drug manufacturer failed to mention that link.

Their research also revealed another troubling tendency. They established a standard for a satisfactory explanation of drug benefits which required the inclusion of both relative and absolute benefits. As the following example shows, it matters greatly what statistic is used. If the mortality rate falls from 4 to 3 percent the absolute difference is 1 percent. But, the relative difference is a whopping 25 percent and seems so much more impressive. The examination of media stories on this issued found that only 15 percent of the stories included both kinds of changes. Relative benefits were presented in over 80 percent of the stories and the authors of the study emphasized that the exclusive use of this presentation method only tends to exaggerate the expectation of doctors and patients.

It is obvious that the way data are presented can influence a person's interpretation of what the data mean. Here's another short illustration of that principle. Imagine the outbreak of an unusual disease that has the potential to kill many people. You are given the result for two treatments used to treat the disease and you must choose which treatment is better. You are told that treatment A can be given to 600 patients and it is certain that it will save exactly 200 lives – no more, no less. You are also told that treatment B is available and it has two possible outcomes. In outcome 1 there is a one-third chance of saving 600 lives. In outcome 2 there is a two thirds probability of saving no lives. If offered this choice which treatment would you choose – A or B?

Most people prefer treatment A, but in actuality treatment A and B are equal. Treatment A will clearly save 200 of the 600 lives – that's a given. What will happen with treatment B is a bit more complex, but the average number of lives that would be saved is also 200. You need to multiply the 600 lives by the outcome's probability and add the results for options 1 and 2 together. In option 1 you multiply the 600 by 1/3 and get 200. For option B you multiply 600 by 0 (no lives will be saved) and you get 0. The sum is 200 lives saved. The 200 saved lives are certain with treatment A. With treatment B there is uncertainty, but on average you also end up with saving 200 lives. Both treatments will, in the end, save the same number of lives.

Advertisements

In 1985 the FDA removed a moratorium on prescription-drug advertisements directed at the public. Prior to this change, drug advertisements could only be aimed at the medical profession. Now drug advertisements could be made to the public, but they had to contain information relating to side effects, contraindications, and effectiveness of a drug. Drugs are deemed to be misbranded if their advertising is judged false or misleading, and the FDA provides pharmaceutical companies guidelines that manufacturers must follow in order to market their products directly to consumers. However, there's a glitch because the FDA does not have the authority to pre-screen advertising messages that drug companies create. They can only stop an ad after the fact. By then, an advertisement that is determined to be misleading or providing false information, could be seen by millions of people. The agency does request companies to submit their advertisements voluntarily before they are run so the agency can determine if they are acceptable, but note that's a request, not a requirement.

There are a number of reasons that support advertising directly to the public. Ads help to create a highly competitive marketplace and that environment can lead to price breaks for the consumer. Proponents of consumer advertising also believe that there is an educational value in having ads seen by consumers, and feel that this practice can improve the patient- physician relationship by causing a discussion about treatment options for the patient. It may even allow consumers to have a more direct role in deciding which treatment regimens are best for them, and patient compliance in taking a medication might also increase because people will feel they have a more direct stake in the treatment decisions. In addition, advertising directly to consumers could prompt people to seek medical care whom otherwise might not be aware that they suffer from a disease for which effective treatment exists.

Critics of consumer ads argue that the marketing programs used are often misleading by failing to adequately communicate risk information in the advertisement. They say that if a patient learns about possible treatments through ads, the patient-physician relationships can be undermined. Patients may attempt to either self-medicate, or dictate to their doctors the specific treatments they want to take. Opponents also fear that direct-to-consumer advertising may lead to excessive demands on physicians, over-medication, and drug abuse as patients demand a remedy for every symptom that ails them. Additional concerns include ads that may not be written in layman's terms and thereby confuse patients. Patients may be duped into believing that a minor difference in drugs represents a major therapeutic advance. Another problem is that pharmaceutical companies may increase drug prices to recoup the costs of expensive promotional campaigns.

When it comes to medical research findings, getting the news right is probably the greatest challenge healthcare reporters' face. U.S. newspapers, TV stations and magazines are a pervasive force that can profoundly influence our beliefs, attitudes, expectations and behavior when it comes to healthcare. Studies have shown that adults obtain much of their health information from these sources. Moreover, research in health communications, demonstrates that the mass media may be more important than interpersonal communication in increasing awareness and knowledge of health issues. Even fictitious TV, starting with Dr. Kildare in the early 1960s to the current hit ER, can affect people's understanding of and belief in medical treatments.

Another widely used medium, the Internet, allows unlimited access to medical news and can provide around-the-clock medical advice and recommendations. Just about every print and TV organization maintains a world wide web site. Hence the concerns expressed about the media in general, apply to their Internet sites as well. Sometimes it is difficult to recognize whether the health information on a site represents an advocacy or commercial position. This means, for individuals searching the web to gain advice on specific diseases and treatments, that the quality of the available online information can be questionable or even erroneous. This may explain why articles in medical journals, that assessed the quality of information available on the Internet, generally find it biased and of poor quality.

As illustrated in this chapter, reporting scientific news is a tough job and medical journalists must both understand and interpret very detailed, technical and sometimes jargon-laden information in order to transform it into interesting reports that are comprehensible to consumers. Errors in this conversion only compound and exacerbate the mistakes that already occurred in the medical research publication phase.

Although the medical profession is quick to fault journalists for unbalanced and misleading news stories, they too bear some of the responsibility. Instead of viewing journalists as inept and preoccupied with sensationalizing health news, medical researchers need to play a more collaborative role. These specialists should work with journalists and assume some of the responsibility for the production of a fair and accurate news story. Through collaboration, the tendency to exaggerate findings, overstate benefits and make inappropriate generalizations can be held in check.

Chapter 20
Product Development – Getting Discoveries to the Market

Abstract The odyssey that drugs travel as they work their way through the development maze on their way to the marketplace is reviewed beginning with the search for a new drug in the laboratory of a company, government or university. The next step, involving the use of animals to screen potentially useful drugs, has a clear-cut advantages over conducting studies in humans because the control and test groups can be almost identical and the test conditions tightly controlled. However, in spite of the advantages differences in the biology of humans compared to other animals may result in different effective doses and disease susceptibility. Overly cautious governmental reaction to negative animal studies is exhibited by rescinding the charge that saccharin caused cancer in laboratory animals. After animal testing the next stage involves human studies which begins with the filing of an Investigational New Drug application and culminates, hopefully, with a Food and Drug Administration marketing approval. The drugs that make it are presumed to be safe and effective, but this cannot be guaranteed because the standards of "proof:" simply cannot identify all the vulnerabilities that permeate clinical research studies.

Keywords Animal studies · drug efficacy · drug safety · new drug application approval · saccharin

This chapter reviews the odyssey that medical discoveries travel as they work their way through the development maze on their way to the marketplace. The steps are similar whether the product comes from the pharmaceutical, biotechnology or medical device industry. Let's consider the hurdles a new drug must overcome as it attempts to receive an FDA marketing approval. Getting over all the hazardous and challenging hurdles of the development process can only be achieved by an exceptional drug, but there is still no guarantee that it will live up to the developers expectations and hopes.

The search for a new drug begins in the laboratory of a company, government or university, with chemists looking for and designing chemical substances that can be developed into safe and effective medicines. After synthesizing and purifying the substance it moves ahead to pre-clinical testing. At this stage studies are conducted in test tubes and animals to see how the compound might affect the human body. On average, out of every 5,000 new compounds identified during the discovery process, only five end up being tested in humans. The flunkout rate during animal testing is high, but it doesn't guarantee that all drugs that make it through and move on to human testing are the best choices, nor does it mean that the preparations that fail are always the inferior ones. An examination of the animal testing process reveals why this is so.

Animals Testing

It should be obvious that animal testing has some clear-cut advantages over conducting studies in humans. In an animal study the control group and the test groups can be almost identical and the test conditions can be tightly controlled. Dosing amounts and schedules can be imposed without fear that the animals will not comply. They can be exposed to painful procedures without the risk of having them quit the study. Animal research can also use germ-free animals with better supervision and control compared to studies conducted in humans.

Animal studies are used not only in the testing of new drugs, but they are also useful for development of new surgical techniques (e.g. organ transplants) and in nutritional research. Animals are especially valuable in research involving diseases in which there is a deterioration of the body such as arthritis or heart disease. Examples of animal diseases that are quite similar to commonly occurring human diseases include emphysema in the horse; leukemia in cats; muscular dystrophy in chickens; hardening of the arteries in pigs; gastric ulcers in swine; diabetes in hamsters and hepatitis in dogs.

Selective breeding can produce a superb specimen for use in animal studies. Animals that possess a particular trait can be mated and this process repeated for many generations. Over time, a strain eventually emerges with a very unique, but well-entrenched trait. This approach has been used to produce alcohol-preferring strains of rats and mice that can be used to study alcohol addiction.

Animal research can also investigate areas that are totally impossible to do in human investigations. A wide range of doses can be administered – and especially valuable are tests using extremely high doses because they can expose the potential harm a drug could cause. After drug administration, animals may be sacrificed and the drug's effect on the animal's tissues and organs examined. Did the kidneys show signs of damage? How much drug ended up in the brain?

In spite of the advantages of using animals in research, there are significant problems as well. There is a major controversy over whether animal experimentation is even humane or not. But for our purpose (understanding research methodology) it will not be necessary to get involved in that issue, although it certainly raises important ethical questions. We will have to be content knowing that there are a growing number of regulations on the care of animals and standard training necessary for personnel involved in animal research.

To begin with, the biology of humans and other animals may be similar, but there can be crucial differences when it comes to a drug's effect on critical elements such as the effective dose, the tolerable dose, disease susceptibility, life span and predisposition to withstand or succumb to different types of adversity. Although researchers can push dosing limits much further in animals compared to humans, an aggressive trial in animals may lead to a misleading conclusion. As an illustration, when animals are subjected to massive doses in a short period of time, there may be no chance for their body to repair damaged cells before they become cancerous. This phenomenon leads to a charge that the drug is a carcinogenetic agent, but that finding would only be true when there is an aggressive dosing schedule, which would never be applicable to humans.

For many diseases there is no useful animal model. For example, a common problem with many drugs is their harmful effect on the liver. The way the human liver functions is exceedingly complex. A drug's effect on the liver is dependent on numerous enzymes, co-factors, and other elements (e.g. the environment). When investigators sought animal models to estimate how drugs would affect the liver, they encountered appreciable differences between rodents and humans.

Governmental reaction to negative animal studies can be overly cautious. For instance, studies published as far back as the 1950s reported that saccharin, the popular sugar substitute, caused cancer in laboratory animals. However, it took a late 1970 pivotal Canadian study in rats to arouse governmental concern. The Canadian study showed high doses of saccharin caused cancer in rats and prompted both the United States and Canada authorities to caution the public about the use of saccharin. In the U.S., labels were required on foods containing saccharin advising consumers that saccharin caused cancer in laboratory animals. Today the consensus among most of the scientific community is that saccharin is not a risk to humans. The way the rats developed their cancer was not possible in humans. In addition the incriminating rat study used very high-doses of saccharin – in humans they were the equivalent of hundreds of cans of diet soft drinks per day for a lifetime. When it was found that the mechanism that induced cancer in rats was not applicable to humans, saccharin was finally removed from the government's list of possible carcinogens, but it took 25 years for that to happen.

In the chapter on usefulness, we worried about how comparable a study done in humans with a narrow set of demographic characteristics (e.g. middle-aged males with a severe illness) would do in predicting what would happen in a broader human population. But when it comes to transferring results from animal studies to man, the research community seems to be far less concerned. Fortunately there are scientists who are skeptical about applying rat and other animal studies to humans. They point out that even if humans and rats once had a common ancestor, the two species today are just so different that it seems ridiculous to extrapolate the experimental results with rats to man. To some, the use of research findings from animals appears to be out of control – it lacks common sense.

An excellent example of what can go wrong is represented by a study reported in 2001 in the journal *Stroke*. Because clinical trials performed with nimodipine did not demonstrate a beneficial effect on outcome following a stroke, researchers wanted to determine whether the evidence from nimodipine animal experiments supported the use of the drug in clinical trials. The condition treated was extremely important – reducing the extent of brain damage in people who had a stroke. In exploring the animal evidence, the authors concluded that their review did not show convincing evidence to substantiate the decision to perform trials with nimodipine in large numbers of patients.

Unfortunately, effective drugs can also be left behind because they did not perform well in the animal screening tests used to evaluate prospective drugs. Their efficacy is missed because the mechanism of action of a drug in animals is simply too different from that in man. Drugs that fail the efficacy screening tests never get a chance to demonstrate their value in human clinical trials. Good drugs may also be rejected from further study because of harmful toxicity results in animal trials that would not be a problem in humans. A good example of this phenomenon is probably aspirin, which if it were an experimental drug today, would be found to be too toxic for human research based on animal experiments. Aspirin can cause gastric problems in humans, but they are manageable and its many advantages far outweigh its risks. However, the rate of bleeding and ulcer development in animals is so high that it would rule out aspirin as a drug worthy of human experimentation.

In general the best animal models for man are primates, such as the monkey. It should be noted, however, that although monkeys are more similar to man regarding certain functions, they might be no better or no worse than other species for other functions. But we are awed when we learn that primates share up to 99 percent of their DNA with humans. Jane Goodall's experiences have impressed millions by the human-like behavior gorillas display. All this surely means laboratory experiments on primates are reliable indicators of what will happen in humans. Unfortunately, the track record using primates as a screen for human drug safety is not always that great.

Indeed, primate research has gotten it wrong when it comes to predicting dangerous side effects of medications. Aspirin produces birth defects in primates, but not humans. It's just the other way around with Thalidomide, the drug that sparked major drug legislation in 1963. An arthritis medication (Flosint) was well-tolerated by monkeys, but in humans it caused deaths. A medication for heart failure (Amrinone) was tested on numerous primates and looked fine. But when administered to humans some hemorrhaged because their blood couldn't clot properly.

These examples indicate that we should not naively believe primate research will always be comparable to human research. Yes, we are impressed when we're told that there's only a 1 percent difference in DNA. But what a difference that 1 percent makes.

Human Testing

In spite of its limitations, many potentially useful drugs survive the animal research process and enter the next stage which involves human studies. Before starting studies on people, all drug sponsors must first file an Investigational New Drug application (IND). The IND allows tests in humans and becomes effective if the FDA does not disapprove it within 30 days. The IND contains the chemical structure of the compound; how it is thought to work in the body, any toxic effects found in the animal studies and how the compound is manufactured.

The IND also includes results of previous animal experiments and plans for future human studies (e.g., how, where and by whom will the first human studies be conducted). In addition, the protocol for all human trials must be reviewed and approved by an Institutional Review Board (IRB) where the studies will be conducted. Progress reports on clinical trials must also be submitted at least annually to the FDA.

The clinical testing of a drug is then done in three phases.

Phase I

Phase I studies are primarily concerned with assessing the drug's safety. This initial phase of testing in humans is done in a small number of healthy volunteers (e.g. 20– 100) who are usually paid for participating in the research. Studies are designed to determine what happens to the drug in the human body – how it is absorbed, metabolized and excreted. A Phase I study will also investigate side effects that occur as dosage levels are increased. A trial in this initial phase of testing typically can take several months or more. There are a number of Phase I studies required so a drug will spend about a year in this phase. About 70 percent of experimental drugs pass this initial testing period.

Phase II

Once shown to be relatively safe, a drug must then be tested for efficacy. This is the second phase of testing in human beings and it lasts for several months to two or more years. Several hundred patients may participate in these trials. Some, but not all, Phase II studies are RABCOT trials. These studies provide additional comparative information about the relative safety of the new drug and begin the assessment of its effectiveness. About one-third of experimental drugs successfully complete Phase II.

Phase III

In a Phase III study, a drug is tested in several hundred to thousands of patients. This large-scale testing provides a greater level of understanding concerning the drug's effectiveness, benefits and a range of possible adverse reactions. Most all of the Phase III studies are RABCOT trials. The length of Phase III studies depend on the condition being investigated, but can typically last several years. On average, around 70 percent of drugs that enter this phase make it to the end.

If the Phase III studies show the drug is relatively safe and effective, the drug's sponsor requests FDA approval for marketing the drug by submitting a new drug application or NDA. The NDA must contain all of the scientific information that the company has gathered and they tend to be massive documents. NDAs typically run 100,000 pages or more.

An outline of the drug development process is shown in the chart (Chart 20.1) which appears on the following page. No one year is like the last year so the numerical information in the chart should be interpreted as rough estimates and not fixed values.

The most critical step in the clinical testing period is the Phase III trials. The concerns expressed in the previous chapters of clinical trial difficulties are clearly at play during these studies. The drugs that make it ands win NDA approval are presumed to be safe and effective, but this cannot be guaranteed. The FDA standards of "proof:" simply cannot identify all the vulnerabilities that permeate clinical research studies. Consequently, approval mistakes cannot be avoided and the post-marketing experience, which is discussed later, becomes critical in further defining the safety and efficacy of a new drug.

Chart 20.1 Drug development process (Adapted from "The Drug Discovery, Development and Approval Process," *Pharma New Medicine* (October 2004)

	Preclinical testing	File an IND	Phase I	Phase II	Phase III	File An NDA	FDA review	Total time	Phase IV
Years	3.5		1	2	3		0.5–2.5	10–12	
Test population	Laboratory and animal studies		< 100 healthy volunteers	100–300 patient volunteers	500–5,000 patient volunteers		Review evidence and approve safe and effective drugs		Additional post marketing testing required by FDA
Purpose	Assess safety and biological activity		Determine effects in humans and estimate useful dosage range	Evaluate efficacy, look for side effects	Verify efficacy, identify side effects				
Success rate	5,000 Compounds evaluated		5 enter clinical trials				1–2 approved		

Chapter 21
Medical Innovations – Regulators, Resources and Results

Abstract The major players that influence the development of medical innovations include the FDA, the chief regulator, and the National Institutes of Health, the primary resource for training the skilled research personnel as well as sponsoring major clinical trials. A historical review of the Food and Drug Administration shows that disasters have been the catalyst that has molded the agency which faces the impossibility of satisfying its many interest groups. Timeliness has been a constant battleground – should product availability or safety be stressed? In the early 1990s the "speed-up-the-process" side won and the agency implemented programs that would lead to quicker drug approvals such as fast tracking and accelerated review. These innovations led to a change to the "substantial-evidence" standard that required only one rather than two well-controlled clinical studies for a marketing approval, providing the product treated a life-threatening condition. For-profit companies are also a indispensable member in developing new products. For decades, new novel and important drugs wended their way through the testing phases and onto the market. But that flow has slowed. Consequently, drug discovery must exploit new opportunities such as that created by the Human Genome project in order to bring more major new products to the marketplace.

Keywords Accelerated NDA review · substantial evidence standard · Food and Drug Administration · National Institutes of Health · pharmaceutical industry

The last chapter laid out the path that drugs and devises had to transverse in order to make it to the marketplace. Let's now consider the role of the major players along the route. The government plays a huge role – the FDA is the chief regulator that defines and oversees the steps and standards of most of the process. Another governmental agency, the NIH, has an important role as well. The NIH makes a valuable contribution because it is a primary resource for the highly skilled personnel needed to conduct the basic and applied research that moves a novel medical product through the system. However, there would be no product development without private industry. Pharmaceutical, biotechnological and medical devise organizations spend millions of dollars funding the discovery and development of promising innovations.

With all the investments on the part of government and industry, it is appropriate to look more closely at the roles these organizations play and ask how well is the operation doing in finding new treatments that truly advance healthcare.

The FDA's Role

The FDA, the primary governmental agency that oversees the drug developmental process, has an enormous responsibility. As other regulatory bodies they come under relentless attacks from all sides. However, their presence is essential. Without the FDA, the drug development process would be out of control and Americans would be the big losers.

Disasters have been the catalysts that have molded the FDA. Shocking disclosures in the 1900s of unsanitary conditions in meatpacking plants, the use of poisonous preservatives or dyes in foods, and cure-all claims for worthless and dangerous patent medicines led to the birth to the Food and Drug Act of 1906. However, federal oversight had begun earlier. In 1848 federal controls over the drug supply had started with the inspection of imported drugs. But attempts to create an actual agency to regulate drugs were unsuccessful throughout the 19th century. All that changed in 1906 when Upton Sinclair authored *The Jungle*, containing sensational stories about the filth in food manufacturing and the unfounded claims for patent medicines finally motivated Congress to pass legislation to prohibit interstate commerce in misbranded and adulterated foods and drugs. This responsibility fell to the USDA Bureau of Chemistry which later became the FDA.

A second shocking disaster struck in 1936, 30 years after creating the agency. A consumer product known as a Sulfanilamide Elixir contained a poisonous solvent and killed over 100 people including many children. The tragedy prompted Congress to pass a new bill that required evidence of drug safety before a drug could be marketed thereby extending the FDA's authority.

A period of insignificant change was followed in 1962 by another devastating event. Thalidomide, a new sleeping pill that also could prevent morning sickness in women, was on the European market and sales were growing. Then tragically it was found that Thalidomide caused birth defects and thousands of deformed babies littered European countries. U.S. citizens were spared the horror because an FDA medical officer had kept the drug off the U.S. market. Still this "near miss" galvanized Congress to change the law governing new medications. First, makers of new drugs needed to demonstrate that their products were effective as well as safe. Second, the effectiveness had to be proved by "substantial evidence." Third, no drug could be marketed until the FDA agreed that the drug had been shown to be safe and effective. In response to the new legislation, FDA established a standard for substantial evidence. To meet the standard there had to be two adequate and well-controlled studies before a drug could win marketing approval.

The next major pieces of legislation affecting the FDA took place in the 1990s when a number of actions designed to modernize the FDA were put in place that allowed the agency to review NDAs much more quickly and order applications so the most important medial advances received priority attention. As the 20th century ended, the FD had become the target of fierce but quite divergent criticisms. However, there was consensus on one issue – the FDA had to change. Nevertheless, one side believed that the FDA was slow to address dangers associated with old drugs and careless in guarding against the hazards of new ones. The other side focused on getting new drugs on the market sooner and believed that the agency was too slow in reviewing and approving new medicines. They argued that new and valuable drugs were delayed in reaching the U.S. public while these same drugs were readily available overseas. The battle lines were drawn – should drug approval decisions emphasize safer drugs which would delay drug approvals or should they emphasize quicker availability and that meant speeding up the approval process?

FDA has always faced the impossibility of satisfying its many interest groups. Timeliness has been and is a constant battleground. It's valuable to learn as much as one can about a drug before it becomes available to millions of people. Approving a drug with inferior efficacy is costly to patients and can jeopardize their health needlessly, especially if a more effective preparation were already available to treat their medical condition. Still the greater cost is often missing harmful or even lethal side effects because the Phase III clinical trials were too short, too small or too few. However, getting additional safety information on a drug can add years to the pre-approval process and hundreds of million dollars to the development costs. Even then, it's likely that some important safety features may be missed. On the other hand, holding back on drug approvals keeps a useful product from reaching needy patients and adds to the price tag of new drugs. Approval delays also cost the drug sponsor because they are not able to start receiving a return on their sizable investment in developing a drug. In addition, statistics had shown that drugs were being approved sooner in other countries and that made the FDA appeared overly cautious.

The "speed-the-process-up" side won out and ways to accelerate drug reviews began in earnest in the early 1990s. There had been just too many pressures to expedite drug approvals. For instance, the lack of drugs to fight AIDS motivated AIDS advocates in the 1990s to demand faster approvals of drugs that could help patients who had been infected with HIV. In addition, the cost of developing new drugs continued to rise because the trial designs, conduct, and analysis of clinical trials became increasingly rigorous and expensive. Approval delays only made a bad situation worse. The need to make the kind of subjects who participated in a clinical trial more like the patients who were likely to use the drug (e.g. by increasing the number of women and minorities) expanded the size of trials and added to research expenditures. The importance of doing studies in pediatric populations also would lead to more trials that had to be conducted.

The agency responded by implementing various programs that would lead to faster drug approvals. For example, by the mid 1990s appropriate drugs could earn "fast track" status or a priority review. This meant the sponsors received early input from the FDA about their development plans, the option of submitting a New Drug Application (NDA) in sections rather than as a complete application and the possibility of using surrogate endpoints in the Phase III clinical trials. In addition, in special cases a priority review was available that shortened review time of an NDA. An even better option was an accelerated review. The program, available for drugs that treated life-threatening conditions, granted approvals with less stringent standards. However, this substantial benefit came with a cost. The sponsor had to agree to undertake studies the FDA deemed necessary to confirm the drug's safety or efficacy following an approval. In addition, for drugs that would be used in children, the FDA could issue a drug approval without all the necessary data, if the manufacturer agreed to do the required trials in children during the postmarketing phase. The agency also relied increasingly on outside medical experts, whose views about the risks and benefits of new drugs were expected to be less cautious than those of the FDA reviewers.

The data indicating that, on average, it took the FDA longer to process new drug applications (NDA) and approve drugs than it did in other industrialized countries had to be dealt with as well. Some NDA reviews took as long as eight years. Often, the cause of delay was not the difficulty of the application, but merely backlog. Applications would sit unexamined for months or even years. The FDA concluded that the process of approval could be speeded up if they had better equipment and more workers to review applications. Congress was unwilling to increase FDA appropriations, however and the solution was addressed by charging applicants a fee for processing their marketing applications. The user fees, charged to manufacturers to have their NDA evaluated, had to be earmarked for NDA activities like hiring and training additional staff to review NDAs.

The stage was set for other profound changes in the FDA operations. The "substantial-evidence" standard for proof of a drug's effectiveness that required at least two well-controlled clinical studies was about to change. The agency announced that it would approve a drug based on a single study under special circumstances. For example, when the drug offered treatment for an otherwise untreatable disease. They noted that it would be unethical to require a second study when an initial study demonstrated a profound effect (e.g. reductions in death). It was argued that large multicenter studies were also convincing, even without replication. In the end the FDA was granted discretion to base a drug approval on a single controlled study if, in addition, there was other "confirmatory evidence" or sound reasons for this action.

To put this change into perspective, realize that even with the prerequisite of two adequate and well-controlled trials, there was the possibility that that requirement would not weed out undeserving drugs. This concern is valid, even though there are often more than two large RABCOT studies included in the NDA, because some studies can result in an inconclusive answer and sponsors would be foolish to run only two major trials. Nonetheless, the criterion of at least two well-substantiated studies is not really as stringent as it sounds, leaving plenty of room for poor drugs to make it onto the market that eventually have to be withdrawn because they are ineffective or unsafe.

What's paradoxical about FDA's emphasis on having a faster approval system rather than pressing for grater assurance on drug efficacy and safety is that it appears to contradict what the American public wants. The results of a 2004 poll published in the online edition of the *Wall Street Journal* showed that more than half the respondents believed that ensuring safe and effective drugs was FDA's most important job. Moving drugs to the market faster was a distant second. However, the FDA could take some comfort from another result – in 2004 a majority of Americans (56 percent) rated the FDA as excellent or good in terms of the job the agency was doing. In spite of FDA's exposure to criticism, the general public did not appear pessimistic about its performance. Unfortunately, for the agency their performance rating fell in later years and was down to 35 percent by 2008.

At the heart of regulatory decision-making are judgments about risks and benefits. Under this philosophy there are arguments to support the decision to accept a single study as evidence of the safety and effectiveness of a drug. Benefits include reducing the number of subjects who must participate in a clinical trial – a major gain in reducing cost and time. In addition, if placebo controlled trials were called for, there was an added benefit – it eliminated subjecting volunteers to an ineffective treatment. However, the most appealing reason for the single study policy was that it made the new drug more quickly available to the public.

There are justifiable concerns with the one-study strategy as well. The down side is an increased risk that an ineffective drug or a drug with unknown harmful effects (the far more likely possibility) would now be accessible to unsuspecting consumers. Even with the two-study requirement that remained in place for most drugs, there is the possibility that a drug approval error could happen. It is just not possible to know all there is to know about a drug before an approval decision must be made even after conducting two adequate and controlled studies. Serious side effects may exist in some cases, ineffectiveness may be present for subpopulations now and then, and a poor harm/benefit ratio may exist as well. Nonetheless, requiring only a single study places increasing pressure on the post-marketing phase to monitor a drug. However, whatever standard is used, the FDA can not do the impossible and approve only the perfectly safe and efficacious drug. They can only strive to approve drugs in which the benefits clearly appear to outweigh reasonable risks. Most of the time the FDA will get it right, but not always. It is therefore left to the post-marketing period to weed out the bad drugs.

In the end, no matter how many studies were done, the FDA must decide if a drug has an unacceptable benefit/risk ratio. However, note that the two factors, benefits and risks, are not measured by the same common attribute so there is no identifiable benefit/risk ratio that can be met. It's only in the eyes of the decider (i.e. FDA) that the right ratio is satisfied. For the consumers the inescapable certainty is that, for some, the risk of a serious adverse event will become a reality.

Even if the agency could calculate a legitimate benefit/risk ratio for a drug when it is approved, that calculation would also certainly be inaccurate. There are many positive and negative effects of drugs that go undetected during the clinical research phase. The greatest threat is hidden safety issues and at the time of approval, the extent of that threat is unknown.

Clinical Research Resources

The NIH, the principal health-research agency of the federal government, is arguably the world's leading biomedical organization. The NIH traces its roots to 1887, when a one-room laboratory was created within the Marine Hospital Service. Congress established the service in 1798 in order to provide medical care to merchant seamen. Today the NIH is one of the world's foremost medical research centers, and the focal point for government sponsored medical research in the U.S. The NIH, which is part of the Department of Health and Human Services, consists of 27 separate institutes and centers. It employs nearly 20,000 people and has a budget of almost $30 million. Its primary goal is to acquire new knowledge to help prevent, detect, diagnose, and treat disease and disability. The NIH conducts research in its own laboratories; supports the research of scientists in universities, medical schools, hospitals, and research institutions and helps to train research investigators.

The NIH has the size, scale, and collaborative culture to advance clinical research in the 21st century. Its accomplishments of the past, promise that it will be a force in the future. The NIH's emphasis on innovation and creativity are essential for the advancement of clinical trial methodology. The greatest hope for advancing medical research and maintaining an adequate level of skilled medical researchers falls to the NIH.

Certainly, there can be no medical advancement without people to do the work. No one in the drug development cycle is more necessary than clinical researchers. For a full time clinical researcher, the combination of time commitment and the daunting challenges of performing research on human subjects often discourage all but the most committed physicians. A career in clinical research did not become broadly accepted in most medical centers until an expanded federal commitment to it was implemented by NIH after World War II. But even then, the federal commitment was largely directed toward basic research.

A 2001 survey by the Association of American Medical Colleges revealed that about one in ten medical school graduates plan careers that have to do with some form of medical research. Nonetheless, most of the graduates tended to favor basic versus applied research. Basic research advances scientific knowledge, but is not directed at commercial objectives. Clinical research, on the other hand, is considered applied research because its purpose is to produce results that are directed at real world problems.

However, even before the survey, applied clinical research careers appeared to be held in low esteem by academic health centers as well as at the NIH. Both institutions seemed to favor basic science. Many qualified to perform clinical trials viewed the road to academic promotion (and higher salaries) steep, long, and rocky. High educational debt and prohibitive costs of housing forced many into a more lucrative specialty practice. Furthermore, the regulatory aspects of clinical research consumed inordinate amounts of time for which there was little or no compensation.

Bach in 1995, the leadership of NIH had recognized that clinical research itself was in trouble. This finding was supported by a survey of senior researchers and department chairs of U.S. medical schools a few years later. There was clearly an insufficient supply of trained clinical researchers currently available to meet the demand. Predictably, there was substantial concern among the leadership at medical schools with respect to the entire clinical trial environment at their institutions. Problems included:

• The pressure to see patients taking time away from research
• Insufficient money for clinical research
• Inadequate supply of trained researchers
• Competition from commercial research organizations
• Problems introduced by the institutional review process
• Lack of research subjects

At NIH, a panel was convened to make recommendations to foster support for the clinical research field and steps were taken to implement the panel's recommendations. In 2003 an NIH report concluded that the steps taken (e.g. clinical training programs and educational loan relief for those who pursue research) diminished the aura of discouragement surrounding clinical investigation.

The supply of researchers for clinical trials is augmented by practicing physicians who have access to many potential subjects The physician may also enjoy the prestige of being involved in research and the intellectual stimulation that the research affords him or her. Doing some thing beyond the usual routine of office practice, the opportunity to be on the cutting edge and contributing to actual improvement of medical care are additional incentives. Furthermore, the physician's patients are given the chance to participate in studies that offer new treatment options. Despite these potential advantages, the incorporation of research procedures such as recruitment and principles of informed consent into an office system requires a delicate balance between the demands of scientific rigor and the clinical mission of the practice. The psychological conflict in the simultaneous roles of the physician as (1) patient advocate and (2) experimental researcher may represent an additional obstacle.

Private Industry

The for-profit companies specializing in health remedies employ numerous health care professionals to discover and assess new products. Major companies have their own resources that can take a product from the laboratory bench to the marketplace. However, there is a trend in the clinical research process that merits our attention. Driven by mounting costs to design and run clinical trials in the mid 1990s, drug makers turned to greater use of outsourcing clinical research. They, therefore, looked to a new developing business venture – contract research organizations or CROs. A CRO can do just about everything involved in the drug development process – carry-out pre-clinical evaluations, design a study, manage a trial, collect data, conduct a statistical analysis and submit regulatory applications to the FDA. Although their most obvious purpose is to provide extra capacity for a drug company, a CRO can also provide expertise in a research area (e.g. pediatric research) that may be lacking within a company. Furthermore, the pharmaceutical industry may prefer to employ the more applied approach of a CRO compared to the theoretical orientation of an academic medical research team, which was the research team of choice for many years.

The industry continues to be one of the most profitable, although in large part that's because the consumption of medications has skyrocketed in recent years and more people are given prescriptions for longer periods of use and at higher prices. Yet the strategies that produced a steady flow of new drugs don't seem to be working to the degree they once did. To make matters worse there's that rise in clinical research costs to test medications. It's been estimated that a new drug costs from $800,000 to $1.7 billion to bring it to market.

The quality of the clinical research sponsored by drug companies has been questioned. Reviews that appeared in medical journals such as the *British Medical Journal* indicate that the clinical research methods and the rigor of industry sponsored trials are comparable to that done for not-for-profit study sponsors (e.g. private foundations and government). However, there is a concern that when a pharmaceutical company funds a trial, the published results are more likely to find their drug superior to the control drug compared to studies financed by the government and non-profit organizations. A number of possible explanations have been offered for this result. For example, a comparison treatment may have been selected that was almost assured to be inferior to the sponsoring drug maker's product. The possibility that the design may have allowed the comparison drug to be given at a less than optimal level has also been suggested. Another reason for the higher number of positive results in industry sponsored studies may be due to the likelihood that negative studies for a company's product simply aren't submitted for publication. Even if they are submitted there could be publication bias, a journal's reluctance to publish studies that end up with inconclusive findings or do not demonstrate statistical significance.

Results – A Downturn in Important New Products

For decades, new novel and important drugs wended their way through the testing phases and came onto the market. According to the FDA, in the 1990s about 14 drugs were approved that were new chemical compounds and had the potential to represent a significant medical advancement. In the early 2000s that number was down to an average of about eight. Considering that 5,000 drugs are tested each year, it is an amazingly poor outcome. Although there are numerous ways to measure how the product development process is doing, there seems to be consensus that it is a downward trend. In the mid-1990s, the FDA received on average close to 50 applications for new drugs in a year but that rate fell by about a third a decade later. A similar downward pattern was reflected in the submissions for novel medical devices.

What is clear is that the overall poor performance in developing major new drugs was not caused by a lack of research effort or funding by pharmaceutical companies. In a 10-year period, starting in the early 1990s, there was a three-fold increase in research and development expenditures. Productivity, measured as the amount spent to find a new drug got worse year after year. The lack of new drugs, and especially "blockbuster" drugs, (so named because of their high profitability) is naturally of special concern to the health care and drug industries.

A study, by J. DiMasi at the Tufts Center for the Study of Drug Development, looked into the question of why drugs, that made it through animal screening, flunkout in the human testing period found that the most common cause was a lack of efficacy. The other two primary reasons had to do with safety and economics. Safety problems stemmed from toxicity found in humans or on-going animal studies. A small and unprofitable market for a drug was the primary economic cause for not pushing a drug along.

The frustration with new drug discoveries is especially visible in the field of antibiotics. Since their discovery in the 1940s antibiotics have saved millions of lives. But the bacteria they are designed to kill have grown more resistant and the number of drug-resistant infections is on the rise. In this instance economic considerations play a major role. There's been a lack of interest on the part of industry to do research in this area for some time. First, the field is very competitive and many of the products became relatively inexpensive. Furthermore, targeting a drug to treat resistant organisms translates into a small market. An added disincentive is the fact that efficacious drugs work quickly, and there is much more profit in drugs that can be used for long periods of time.

To stimulate more antibiotic research and development, the FDA, in recent years, has provided incentives to private industry to pursue new novel products. For, example one of their strategies is to provide an expedited NDA review. It would appear that from an industry perspective, finding new antibiotics should be an attractive option. However, only a few major corporations have taken up the challenge. Conversely, many small biotech firms have shown an interest in this area.

The Future

Drug research has contributed magnificently to the progress of medicine during the past century. The failure of the current drug development system to come up with major new treatment breakthroughs is an ominous sign. The current trend suggests that the drug discovery enterprise must exploit new opportunities to restore momentum. The Human Genome project provides an unprecedented opportunity to understand diseases and provides medical science a new avenue to find useful pharmaceutical agents. For instance, consider a genetic database that can be searched for causal associations between genetic traits and disease states. With this model, it may be possible to identify a particular patient type and know, in advance, if the drug is suitable. Asthma, migraine headache, Alzheimer's disease, depression, psoriasis, and arthritis will be among the diseases that could profit from this approach. Most pharmaceutical companies are building or buying access to genetic databases to achieve these ends. Genetic information can also aid toxicological investigations. How genes influence adverse drug events and what is the genetic pathology in some kinds of cancer are also promising avenues of investigation. Even though these dramatic gains are years away from realization, and some may not succeed at all, it's hard to resist visualizing a new golden age of drug discovery.

The study of how genetic variation between individuals affects their response to medicines also has the potential to revolutionize clinical trials. New compounds that are developed, based on the genetic make-up of patients, could allow investigators to restrict the type of subjects selected for a clinical trial. If the genetic profile of potential subjects indicated the experimental drug would be harmful or ineffective, they would not be chosen as participants in a trial. Not only would unresponsive patients be spared the ordeal of a clinical trial, but by removing these patients from a study, fewer subjects would be needed and time could be saved as well. This would in turn reduce the overall costs of clinical development as well as shortening its duration.

There are no calls to make major modifications in the steps that drives drug development. The use of animal experimentation early on to find drugs that may be effective and to root out those that would be harmful to humans, is far from being a perfect system. Still, much is learned using animals, and even if some of the information is misleading, the insights gained far offset the liabilities. In the future, alternatives to using animals such as computer simulations or the use of cultured cells may turn out to be practical and better predictors of human reactions, but for the present animal testing remains an essential part of the progression needed to seek safe and effective drugs.

What is clearly needed is the development of better predictive tools. Pharmaceutical research could improve change dramatically if scientists could come up with better methods to predict success such as computer modeling techniques and finding biological markers (a physical sign or laboratory result that can tells us something about that state of an illness). As this happens, there will be corresponding improvements in the selection of drugs.

The discovery process of medical science is a cumulative one; each discovery, no matter what its source, informs us in many ways. A single trial can only give us a portion of the total picture. Progress comes from researchers building on the work of others. With each new answer, it seems, new questions arise. And with them come new clinical researchers who pursue new knowledge. We have progressed from individuals making magical potions at home to thousands of scientists contributing to the highly complicated drug development process of today. Along the way many incorrect beliefs have been tossed out and new information has taken their place. History can repeat itself and many of the current drugs are destined to be replaced with more effective and safer agents in the future.

Chapter 22
Science and Politics – A Troubling Mixture

Abstract An analysis of the prominent role of special interest groups in medical research reveals that these groups can indeed be influential. Congressional involvement is also evident, especially when it comes to ideological issues such as abortion drugs, condom use, and concerns regarding sexually transmitted diseases. The far-reaching power of the drug industry to shape clinical research is also extraordinary. The industry preference to compare their drugs to placebo, and therefore avoid studies that use competitive products as the comparative treatment, has been unusually successful. The healthcare field is also laden with all sorts of advocacy and support groups that seek ways to influence medical research. For example, cancer patients have been successful in getting priority attention for oncology drugs and AIDS advocates were instrumental in getting the FDA to modify their regulations to make drugs that treat HIV available sooner. However, there are examples, such as the unsuccessful cancer drug Iressa, that indicate that changes in FDA approval standards have also had untoward consequences. Involvement in medical research by independent groups and citizens has also been noteworthy. For instance a Lyme Disease association and a breast cancer survivor have been able to change the policy and recommendations of professional medical societies concerning medical treatment.

Keywords Advocacy groups · congress · interest groups · pharmaceutical industry · politics

Medical research is not immune from the political process. On top of the difficulty medical science faces to find the truth lays the additional burden of possible political meddling. Political intervention is often done for a noble reason – a belief that it will help to promote better science and public policy. Because the decisions made by the FDA cannot guarantee that all the drugs it approves are safe and effective, there is constant debate about what should be done to improve their decision-making process. But politics can play an intrusive role and Congressional actions can trump FDA's authority to reshape the standards for new drug approvals.

Because health care is an issue that affects everyone, an array of special-interest groups gets involved in the selection of issues and solutions that are pursued by Congress. One of the largest and most influential of the groups is the pharmaceutical industry. In addition to the pharmaceutical lobby, other influential special-interest groups are active and include patient advocacy groups for almost every conceivable illness, the insurance industry, medical schools and professional health societies. The energetic participation by all parties makes reaching rational decisions on research subjects extremely difficult.

> *The FDA has an almost impossible task in supervising a multimillion dollar industry in the face of public criticism and political pressure.* (E. Gale, *Lancet*)

Political Intervention

Because of its power to approve drugs and devices, the FDA has become a major pawn in political struggles based on ideological beliefs. Some of the issues legislators have gotten involved with include abortion drugs, condom use, free needle exchange and concerns regarding sexually transmitted diseases.

Abortion, one of the most controversial issues in America, polarizes Democrats and Republicans. It is a major question in vetting Supreme Court candidates and a subject that produces legions of proponents and opponents. It makes for an ideal flash point for a confrontation between science and politics.

Abortion-rights supporters hailed an FDA decision to approve a unique contraception drug in 2006, but only after a series of unbelievable delays. Plan B, a novel name for a drug, was often referred to as "the morning-after pill". Plan B mainly acts by preventing fertilization, but it could occasionally dislodge an hours-old fertilized egg and therefore abort it. Barr Laboratories, the Plan B manufacturer, had been selling the drug in the U.S. for years on a prescription-only basis. The FDA rejected their first application to sell Plan B over-the-counter (i.e. without a prescription) in 2004. The drug had adequate data on its safety and efficacy in adults, but there was little information on its effect in young women. Barr then submitted a revised application offering to sell Plan B to adults without a prescription, but requiring a prescription for women younger than 18.

The revised application went before an FDA expert advisory committee and received a favorable judgment. The vote was 23 to 4. An internal FDA review by its professional review staff also recommended approving Plan B. The Acting Commissioner of the FDA, L. Crawford, who had had to get past a Senate Committee before he became the official commissioner, had also signaled his intention to approve the drug during his confirmation hearings. He promised the Senators that a decision about the drug was forthcoming. Approval seemed imminent. There were, as would be expected, socially conservative groups opposed and close to 50 members of Congress representing their interest, joined together and wrote a letter to President Bush asking that the application be rejected.

The storm broke in May 2004 when the FDA sent Barr a non-approval letter rejecting its application. A top FDA official said politics had had no part in the FDA decision, but Plan B proponents charged foul. A U.S. representative announced that a bill would be introduced requiring the FDA to review their negative decision. The FDA's Assistant Commissioner for Women's Health resigned her position in protest and charged the Commissioner with pandering to conservative interests. Newspapers across the country carried the story and a biting editorial in the *Washington Post* condemned Crawford's refusal to approve the drug claiming science was being trampled by politics. A coalition of women's health and pro-choice groups also protested the decision and another group of Congressmen wrote a letter to Crawford asking that the decision be reviewed and overturned.

Although the non-approval letter did not outright reject the application, it clearly delayed its approval by telling the company that they had not provided enough information to ensure that the drug could be safely used by girls 16 and under. The FDA position, that there were regulatory problems with availability based on age, meant there would now be further study and public comment and that could take years. To many, politics had triumphed over science.

A short epilogue deserves inclusion. Crawford resigned shortly after his Plan B decision. He had served as Commissioner for less than two months. He denied his decision to leave had anything to do with his failure to approve Plan B. Speculation about reasons for his early departure (he was Acting Commissioner for close to two years before becoming Commissioner) varied. One possibility was that Plan B was too much and he wanted out, given all the unfavorable publicity heaped upon the agency highlighted by the Vioxx debacle some months earlier where the FDA was assailed for not acting quickly enough. Another likely reason was the possibility that he would face legal and ethical challenges because he had not fully disclosed financial holdings prior to his appointment at the FDA. Incidentally, under a new Commissioner, the application was approved.

Another touchy subject involves the use of condoms to prevent the spread of sexually transmitted disease (STD). In way of background, a virus called HPV (human papilloma virus) produced genital warts, which could lead to cervical cancer. Since HPV was transmitted during sexual intercourse, an HPV infection was considered a sexually transmitted disease.

During the 1990s, condom use was recommended in order to prevent sexually transmitted diseases, but a few preliminary studies appeared late in the decade suggesting that condoms might not protect against HPV. Conservatives seized on the findings to support their campaign for abstinence. The NIH convened an expert panel to assess the evidence on condoms' effectiveness and found that condoms offered substantial protection against HIV, the virus that causes AIDS, but there was not enough data to draw conclusions about other sexually transmitted diseases such as HPV. However, the NIH report cautioned that the absence of definitive conclusions was a result of too little data and should not be interpreted as proof of the adequacy or inadequacy of condoms. Nonetheless, the HPV issue quickly became a rallying point for social conservatives to challenge the claim that condoms could help contain the spread of sexually transmitted disease. In fact, a U.S.

Representative, T. Coburn who later became a Senator, engineered the passage of legislation that mandated the FDA to reexamine condom labels "to determine whether the labels are medically accurate regarding the overall effectiveness or lack of effectiveness of condoms in preventing sexually transmitted diseases, including HPV." The transparent goal of the abstinence lobby was to force condom manufacturers to add a warning on their condom packages. The warning would note that condoms might not prevent the HPV virus that could lead to cancer. The FDA was now expected to make a "scientific decision" with only limited data at their disposal and an influential politician pressuring them to imply that condoms were not particularly effective.

In 2006, the FDA issued its proposed rules: condom packages should say that condoms are thought to be less effective against certain STDs, including HPV, because those diseases can be transmitted through skin-to-skin contact in places not covered by a condom. In addition the labeling should add that studies have shown condom use does reduce the chances of a person suffering from some of the worst effects of HPV, which include genital warts and cervical cancer. Senator Coburn, who was also an M.D. responded with a press release berating the FDA for refusing to use its authority to ensure the "scientific accuracy" of condom claims and taking five years to issue the proposed guidelines.

This contentious issue was resolved by a 2006 study published in the *New England Journal of Medicine* showing that consistent condom use offered protection against HPV. The study, conducted by an epidemiologist at the University of Washington and published in such an influential journal, appeared to be the most serious blow yet to the campaign to promote abstinence until marriage as the only responsible way to prevent sexually transmitted diseases. Fortunately, the FDA did not let a politician with strong ideological beliefs sway their medical judgment.

Interest Groups – The Powerful Drug Industry

An impressive example of the potency of the drug industry on capitol hill is illustrated in passage of the Medicare Prescription Drug Bill which was to be the cornerstone of the Republican Party's domestic agenda. The 2003 bill, designed to help senior citizens pay their prescription drug bills, is distinguished by the massive lobbying effort by the pharmaceutical industry to secure its passage. Because of the pharmaceutical lobby, the law included a provision barring the government from negotiating with the pharmaceutical industry for lower prices. This provision keeps drug prices higher in the U.S. compared to other countries. For instance, prescription drugs cost, on average, are 30–50 percent higher in the United States than in Europe. The major argument for the negotiation exemption was the need to keep the industry financially healthy so it could continue to discover new and effective treatments. That argument has some validity, but without a doubt, Americans have ended up underwriting the costs of drugs that are sold worldwide. Surly a benevolent act, but it comes about through political manipulation not generosity.

In 2004 it was estimated that the drug industry spent over $150 million on lobbying the federal government and gave almost 20 million more to federal politicians as campaign contributions. It is not surprising that many feel they are one of the most powerful groups in Washington and frequently get what they want from federal agencies.

Their interest in what goes on in the halls of Congress makes sense. They have a significant investment in the health care field. Most drug research is financed by the pharmaceutical industry. For many years drug companies did a large share of their research at academic medical centers and teaching hospitals. However, the current trend is to place more studies in private practice settings. As the 21st century began, the percentage of industry-sponsored trials conducted in academic medical settings dipped below 50 percent for the first time.

When being criticized, drug makers are quick to point out that their research costs grow each year and they invest a greater percent of sales in research than any other American industry. They boast that they spend more on research than NIH spends on its total operation. The industry believes drug development costs keep going up because the scientific measurements used in research become more sophisticated and expensive. Furthermore the research areas they pursue represent more difficult diseases that are not as amenable to drug therapy. In particular, finding ways to treat degenerative diseases such as cancer or a mental illness (e.g. Alzheimer's) are exceedingly difficult and costly.

On the other hand, there has also been a corresponding rise in the use of medications produced by the industry. The industry attributes the rise to the development of better drugs that prolong lives, alleviate suffering, and improve the quality of life. Drug costs are often defended on the basis that they replace the need for other more invasive and expensive treatments as well as reducing the length of hospitalizations. They argue that a narrow focus on the cost of drugs, without regard to their value and their role in the health system as a whole, would discourage innovation.

In spite of their many success in the economic and political arenas, drug makers face difficult choices. Firms that do not invest heavily in the drug discovery process run the risk of falling by the wayside. Those that push for extensive drug research may not succeed and end up with a poor return on investment. Overall the industry has an outstanding record of developing useful and important drugs, but in their effort to be highly profitable, they also incurred bad publicity and blame for errors of omission and commission. Thus, it is not surprising that a 2004 Harris poll found that only seven percent of the public polled do not trust the prescription drugs they take compared to 41 percent who do not trust pharmaceutical companies. Another Harris poll asked the public if the industry was doing a good or a bad job in serving its customers. Starting in 1997 with a 60 percent plus rating, the industry fell to a minus 4 percent rating by 2004. The numbers improved a bit in the next two years, but the drug makers still trailed the automotive industry. For company scientists and for the industry as a whole, the trend shows the quandary they face. No doubt, pharmaceutical firms must operate as a profit-making businesses, but the effort to maximize profits can make conducting research in the public interest an elusive goal.

Another example showing how business interests can influence medical research deals with learning what marketed drug is best and safest. When there are several drugs available to treat a given condition, it's only natural to wonder which one is the wisest choice. From a research perspective, the answer to that question comes from the head to head equivalence trial.

There is growing concern in the medical and insurance communities about the lack of comparative studies for marketed drugs. After a drug is approved, key questions remain such as how different is the new drug, compared to the current standard in respect to effectiveness and tolerance? How much does the new drug cost and is the cost commensurate with the drug's efficacy and safety? Those who pay a sizeable portion of the bill, government and private insurance companies, have a stake in this as well. They'd love a more rational basis for deciding what drugs merit a reimbursement. However, drug companies are not eager to have their drugs compared to a competitor's and they've been extremely successful in avoiding comparative trials. To overcome the reticence on the part of the drug makers, it has been suggested that there should be an independent unit within the NIH for testing prescription drugs against each other without involving the industry. This idea faces a major hurdle because the drug industry would lobby against such a move and, as we've seen, they have a very successful track record when it comes to influencing Congress. A drug ally, fiscal conservatives, might also have trouble with this role for the NIH because it would be one more intrusion into private industry by a federal agency and the enormous cost of such trials would have to be paid by the government.

Under the current legal and regulatory environment, head to head tests won't be done unless the pharmaceutical companies agree to do them. It's hard to believe that the drug manufacturers would go along with such testing of their products because results showing a company's drug to be inferior to a competitor's product would be disastrous for the company especially if it turned out that they were the ones sponsoring the study.

There is also a practical aspect to this discussion. Would the results from equivalence studies change the prescribing practices of doctors? A very interesting comparative drug trial, conducted by the NIH, sheds some light on this question. The clinical trial, a 33,000 patient, eight-year, $125 million study, compared the effectiveness of blood pressure medicines. The trial found that diuretics (50-year-old drugs that cost around 10 cents a pill) worked better than a relatively newer drug that costs about $2 a pill. As you might guess, the study design was criticized and the debate over the best way to treat high blood pressure was not resolved. One of the study's problems was, as usual, its rigidity. All subjects had to take the drug they were originally assigned. They could not switch to the other comparison drugs even though patients suffering from hypertension routinely change medications until one that really works is found. Yet allowing treatment switches creates a mess for the researchers because it becomes almost impossible to know what outcome should be assigned to what treatment. What's ironic, however, is that after publication, instead of the newer drug's sales eroding, they grew. The following year sales were up by 13 percent, to over four million making it one of the top selling drugs in the world.

In a confrontation between interest groups, the drug industry took on a coalition of organizations pushing for comparative studies that also had the backing of Consumers Union, AARP and many other consumer-oriented organizations. The contest centered on a budget provision to be added to a Medicare bill that provided $50 million for head-to-head trials of comparable drugs. The winner was .....? You guessed it, the pharmaceutical industry. They succeeded in eliminating the full amount required to run the comparative tests from the President's 2004–2005 budget. Opposing groups pushed to restore some funding with little success.

Another illustration of the power of pharmaceutical companies was evident when they were able to persuade Congress, in the 2003 drug entitlement provision under Medicare, to remove a provision known as "functional equivalence." Under this provision, a new drug deemed equivalent to an existing one would be reimbursed at the rate of the older drug. For example, a newer more expensive drug would be reimbursed at the lower price established for the older drug. The industry argued successfully that without removal of the provision, the industry would be discouraged from developing new innovative drugs.

It's easy to criticize drug companies, they make so many decisions that give them an awful reputation. However, we should not lose track of all the good things they do and have done. Some of the most powerful weapons society has are effective drugs created by the industry. The first antibiotics, developed during World War II, were called wonder drugs and changed history by subduing many deadly infections. Pharmaceutical research ushered in the modern age of vaccines, and progress continues as new technologies, rather than just curing an infection, actually teach the human immune system how to prevent the infection in the first place. The accomplishments of the industry are amazing and include anti-hypertensive preparations facilitating control of high blood pressure to effective psychotherapeutic medicines such as tranquillizers and antidepressants. Countless people have been helped by anti-inflammatory medicines for rheumatism and arthritis as well as beta blockers and ace inhibitors for heart disease. Thanks to drug companies, millions of people's lives improved following the introduction of oral contraceptives and medicines that treat ulcers. In a disaster the industry is one of the first to respond, donating life-saving products such as vaccines, antibiotics, antiseptics, and other drugs. Insulin, wound-care products, surgical equipment, millions of cans of infant formula, tens of thousands of personal care kits, plus a wide range of other supplies and large amounts of cash are also provided. Criticizing the drug industry without also acknowledging all the good it has done for mankind would be a serious oversight.

Citizen Advocacy

The healthcare field is laden with all sorts of advocacy and support groups that want to influence medical research. Some are large and well known (American Association for Retired Persons), others are professional organizations (American Medical Association), There are groups for any kind of illness (National Down

Syndrome Society) or condition (Spina Bifida Association of America). There's even a non-profit, organization dedicated to the continuing education and development of clinical researchers, the Society of Clinical Research Associates. Each group has a mission and goals and an essential method to reach those goals is by being politically active.

A notable success story of what these kinds of groups can achieve in the health-care field involves the plight of people with AIDS. The terror of AIDS dominated the last two decades of the 20th century. Because there were so few approved AIDS drugs, there was an enormous drive for more drugs, and that made the FDA the center of attention. AIDS activists wanted to be heard and for a full day they managed to paralyze operations at the agency's headquarters. They demanded immediate approval of drugs that were still considered experimental, if they offered any kind of hope for those otherwise facing death. The pharmaceutical industry also saw this movement as an opportunity to expedite an array of new products to the market. The companies and the AIDS advocates pressed the FDA and Congress to take action. If freed from the usual standards required for a drug approval, these groups felt that more drugs could be available sooner. Their efforts paid off, and as noted earlier, in 1998 the FDA put in place procedures to accelerate approval of certain new drugs that served an exceptional medical purpose.

AIDS groups also wanted access to drugs sooner, even before they had FDA approval. They pressured the FDA and drug companies to supply investigational drugs while they were still in the clinical testing phase. Again they met with success and under the FDA's Investigational New Drug (IND) Treatment Program the agency accepted many applications so that experimental drugs could be taken by patients with an HIV infection.

Cancer patients have also been successful in getting priority attention for their disease. For instance, the number of cancer support groups over time has grown to several hundred, and they have become increasingly educated about the intricacies of clinical trials. Inspired by the accomplishments of AIDS advocates, they successfully pressured drug companies, FDA and their local representatives into allowing cancer patients to also take investigational drugs, thereby allowing thousands of patients with cancer to be treated with a drug prior to its approval. Many new cancer treatments were also eligible for FDA fast tracking and sponsors eagerly took this route to hasten their products entry into the marketplace.

Unfortunately, these "accomplishments" didn't always turn out happily. Given how vulnerable medical research is to errors, the reduction in clinical trials usually required by the FDA, opened the door to possible disasters. Take the case of a drug to treat lung cancer called Iressa. It was approved through the accelerated program. The approval, based on small clinical trials, didn't include placebo controls. The available data indicated that the drug shrank tumors (a surrogate endpoint) in about 10 percent of the patients. After approval, the results of a confirmatory study designed to see if the drug prolonged lives (a more meaningful measure than tumor shrinkage) became available. The results failed to show a statistically meaningful survival advantage for the drug compared with placebo. Questions arose – was the FDA program allowing ineffective drugs on the market? Public Citizen, a consumer group founded by Ralph Nader, filed a petition urging that Iressa be removed from the market. The petition pointed to the failed survival study and deaths in Japan and the U.S. that were linked to the drug. Public Citizen also noted that patients now taking Iressa could continue to receive it through the investigational clinical trial program or they could switch to an alternative drug that was similar, but shown to be more effective.

The drug nevertheless had a strong number of backers since it had been on the market and benefited a select minority of patients. A cancer support group said it was unrealistic to expect a drug to be proven effective for the entire lung cancer population when it provided striking benefits for a small subset of patients. Patients were distressed at the possibility that the drug might be withdrawn. With their backs to the wall, the drug's manufacturer offered up irrational arguments. It said that the confirmatory trial barely missed statistical significance and, based on sub-group analysis, the results suggested the drug was effective in those who never smoked and in those of Asian descent. Clearly further studies that might predict which patients would benefit from the drug were needed, but the damage had been done. In the end, the manufacturer pulled the drug from the European market and, although it remained available in the U.S., its access was severely limited. For FDA's critics, the agency appeared to have acted recklessly.

The experience with Iressa focused attention on the practice of issuing faster and less detailed NDA approvals. Critics of the accelerated program noted that in many cases only a few dozen patients were actually helped by drugs that were granted a fast approval. Even worse, 25 percent of the accelerated cancer drugs were on the market for less than 18 months before serious side effects were observed. The FDA, in turn, supported its actions claiming that since 1996, 68 drugs for cancer therapies had received priority review and approval adding that, in some cases, the reviews were completed in less than six months.

Controversies over the accelerated approval process will certainly continue. Has the agency's energized approval process become too widely used, potentially allowing some drugs on the market with only limited evidence of efficacy and safety? In the case of Iressa, the answer was "yes". But the Iressa case must be considered in light of the fact that effective and reasonably safe drugs have also been made available sooner to people with serious diseases. Patients with deadly illnesses want a chance at recovery and are willing to band together to make their case. They are often quite willing to take high risks that may seem unacceptable to others, but their desperation should not be exploited. The only thing that seems certain under the accelerated program seems that there will be both impressive successes and dismal failures.

Involvement in medical research by independent laypeople has been especially beneficial when it comes to influencing professional medical groups. For instance, the Lyme Disease Association, a national nonprofit group of patients who suffer long-term problems with the disease pressured the Infectious Diseases Society of America, a national doctor's association, to review its guidelines for the long-term use of antibiotics in treating the disease. Even more stunning was the role R. Kushner, a breast cancer victim, played in changing the common practice of performing a radical mastectomy. She boldly took on the American Cancer Society and openly criticized surgeons. She wrote articles and attended professional medical meetings to challenge the medical establishment. Her campaign paid off and surgeons revised significantly the conditions under which radical mastectomy would be recommended

Finding a Balance

There are many stakeholders in the product development process: researchers, healthcare providers, corporations, governmental funding organizations, citizens with a shared interest, public health officials and legislatures who count on votes from concerned constituents. Each seeks political leverage to secure decisions that favor their interests. The FDA is clearly in the center of the interaction between politics and medical science. The agency is faced with a controversy almost every time they take any kind of action. Whenever there are important changes in their regulations, the impact almost invariably has positive as well as negative results.

Due to their past effectiveness, major parties involved in the political-regulatory interaction are likely to remain dominant players. Well-organized patient advocacy groups that enter the fray tend to do well and their accomplishments suggest that their participation will grow in the future. On balance, grassroots organizations have a positive effect and their participation should be encouraged. Many politicians play a key role in health matters and use their office to influence agencies such as the FDA. Some have advanced medical research and regulatory control, but others have had a damaging effect through their ideological and partisan behavior. The FDA has become a politicized bureau with Commissioners chosen on the basis of their conservative or liberal credentials. Due to the political climate, in Congress there will continue to be staunch defenders and unyielding critics of the agency. The powerful pharmaceutical industry is quite successful by many standards, but its negatives are also high. To correct the self-serving behavior of the industry there are those who advocate that nonprofit drug developers, either government or foundations, will serve the public interest better than the pharmaceutical industry. This may be so, but it is unlikely or impossible to believe that the record of major drug discoveries in the last 50 years could have been accomplished under the aegis of the not-for-profit sector. The vigor, determination and sense of urgency of the private sector cannot be matched. It's wiser to find ways to check its power than solve the problem by its elimination.

The FDA has a tough enough job and doesn't need the distractions and pressures caused by organizations and individuals with self-serving agendas. The current environment accepts lobbying efforts from all sorts of groups and creating the best policies and practices for making scientific decision is a tremendous responsibility. For both Congress and the FDA, how to come up with the right legislative and regulatory approach is an awesome challenge. Strong regulatory policies lead to a lack of incentive to develop drugs. Weak policies lead to an abundance of mediocre drugs. Strong regulations lead to fewer drugs. Weak regulation leads to more drug failures. Strong enforcement leads to greater cost and time delays. Weak enforcement leads to dishonesty and manipulation. Looking ahead, the path the FDA will take will continue to be determined by politics, not medical science.

Chapter 23
Research Misconduct – Irresistible Temptation

Abstract Temptation is ever-present in the clinical testing environment, and a conflict of interest can turn that temptation into an unacceptable moral act. Impropriety may also take the form of outright fraud as a researcher tries to profit from the lucrative medical research field. When it comes to safeguarding subjects in a clinical trial, the most important body that can insist on ethical behavior are Institutional Review Boards, which review and monitor research studies involving human subjects. There has always been concern over the relationship between clinical investigators and pharmaceutical companies. With all the complex financial relationships between drug companies and researchers, concerns about imprudent behavior cannot be overlooked. A series of case studies show how personal greed can disgrace the proud research profession. The brilliant academic who authored numerous articles in very good journals until it was discovered they were based on fabricated and falsified data. The successful entrepreneur in California who was caught conducting fraudulent research, exposed by his own employees. The phony physician overseeing clinical trials charged and convicted of fraud and criminal negligent homicide, ending up with a six-year jail sentence.

Keywords Conflict of interest · ethics · fraud · misconduct · whistleblower

In the creation, study and promotion of drugs, personal and professional decisions play a key role all along the line. As in other professions, medical researchers can be guilty of flagrant and criminal behavior or more subtle misdemeanors because of their decisions. Intriguing case studies illustrate how researchers destroy their careers and disgrace their proud profession. Often the victim of an unethical act is an unwary subject who volunteered for a clinical trial. Medical investigators can lose sight of their professional obligation to safeguard these individuals. Temptation is also abundant in the clinical testing environment, and a conflict of interest can turn that temptation into an unacceptable moral act. Impropriety may also take the form of outright fraud as a researcher tries to profit from the lucrative medical research field.

Kickbacks, fraud and misconduct are rife among American medical researchers, according to a scathing critique published by a US Congressional committee this week. (C. Joyce, *New Scientist*)

Ethical Concerns

Many of the news stories about clinical trial misconduct receive headline coverage in the media. But there are also more subtle types of transgressions that degrade the value of research studies that the public never hears about. Take the survey, published by *Nature* in 2005, of almost 3,500 U.S. scientists who received NIH support. A listing of conduct exhibited by this elite group of researchers is shown in the table below and provides important insight into the extent of poor ethical behavior that takes place in American science (Table 23.1).

Table 23.1 Unethical behaviors of health scientists

Behavior	Percent
Inadequate record keeping related to research projects.	28
Changing the design, methodology or results of a study in response to pressure from a funding source	16
Dropping observations or data points from analyses based on a gut feeling that they were inaccurate	15
Using inadequate or inappropriate research designs	13
Overlooking others' use of flawed data or questionable interpretation of data	12
Withholding details of methodology or results in papers or proposals	11

Gross misconduct such as falsifying data and plagiarism was also reported, but occurred infrequently (2 percent of the time or less). Noticeably, there are sins of omission and commission included in the table. Some events may simply be carelessness, but others are more serious such as changing the trial design and results to suit the study's sponsor. Taken as a whole, the survey results indicate a surprising number of scientists engage in bending the truth and purposely deceive others. These deceptive actions certainly damage the reputation and integrity of the healthcare research profession.

Investigational Review Boards

The most important institutional unit that can insist on ethical behavior in medical research is the Institutional Review Board (IRB). The IRB authority to approve, require modifications or disapprove clinical trial plans as it reviews and monitors research involving human subjects is an effective method to safeguard study volunteers.

The concept of an IRB was the direct result of a 1966 article in the *New England Journal of Medicine*, by H. Beecher a Harvard Medical School professor. The article focused on the conduct of U.S. human experiments since 1945. It included examples of studies that were out and out unethical or had questionable ethical properties. The criticism was somewhat subdued: the offences often described as thoughtless and careless acts by responsible investigators. Nevertheless, Beecher took a tough stand when it came to a remedy for the problem. He suggested that medical journals not publish results of studies unless the researchers had properly weighed the risks and gains for trial participants prior to starting the trial. In addition, researchers should not have begun their trials until they had obtained informed consent from the subjects. He also wanted these functions reviewed by an independent committee before the investigation began. In addition, at the time the researchers' sent their manuscript to a journal, the names of the committee members would be included in the submission.

Prior to the middle of the 20th century, research ethics were primarily governed by individual conscience and professional codes of conduct. However, in 1966, the Public Health Service (PHS) established a set of rules and regulations for medical research studies. No research grant would be issued under the PHS policy unless the researchers requesting the grant obtained prior review of their intended study by an independent committee of "institutional associates". Today there are hundreds of IRBs, located in the U.S. and overseas. Some boards are dedicated to a specific organization such as a medical school, but there are others that serve independent investigators who conduct trials for private organizations (e.g. pharmaceutical companies). Currently, IRBs must have at least five members with varying backgrounds and no IRB can consist entirely of members of one profession. Furthermore, if the research calls for a vulnerable category of subjects, such as children, prisoners, pregnant women, handicapped or mentally disabled persons; then the possibility of including one or more individuals to represent these subjects must be considered.

Researchers, while appreciating the importance of protecting subjects from harm, express concerns with the effect the IRB process has on clinical research. For many years most clinical studies were conducted at a single facility, but the demand for large number of subjects means major trials must be conducted at multiple locations as multicenter trials. The result is a much more complex review process because of the potentially large number of IRBs (one per study location) that need to be involved. Different local reviews may also result in different required changes causing the trial plan to be in a constant state of flux. To be sure, all investigators do the research in a common way, additional requirements by one IRB may trigger a resubmission to the other IRBs which is time consuming and frustrating.

There is a concern that IRBs spend too much time scrutinizing the informed consent document and requiring exceedingly long detailed forms. The well-intended efforts of an IRB may even distort the methods planned for a trial and thereby threaten the validity of the trial. The growth in the number and complexity of clinical trials has also placed a strain on the availability of review boards. The net result is that researchers have to overcome yet another hurdle in their efforts to conduct a sound clinical study.

The effectiveness of the formal IRB system to ensure ethical conduct of clinical research is limited. Attention also needs to be focused on the actions by the physician-investigator. The professional integrity of these physicians is vital to an ethically sound clinical research system. A typical issue is how far should they go in explaining the nature of a clinical trial that a potential subject may enter? A good example of this dilemma occurs in early cancer trials.

In the first clinical trials for a new drug, the primary goal is to gain scientific information about a drug's actions rather than help a subject suffering from the illness. Nevertheless, desperate subjects seek out these trials as a last chance because other conventional treatments have not worked. Yet the purposes of an early clinical trial may be to identify a dose of an experimental drug that can be tolerated by patients. In that setting, curing or even retarding the disease is not a goal. And still it would seem unnecessarily cruel for the research physician to destroy all hope for subjects by insisting that they understand that the purpose of the trial has nothing to do with giving them a chance at therapeutic relief.

Patient risk rises enormously when the experimental treatment is unusually novel. Under this condition there is added incentive to be cautious and safeguard the health of a subject. Here's a tragic case that clearly violated that moral standard. Jesse Gelsinger was 18 and a subject in a clinical trial at the University of Pennsylvania and about to become famous. He was the first person known to die as a result of being treated with a brand new experimental approach to curing disease – gene therapy. Investigations into the death disclosed that Gelsinger became extremely ill, but his gene treatments were continued when he should have been withdrawn from the trial. It was also revealed that the researchers concealed from the subjects the fact that monkeys had died from treatment similar to the one they were receiving. The head researcher also claimed he had no financial conflict of interest, but it turned out that he had a strong financial interest and stood to profit if the treatment turned out to be successful.

Conflicts of Interest

There has always been concern over the relationship between clinical investigators and their private sponsors, such as pharmaceutical companies. The ties between clinical researchers and industry include not only grant support, but also a host of other financial arrangements. Researchers serve as consultants to companies whose products they are studying. They join their advisory boards and speakers' bureaus. They can be involved with patent and royalty arrangements. Researchers may also help promote a company's drugs at a symposium sponsored by the company. These events may involve expense paid trips in lavish settings. Many researchers also own stock in pharmaceutical companies with whom they work.

The relationship between researcher and a drug company might also take the form of a partnership. Universities set up research centers and establish teaching programs in which students and faculty members often carry out research projects sponsored by a drug company. Many research institutions, strapped for cash as a result of events beyond their control (e.g. reductions in Medicare reimbursements), find it hard to pass up these opportunities. It's a symbiotic arrangement. For an academic medical group, it means a source of funding; for the drug companies it means access to research talent, as well as affiliation with a prestigious school.

With all these complex financial relationships between drug companies and researchers, concerns about a conflict of interest cannot be overlooked. Many editorials and articles in the medical press address this topic and can agree on at least one common conclusion: the relationships among industry, scientific investigators, and academic institutions are pervasive. One investigation led by S. Krimsky, a Tufts University professor, reported that lead authors in one of every three articles published hold relevant financial interests in a company that would be affected by the outcome. Another investigation reported in a 2003 *JAMA* article, cited a survey by the Association of University Technology Managers that found that approximately two thirds of academic institutions held equity in "start-up" businesses sponsored research performed by their faculty. This same paper also noted that about one fourth of biomedical investigators at academic institutions receive research funding from industry.

Even if investigators involved with healthcare companies do not let that relationship influence their research, there is the perception that it has and that impression has a negative impact on the public's image of the integrity of the clinical research enterprise. The issue prompted a joint editorial, co-authored by the editors of a dozen of the world's most influential journals. The editorial noted that contract research organizations or CROs, the commercial organizations that run clinical trials and perform other duties for a sponsor, had become very competitive with academic research institutions when it came to conducting lucrative clinical trials for commercial companies. The editors complained that too often the competition had a detrimental effect on the independence of academic researchers because CROs were more willing to accept terms laid down by a company. The negotiated agreement could limit the academic researcher's input on the trial design, access to the raw data, and participation in data interpretation. In addition, the editors strongly opposed contractual agreements that denied investigators the right to submit a manuscript for publication without first obtaining the consent of the sponsor.

However, researchers deny that their financial attachment to industry has an effect on their work. They insist that, as scientists, they can remain objective. They resent the idea that they can be bought. To support their position, they like to point to double blind studies arguing that double blinding keeps them from showing an unwarranted preference for any outcome. Nevertheless, a concern over the financial ties between industry and researchers led to an editorial in the *World Health Bulletin* that said the reliability of clinical trials was seriously threatened. The WHO worried that study bias could take place by inappropriate involvement of research sponsors in the design and management of trials, as well as incomplete dissemination of study results. Furthermore, new editorial policies adopted by the *JAMA*,

New England Journal of Medicine and other major medical journals, require authors submitting a manuscript for publication to sign a statement verifying that their results and conclusions have not been influenced unduly by an industry sponsor.

A potential conflict of interest is also present at another level for the researcher who also sees private patients. The person trained in medicine, who wants to do clinical investigations, faces a schizophrenic life. The relationship between investigator and patient differs in important ways from the traditional patient-physician relationship associate with a clinical practice. Clearly, the physician-researcher has two roles – that of a clinician and that of a scientist. The physician–researcher ends up trying to integrate the clinician roles (e.g. do no harm to the patient) with the scientist's goal (e.g. optimizing the research setting by giving placebo treatment, curtailing concomitant drugs, etc). A conflict of interest between these roles cannot be avoided. In the end, medical investigators may have to sacrifice scientific rigor when the health and welfare of a subject is at risk. For example, what if a subject experiences potentially harmful side effects while in a clinical trial? Withdrawing subjects prior to the study's termination can reduce the scientific validity of the trial. In this situation the physician–researcher is in a quandary: sacrifice scientific purity by dropping the subject from the trial or waiting a while longer hoping that the dangerous side effect subsides?

Government Agencies

Prior to 1995 NIH had, what many felt was a very conservative conflict of interest policy. An NIH scientist could earn no more than $25,000 annually from any single outside source and not more than $50,000 per year in total. Stock or stock option payments were prohibited, and senior NIH officials could not accept any payments from outside sources. That changed in 1995 because it was believed that the rules were more stringent than those of other federal agencies. The change required senior NIH officials to file public financial disclosure forms revealing their incomes as well as any stock, fees, and payments from pharmaceutical and biotechnology companies that had dealings with the agency. Whereas the pre-1995 policy may have been overly restrictive, its replacement was viewed now viewed by some as too permissive when it came to a conflict of interest.

In 2003, a Pulitzer Prize-winning journalist at the *Los Angeles Times* broke a front-page story accusing top NIH scientists of receiving massive consulting fees from major pharmaceutical companies. The problem came to light when it was found that a test drug was the probable cause of a death in an NIH study. The trial had been supervised by a physician who energetically defended the drug, but then it was revealed that the NIH sponsored physician also received consulting fees from the drug manufacturer. The newspaper's story prompted hearings on Capitol Hill and forced the NIH to redefine their conflict of interest rules. In response to the *Los Angeles Times* article chastising almost all of the top-paid NIH employees because they failed to file public income-disclosure reports, the NIH approved more stringent standards and transparent policies in 2005. However, the revised rules that used the model designed for medical schools, were considered by many as too lenient for an organization such as the NIH. In fact, it rekindled concerns about a 1980 Congressional Act that allowed medical schools and their faculty to patent their discoveries. The argument was made that the NIH was not just another medical school. As a flagship governmental institution it was expected to meet higher standards. The premier scientific institution should have its scientists pursue promising leads no matter where they go and not be distracted by how much money they could make privately from patents they might secure.

The conflict of interest issue is also relevant to the FDA's advisory committees that provide advice to help the FDA make sound decisions about new drugs. There are committees for all drug classes and typically range in size between 10 and 15 members. Committee members, mostly scientific experts in a field, greatly enhance the level of expertise that goes into the decisions made by the FDA. The downside to this arrangement is that these same experts are in demand by the pharmaceutical industry, which also wants the advice and consul of research leaders. Committee members must disclose their financial ties to industry, but such relationships do not exclude their participation as FDA advisors. However, just the perception of a conflict of interest can affect the credibility of FDA decisions and a case that illustrates this principle is given below.

Generally, the advisory system works well, and a committee's advice to the FDA invaluable, but there can be embarrassing controversies. At a joint meeting of the FDA's Arthritis and it s Drug Safety and Risk Management committees in 2005, the retention or removal of three drugs from the market was under discussion. The drugs belonged to the same chemical class (Cox-2 inhibitors), were for the relief of pain and had done extremely well in the marketplace. There were 32 expert committee members in attendance. Ten had declared ties to drug manufacturers leaving only 22 without any possibility of a conflict of interest. Votes cast on each of the three drugs determined whether the committee's recommendation would be to retain or remove the drug from the market. Breaking the vote down by those with and without a possible conflict of interest showed that there was a total of 30 votes cast by those with industry ties (10 experts and votes on 3 drugs). Of the 30 votes, 28 or 93 percent favored the drugs. For the members without industry connections, 66 votes took place (22 experts and votes on 3 drugs). In this case there were just 37 (56 percent) of the votes that favored the drugs. There is clearly a substantial difference in the percentages (93 versus 56) and it put the FDA in a bad light. The agency looked particularly weak because prior to the meeting they had claimed that due to the "general nature of the discussions before the committee" any potential conflicts were mitigated and all committee members could therefore take part in the vote. Unfortunately for the FDA, many felt that whether a drug would remain on the market wasn't a trivial issue and allowing the 10 experts who received money from the industry to vote was a mistake. In the end, no one claimed the 10 pro-drug members were dishonest or prejudiced, but the notoriety of the case contributed to a commitment by the FDA to revise its conflict of interest rules.

Fraud in Clinical Research

Fraud has been part of science for a long time and may be present in the work of some of the world's great scientists. Mendel, the founder of genetics, had results that today are felt to be just too good to be true. Pasteur's notebooks, long kept secret, revealed that he misled the world and his fellow scientists about the research behind his most famous experiments. It is also alleged that Freud fabricated many of the case studies on which he built his psychoanalytic theories.

One theory about scientific fraud maintains that fraud is common because it is the inevitable product of the elevated status given to science in our culture. Scientists enjoy a privileged place in society because they are seen as seekers of truth and creators of progress. After all, medical research has produced numerous "miracle drugs" and saved thousands of lives. However, the opportunity to commit fraud is too available in institutional cultures such as scientific research organizations that are characterized by secrecy, privilege, and a lack of accountability.

Probably the most common form of fraud in science is the submission of papers to journals in which the data have been faked, numbers fudged, and ideas stolen. As mentioned before, the pressure to publish findings is intense. Researchers can gain prestige from publication in top journals and that can lead to better positions and more funding for their projects.

There's no way to know how common fraud is in medical research. However some form of it may occur more frequently than one would think. A confidential survey of medical statisticians by the International Society for Computational Biology was published in 2000 and found that half of the interviewees knew of at least one fraudulent project, 25 percent reported knowledge of fabrication and falsification, one in five were aware of deceptive reporting of data and 20 percent knew of cases in which data were suppressed.

Research misconduct can occur in any research setting and involve almost any member of a research team. Even well know and respected researchers can become ensnarled in a controversy. There are numerous ways to expose a guilty party, but whistleblowers who usually are support personnel in a research project, are often in the best position to reveal and document the unscrupulous behavior of a researcher. The following case histories illustrate the depth, breadth and seriousness of fraudulent behavior.

The Brilliant Academic

In 1981, Dr. Jon Darsee was regarded as a brilliant student and medical researcher. His affiliation at four well-regarded universities (Notre Dame, Indiana, Emory and Harvard) added to his stature as an important investigator in the evaluation of heart medications. In less than two years at Harvard, he authored seven papers in very good medical journals and his future looked bright.

Unfortunately, for Dr. Darsee, assistants saw him recording data for observations that he had never made. When confronted, Darsee admitted he was guilty of fabrication, but he said he did it because he had been under intense pressure to complete the study quickly. He asserted his innocence and claimed this was the first and only time he falsified data. However, over the next months, other research conducted by Darsee was examined and that raised more questions. One result showed the data he recorded was unbelievable consistent. His data simply looked too good to be believed and an analysis of the data showed this to be the case. There were strong suspicions that Darsee had been fabricating or falsifying data for some time and his work lost its credibility. His research fellowship was terminated and an offer to join the Harvard faculty withdrawn. Darsee's career was ruined, but there was also a major impact on the organizations that utilized his services. Because of his actions, the NIH required the return of over $100,000 of their grant money from the institutions where he had worked.

The Successful Entrepreneur

Dr. Robert Fiddes earned his medical degree in 1970 and went to Long Beach, California as a hospital intern. He joined a medical practice and then opened his own office. The practice did well, but managed care became an impediment in the delivery of health care and Fiddes resented the limitations the rules placed on his discretion to treat patients. His best option was to find a new area to apply his medical skills. He saw, in the growing clinical research business, a chance to be an independent businessman and continue treating patients at the same time. Many of his patients would now become subjects in the clinical trials he contracted to do for pharmaceutical companies.

His clinical trials business grew rapidly, and he built a large staff of assistants to help him conduct the trials. Fiddes had successfully changed his restrictive medical practice into a thriving research business and he became a major research arm for the pharmaceutical industry, ever searching for clinical investigators with many patients. Companies large and small turned to him and he ended up running almost 200 studies making millions of dollars in the process. Then it all came to a sudden stop.

Fiddes was caught conducting fraudulent research, exposed by his own employees. The subsequent investigation found that he cut corners and invented data. Fictitious patients were created and "enrolled" in his studies. If the rules called for excluding smokers from an asthma study, Fiddes' employees were told to enroll them anyway and not to mention their smoking habit in material sent to the sponsoring drug company. If a certain blood pressure was required for patients to participate in a study, employees recorded the required value regardless of the actual reading. If certain bacteria had to be present in a person's blood sample, Fiddes bought the bacteria from a commercial source and added it to the subject's blood specimen. If patients' medical records included information that precluded them from acceptance into the trial, the data were destroyed and the patients participated in the study is spite of the possibility that they could be injured by doing so.

Even though the data from his studies were audited for many years, no suspicion of deceit was apparent until a number of Fiddes employees, who realized what was going on, no longer wanted to be a part of his illegal behavior. One employee was particularly critical and wrote a letter to Fiddes declaring she would no longer participate in his fraudulent activities. Fiddes' response was to order her to clean out her desk immediately, and she was escorted from the building. The spurned employee went to the FDA and contacted other former employees to try to convince them to also speak with the FDA. Meanwhile Fiddes and his top aides planned a cover-up that entailed the destruction of incriminating evidence and the preparation of new false records so the blame for the corrupt practices could be placed on the whistleblower herself.

The case came to a close shortly after federal agents swarmed into Fiddes' offices and video taped every employee's face for use in future identifications. The drama had its intended effect – employees decided to tell the FDA what was going on. In the end Fiddes and three of his employees pleaded guilty to fraud. Thus ended one of the most flagrant cases of dishonest research that required all sponsors to re-evaluate any drugs that used Fiddes as an investigator to see if the elimination of his data would alter the safety and efficacy of the drug.

The Phony Doctor

Paul Kornak was hired by the VA hospital in Albany, NY as a research coordinator for a large cancer drug trial in veterans. He seemed especially qualified because he had attended medical school and although he did not finish, he was well versed in medical terminology and clinical research methods. However, he clearly was not a physician and was not hired to function as one. In his role as a study coordinator, Kornak reviewed prospective subjects' medical records to see if they qualified for the cancer experiment. For the four years he worked at the hospital, many subjects were enrolled in the studies under the assumption that he was a physician, an impression Kornak did not try to correct. Scores of the veterans who were admitted to the study were, in fact, not eligible according to the protocol specification. Because of the nature of the trial, some of these individuals were placed at great risk, especially those who were already very sick.

When hired, Kornak claimed he had been a doctor, but lost his medical license because he could not document a year of medical school in Poland. That didn't matter one way or the other since, except for physicians and dentists at that time, the VA did not require much background information for health workers. But a thorough review of his history would have discovered that Kornak had obtained and lost medical licenses in several states by forging credentials. In fact, he once had been charged with and pleaded guilty to a felony fraud charge.

A drug company, that offered $2,500 for each study subject, sponsored the project Kornak worked on. The money went to the Albany VA hospital not Kornak, but securing a high enrollment clearly advantaged him as well. On a routine visit to the hospital by a representative of the drug company, some paperwork reviewed by the representative raised suspicions – some dates simply didn't look right: the date of a biopsy was later than the report of the biopsy results. How could you have results before the biopsy was taken? As a result, the drug company conducted an audit and the hospital carried out an internal review of the study. Based on what was found the drug company stopped its study and alerted the FDA. By the time the FDA was through, there was more than enough evidence to accuse and convict Kornak. He was dismissed and charged with fraud, making false statements and criminal negligent homicide in the death of one of the subjects. With no where to turn, he pleaded guilty to the charges and in 2005 was sentenced to almost six years in jail.

Medical research is inherently difficult to conduct properly. But there is no question that breeches in ethical behavior by medical researchers contribute to clinical trial misinformation and a general mistrust of published results. It is disheartening that this noble profession must bear the damage brought by unscrupulous individuals. Fortunately, this small minority is overwhelmed by the hundreds of honest investigators who do their best to get at the truth.

Chapter 24
Postmarketing Surveillance – An Imperfect System

Abstract The FDA does not and cannot guarantee that all the medical treatments it approves are safe and effective. Thus, it is left to the postmarketing period to identify inferior products, especially those that have deadly side effects. Finding and removing inferior products falls to FDA's post marketing surveillance (PMS) program, but unfortunately the current system is inadequate. The PMS relies primarily on the lowest level of research methods – case reports, which are sent to the agency where they are analyzed and remedial steps taken if the evaluation shows there is an unanticipated problem. However, it was taking the FDA too long to identify a significant problem and decide what to do about it and in the interval; people were suffering and dying needlessly. There were numerous suggestions on how to improve the system, but FDA's response tends to be judged as unresponsive by its critics. To meet the postmarketing challenge the FDA needs the authority to require (1) independent teams to investigate serious adverse reactions; (2) the use of cohort studies to monitor the performance of newly approved drugs and (3) the employment of clinical trials to investigate unresolved efficacy and safety issues.

Keywords Adverse reaction · drug labeling · drug safety · market withdrawal · postmarketing surveillance

Launching a new product provides hope for many patients and new options for numerous physicians. For a pharmaceutical company it's almost certainly its biggest event of the year. There is no question that a successful launch offers the company a chance to recoup years of expensive and risky research and development – the opportunity to add profits to the bottom line for years to come. It also marks the beginning of a crucial FDA function – instituting the postmarketing surveillance system (PMS) where the FDA monitors drugs in the marketplace to see if they are living up to expectations.

How to protect the public from previously unrecognized harmful adverse drug reactions is a most demanding assignment. Phase III studies, the final stage of pre-marketing research leading up to FDA approval, provide relatively little information about long-term safety because they are not run long enough.

Financial considerations make it impractical for sponsors to run long-term trials in Phase III. Extending the length of Phase III clinical research almost certainly would make the development of drugs even more expensive, and delay their entry into the marketplace.

In addition, the controlled nature of the Phase III clinical trials decreases the ability of researchers to find all relevant adverse events that could occur with a new drug. Sending the drug into the public marketplace opens up a vast range of new situations that were not examined in the pre-approval research period. Clinical studies could not investigate all the new situations a drug faces once on the market, e.g. different dosage schedules, drug interactions, diet variations, geographical environments and effects from use in broader age groups. Exposures to these new conditions creates the opportunity for new safety problems. When we add in the fact that the number of treated subjects in the premarketing period is too small to identify the rare, but serious side effect, the situation is ominous for patients. This depressing picture only gets worse when we learn that information about drug safety in under-reported in medical reports. Articles in medical journals allocate results concerning safety issues an average of about one-third of a page which is equivalent to the space they devote to the authors names and affiliations.

According to a 2002 report from the Medical School at Harvard University, over half of all approved drugs had serious adverse effects that were not detected in the clinical testing period. Worse yet, seven drugs approved in one 10-year period (1993–2002), were withdrawn from the market and may have contributed to over 1,000 deaths. The study found that less than 10 percent of drug reactions are reported to FDA's voluntary postmarketing surveillance system. Another finding showed that drugs frequently had to be removed from the marketplace or required a warning label because of newly discovered adverse drug reactions after they were marketed. Between 1975 and 2000, the investigation discovered that ten percent of all drugs marketed subsequently required the addition of a serious warning and three percent had to be withdrawn from the market altogether. Clearly, the data provided for drug approval too often does not detect important and even life-threatening problems with a drug. This accusation is not confined to the U.S. A U.K. physician and pharmaceutical consultant, R. Shah stated in a 2006 paper that during the past 16 years, 38 different drugs had been withdrawn from major markets world-side due to safety concerns.

A tragic example of what can happen is illustrated by the use of Propulsid, a drug for a rather insignificant problem (heartburn). At the time of approval the FDA was aware of only minor side effects caused by the drug, and certainly nothing life-threatening. Although approved for adults in 1993, there was no warning about the drug's use in children. Although children died in the clinical trials, the data apparently were not sufficient to include a warning in the labeling against use in children. Once on the market pediatricians prescribed it for infants. The number of deaths led to the removal of Propulsid in 2000, but not before the heartbreaking loss of 24 children under age 6.

The Postmarketing Surveillance System

It is not just important, it is essential to monitor the safety of marketed drugs with the utmost care. Learning more about a drug becomes a mandatory public responsibility that falls to primarily to FDA's postmarketing surveillance system (PMS). How to protect the public from previously unrecognized harmful adverse drug reactions is a most demanding assignment. The crucial question becomes; is the FDA up to the challenge?

After drug approval and marketing, the FDA uses different mechanisms to gather information about a drug's performance in the real world. One requirement for an approved drug is for manufacturers to submit all the adverse reaction reports they receive to the FDA. In addition to industry reports, the PMS program also allows health professionals and the public to voluntarily report adverse reactions and problems. The FDA's voluntary reporting system is far from perfect because it expects others (e.g. busy doctors) to send information to them using a cumbersome process. Predictably, instead of a big jump in the number of non-industry reports, there is only a trickle. Healthcare professional submissions account for less than 1 percent of the 300,000 accumulated reports FDA receives each year. Not surprisingly as few as one percent of all the adverse reactions physicians see are sent on to the FDA. Regrettably, the quality of the information collected tends to be low as well.

FDA physicians and epidemiologists evaluate the reports to identify safety issues. When the agency discovers a problem it informs the drug manufacturer that a warning should to be added to the product's labeling. It may also decide that the manufacturer should send a "Dear Doctor" letter that warms doctors and others of a new drug risk. If there are alarming or life-threatening effects, the agency may conclude that a drug's risks outweigh its benefits and it is too dangerous to remain on the market.

The PMS effort focuses on safety and that is as it should be. The presence or absence of safety issues is much harder to investigate in Phase III trials than efficacy. Furthermore, once on the market an ineffective drug can be discovered more quickly than an unsafe drug. A drug that fails to help a patient isn't going to be tried too many times before a physician stops writing prescriptions for it Thus, the market has a way of relegating inferior products to an obscure market share. As a result, postmarketing surveillance concentrates on establishing safety, especially finding the uncommon but deadly adverse event.

A 2002 survey asked FDA scientists what they thought about the about the agency's program to monitor marketed drugs. Conducted by the Health and Human Services Department's Inspector General, the results revealed that the majority of workers had significant doubts about its adequacy. In addition, a third of those polled were not even particularly confident of the FDA's ability to assess the safety of drugs in the first place.

The judgments and actions by the FDA were also challenged by a survey conducted by the Union of Concerned Scientists that was released in 2006. Approximately one-fifth of the nearly 1,000 FDA scientists surveyed said that they had been asked, for nonscientific reasons, to exclude or alter technical information as well as modifying the conclusions they had reached. Twenty percent said that they were asked explicitly by FDA decision-makers to provide incomplete, inaccurate or misleading information to the public, industry, the media and government officials.

In addition, external FDA critics add their claims concerning the quality of FDA's postmarketing surveillance system. Their complaints include:

- Too much reliance on voluntary reporting by health care professionals.
- Poor quality of the reports submitted.
- Under reporting of adverse reaction outcomes.
- Difficulty in calculating rates of adverse events because of incomplete data.
- Limited ability for spontaneous reports to establish causal relationships.

Other concerns about PMS is that it is slow to react and requires expensive resources to come to a conclusion. There's no question that analyzes of post-marketing data are time consuming and tedious. However, information technology improvements that might fill some of the gaps have not always been exploited. There have been organizational concerns as well. Staff, who had a role in approving drugs, also participated in decisions about keeping drugs on the market that they may have approved in the first place. Could they render an impartial judgment in that situation?

The answer came in 2005, when the FDA, responding to its critics, announced the creation of a new safety board – an "independent" body to more aggressively monitor the safety of drugs on the market. The Drug Safety Oversight Board would include FDA officials, but none who approved new drugs. The omission of new drug reviewers on the board made sense because as noted above, these individuals might be hesitant to take tough positions on marketed drugs since such actions implied they made a mistake when they approved the drug in the first place. Generally, the new body was met with approval, but an editorial in the *New York Times* complained that although no drug reviewers would be allowed on the board, the board was not fully independent since most members would be FDA staffers. They also lamented the fact that too little money was allocated to upgrade the monitoring effort. The absence of a commitment to give the FDA the power to act against drugs that had already won marketing approval was even more disturbing. The editorial also chided the administration for not seeking greater legal authority to force manufacturers to conduct postmarketing tests when safety concerns arose.

The medical community also reacted to the FDA plan. The FDA move appeared to some as being too little too late. One of the most prestigious medical journals published an unusually harsh editorial opposing the board. According to the *New England Journal of Medicine*, the creation of the board was just more internal restructuring by the FDA. The editorial took the agency and the pharmaceutical industry to task for not adequately protecting the public from unsafe drugs.

Back in 1998, the *Journal of the American Medical Association* and the *New England Journal of Medicine*, arguable two most prominent journals in the U.S., had called for a truly independent drug safety board to monitor the drug safety program. The proposal visualized a board fully detached from the FDA. It was felt an independent board was essential to ensure objectivity and avoid conflicts of interest. A recommended alternative would use the model followed in the airlines industry. In that approach, the Federal Aviation Administration (FAA) set standards for airlines and the National Transportation Administration investigated airline accidents and identified flaws with FAA standards.

Behind the uproar was a belief by FDA skeptics that until drug safety became as important as approving drugs quickly, the fundamental monitoring problems would remain and the availability of unsafe drugs would continue on the market too long. From the FDA perspective, establishing an independent board would amount to an admission that the FDA had paid too little attention to drug risks, focusing instead on speeding new products to market. Support for this contention came from an analysis that appeared in the *Journal of Law and Economics* on the effect of the policy reforms put in place to accelerate the evaluation of new drugs. The article noted that by 2002, review time had fallen by as much as 50 percent, but that improvement was associated with an increase in adverse drug reactions resulting in deaths and patient hospitalizations.

A 2005 conference at NIH with the imposing title of "Moving from Observational Studies to Clinical Trials: Why Do We Sometimes Get It Wrong?", highlighted concern over the inability to identify harmful drug effects in a timely fashion. The warning by Dr. E. Zerhouni, Director of the NIH was clear – failure to spot serious side effects of drugs was eroding public trust. The FDA was essentially censored for its failure to give equal weight to safety as it did to the efficacy of medicines.

Analyzing the System

By 2006, disturbed by the run of bad news about drug withdrawals and poor oversight of pharmaceuticals companies, a number of reports appeared aimed at both changing the FDA and improving the integrity of clinical research. Each report shed light on issues pointing to unsatisfactory FDA performance.

A report by the Governmental Accounting Office (GAO) took the FDA to task for disorganization, infighting and failure to force drug makers to conduct needed safety tests. In addition to the FDA's weak emphasis on the postmarketing drug-safety program, the general quality of clinical trials sponsored by drug manufacturers leading up to drug approval were also criticized. The spotlight fell on the failure to detect serious adverse drug reactions. The GAO report confirmed many of the handicaps that led to the need for a strong PMS – there were too few subjects in clinical trials to detect serious adverse reactions in the clinical trials leading to an approval and that too often, the studies were carried out on homogeneous population that did not reflect the full range of patients who would eventually take the drug.

The next report appeared in September, written by a committee of the distinguished Institute of Medicine (IOM). This evaluation titled "The Future of Drug Safety" called for a stronger system of drug regulation. The authors, skilled researchers in multiple disciplines, charged that speedy approvals and poor safety oversight had made the U.S. patient population the world's testing ground for new drugs. Among the many recommendations, there was an urgent call for a more timely use of side effect information throughout the entire drug approval process so harmful drugs could be identified and eliminated before they could harm people. The authors argued that under current operations, after a drug was approved there appeared to be little effort to follow up with informative postmarketing studies. It was easy to interpret the implications of the assessment – a drug approval came with many unanswered question about the drug, especially its safety. Additional active research following approval was necessary to answer the unresolved issues.

In October the next commentary appeared, authored by members of FDA's own Drug Safety and Risk Management Advisory Committee. It called for Congress to step in and overhaul the agency. The authors repeated many of the criticisms directed at the FDA by the other reports, but added some new important ones as well. Some typical examples included accusing the FDA of allowing massive under-reporting of adverse reactions, having an ineffective safety oversight structure and a lack of expertise and resources to insure drug safety.

The FDA responded to these critical reports pointing out the strategies they had and were implementing to improve the PMS operation. For instance, they would continue to develop ways to increase the frequency of adverse reports from health care professionals. Reports would be filed by fax, telephone and the Internet as well as the conventional mail system. The FDA also created ways to expand the base of potential reporters. It reached out to the health care professionals stressing the importance of recognizing and reporting serious adverse events. The outreach program included Internet appeals, speeches, articles and exhibits. The FDA developed educational programs directed at the public that emphasized the importance of patients sharing drug problems with their physicians and urging the doctors to send in reports. The FDA also worked with health maintenance organizations and governmental agencies that had large databases (e.g. Medicare records) to tap into the rich resources they had to detect drug safety problems in a timely manner.

In January 2007, the agency made its initial response to the IOM assessment describing plans to improve its operations. The reaction to the FDA plan was mixed. A positive assessment said that the plan was an important step in the right direction. Others were dismayed because what the FDA had in mind fell short of expectations. For example, frustrations were evident with the FDA's reaction to the IOM's recommendation to conduct an in-depth analysis of adverse drug reaction reports within 18 months of a drug's launch. The FDA answer to this was a pilot program that would take a year to create, 18-months to gather data and then additional time to conduct the analysis.

The *New England Journal of Medicine* reacted to this plan with an article entitled, "Sidelining Safety – The FDA's Inadequate Response to the IOM," in which it said the FDA's response once again highlighted the low priority it assigns to its responsibility for arbitrating drug safety. They concluded that the FDA's response to the IOM report demonstrated a lack of understanding of the magnitude of the changes required to create a culture of safety.

A New Approach to Post Marketing Surveillance

The system in place for post marketing monitoring relies primarily on one method; gathering case reports and then trying to make sense out of them. The truth is we need all our arsenal of research methods to help us meet the postmarketing challenge – the cohort study, the clinical trial and case reports. I believe the best strategy requires the use of each method.

Cohort Trial

By virtue of its unique advantages, the cohort trial could be a powerful tool in a new postmarketing environment. As new drugs enter the marketplace, patients with the target illness or condition would be encouraged to join a cohort group. For instance, there would be a cohort for patients with diabetes, rheumatoid arthritis, AIDS, etc. Initially new cohort groups would have to be established for each disease, but over time it would only be necessary to maintain the cohort. Obviously, members of a cohort will be on different treatment, and perhaps some receiving no treatment at all. They are therefore an excellent source to maintain, investigate and evaluate adverse reactions and other issues related to marketed drugs. The cohort trials would need to be run by research centers not directly connected to either the pharmaceutical industry or the FDA. An excellent example is the Center for Education and Research on Therapeutics (CERT) an organization currently consisting of 11 research centers and a coordinating center. The CERT organization is administered by the Agency for Health Care Research and Quality, an agency within the Department of Health and Human Services. The lion share of costs for the cohort program would be paid by the drug company on a prorated basis based on the proportion of patients in a cohort taking its drug.

This approach takes advantage of the cohort's ability to find potent adverse reactions in a reasonable amount of time. Confirmation of the findings might require clinical trials or other means to support a cause and effect relationship, but at a minimum there would be an early alert about possible harm and allow the medical community to take appropriate action.

A good example of what can be accomplished using the cohort paradigm involved a multicenter safety study of three different drug as well as patients who received no treatment. The study, conducted by the Ischemia Research and Education Foundation, enrolled over 4,000 patients from many medical practices in various parts of the world. The data showed a clear-cut connection between one of the study drugs, aprotinin, and serious end-organ damage. A *New England Journal of Medicine* editorial praised the study as an example of what can be achieved in a postmarketing setting. Subsequently, the FDA performed a review of aprotinin, which culminated in the manufacturer suspending marketing of the product.

Clinical Trial

One place for a clinical trial in the post-marketing period would be to investigate a major health risk discovered by a required cohort trial. Such trials would have to be carefully justified because of their the cost and length. However, as illustrated by the hormone replacement confusion, they may be the only way to settle a controversy that has huge health ramifications.

A more common role will be to provide the assurances needed for drugs that have received an accelerated approval. These Phase IV trials would be mandatory and sponsors must be required to perform them in a timely manner in order to address problems left unanswered during the premarketing research phase.

Another category of clinical trials should also be mandated. For patients, their doctors, and health insurers it is critical to know how the efficacy and safety of a new medication measures up to the best available alternative. Again, these competitive drug studies should occur post-approval and be paid for by the companies whose products are tested. The design and execution of such trials are best left to impartial research centers. Again CERTs, mentioned previously, could be the type of research groups that would be able to carry out these trials.

CASE REPORTS. Collecting case reports is crucial in sifting out adverse reactions and cannot be abandoned. The FDA needs to continue to enhance their case report system and improve the drug safety monitoring system. For example, as recommended by Congress new drug applications should contain a risk evaluation and mitigation strategy that would lay out a post-marketing safety surveillance plan. In addition, a public-private partnership should be established to speed the development of a new generation of predictive tools to increase safety and speed product development

A prototype of what can be accomplished in the surveillance of case reports merits attention. There are impressive results from a project called RADAR (Research on Adverse Drug Events and Reports). A multidisciplinary team of independent researchers work together to evaluate initial reports of previously unrecognized, but serious reactions. They develop possible explanations on data collected from multiple sources (e.g. case series reports, physician correspondence, published trials, unpublished trials, FDA databases and manufacturer sales figures). Core investigators located at various centers throughout the U.S. hold meetings to discuss issues that surface. The teams, funded by NIH and the American Cancer society, prepare summary safety information and send it to the FDA and drug maker. The results may also appear in medical journals or at medical conferences.

In addition to these steps, international cooperation is another avenue that needs to be pursued. The WHO is in the position to be a pivotal player in gathering drug related problems from multiple sources and sharing the information with participating nations. The FDA must continue to innovate and be mindful of ways to enhance the case reporting system using worldwide resources.

In conclusion, the book's title, *Its Great – Oops No It Isn't*, emphasizes that there are still many unknowns when the FDA approves a new medical treatment.

Based on what they know at the time of approval a new product looks .... well *great*. The FDA declares it to be safe and effective, the manufacturer emphasizes its strengths and its researchers highly recommend it. Then we run into the post-marketing phase and the *oops* begins.

It is important that interest in medical research not be focused primarily on the pre-approval period. Look at all the things we don't know about a drug when it hits the market and only find out later – months and years after a drug is released. Some of the news is going to be bad. When a serious problem is revealed, perhaps we should be grateful. The recommendations of this chapter are designed to find severe problems that went unrecognized at the time of a drug's approval as quickly as possible. The sooner we discover unsafe reactions, the sooner we can reduce pain and suffering. The quicker we identify harmful effects, the more lives we save.

Chapter 25
Regulatory Reform – Changes Needed

Abstract The weaknesses of the postmarketing surveillance (PMS) system weren't the only problem the FDA had. Another burning issue was poor supervision of postmarketing studies that were to be conducted in return for an accelerated product review and approval. It was found that the agency had allowed drug companies to renege on performing the postmarketing trials. Analyses indicated that almost half of the promised studies remained unfinished. While the FDA had made enormous strides in improving the time to approve products, it had neglected its postmarketing responsibilities. This situation occurred because under a user-fee agreement, the industry paid the FDA to review their marketing application, but the money was only for functions related to those applications. In the meantime, the overall FDA budget was being cut and those reductions had a serious effect on other programs such as PMS. The downfall of Vioxx, a top selling pain drug illustrated the deepening negative image of the FDA. Congressional hearings and press stories painted a picture of overly aggressive drug marketing and negligent regulation by the FDA. Corrective action by Congress led to passage of the FDA Revitalization Act giving the agency the power to deal with many of the postmarketing problems it faced.

Keywords FDA budget · FDA Revitalization Act · postmarketing studies · prescription drug user fee · Vioxx

The weaknesses of the PMS system that could delay detection of harmful medicines wasn't the only problem the FDA had when it came to the post-marketing period. Another burning issue arose that could be traced to the early approval of promising products for life-threatening diseases. The regulatory reforms, that led to NDA fast tracking and accelerated approvals, were instituted by the FDA for a very sound reason – speeding up the approval of these vitally useful drugs. The steps the FDA had taken were considered highly successful since they made valuable drugs available to consumers sooner than if they had to meet the usually NDA approval requirements. The clinical trials, that would normally have been required as part of an NDA for other drugs, were allowed to be conducted as Phase IV trials after a fast track drug was on the market. However, the FDA's performance came under attack in 2005 when extraordinary news broke that the agency had allowed drug companies to renege on performing the Phase IV trials they promised to do if they received an early approval.

There were early signs that there could be trouble in the accelerated approval program. A 1996 report by the Inspector General of the Health and Human Services Department showed that that the percentage of new drugs with postmarketing study commitments was increasing. An FDA report to Congress in 2002 found a similar trend. However, the 2005 finding of a low level of completion of the postmarketing studies commitments came as a shock. Congress was especially alarmed and reasoned that the deficit in completed post-marketing trial commitments was due to lax regulation by the FDA. Lending fire to the criticism was a chilling detailed report by C. Bennett, and other Northwestern University researchers, that appeared that same year. They found that the FDA had requested follow-up studies for 26 drugs, but a disturbing two-thirds of those had not been carried out. Some of the delinquent trials had been pending for over a decade. Nevertheless, those studies were not classified as "delayed" because the agency had never set a specific time for the studies to be performed or completed. The Northwester researcher's report also pointed out that the FDA had yet to rescind an approval even when the follow-up findings from a Phase IV study were disappointing. In the eyes of an increasing number, the FDA was too soft. Critics argued that if a follow-up study was not done by a designated time, the sponsor should lose its drug approval designation.

In addition, there was also concern about the low number of subjects treated at the time of an expedited review. Almost two-thirds of cancer drugs receiving an accelerated approval included less than 200 patients, a number most would consider quite inadequate for drawing conclusions about safety. Four of the drugs approved for cancer treatment had a total of 472 treated patients for an average of 118 subjects per drug. Again, a woefully inadequate sample size to detect a rare but deadly adverse reaction.

Criticism of the agency continued to roll in. One 2005 report from a U.S. Congressman (E. Markey) was particularly damaging. He independently conducted a detailed analysis of FDA's postmarketing records and found that 42 of 91 promised postmarketing studies remained unfinished. Even the Department of Health and Human Services, the governmental agency that housed the FDA, faulted the agency. An Inspector General report in 2006 said the FDA simply did not know the status of many post-approval studies promised by drug makers. The Inspector General went on to say that the FDA needed to improve its monitoring of the studies by upgrading its tracking systems and, based on interviews with FDA staff, it concluded that monitoring the committed studies was not considered a top FDA priority.

From the industry point of view, there are mixed feelings about conducting clinical trials after a drug is granted marketing approval. Pharmaceutical firms eagerly conduct many offensive trials after a product is approved. Offensive trials are undertaken to expand the drug's sales (e.g. acquire a new indication or a new formulation). Most defensive trials commence because there is a potentially serious problem with a drug, and are frequently forced upon a company by the FDA. Defensive studies are also carried out when pressure from the medical community compels a company to act. For the industry, the "best" result from a defensive trial is a negative finding – the drug does not do this or cause that. At best, the study maintains the drug's market share, but at considerable cost and consternation.

Pharmaceutical companies are well aware that research isn't perfect and an untoward finding in a defensive study could do irreparable damage to a perfectly good product. Add to that, the trial expense, estimated on average to be about $4 million per trial, and it's easy to see why drug makers are reluctant to invest in post marketing studies. Furthermore, ambitious researchers aren't interested in the studies because the benefits to them pale compared to the chance of studying a new breakthrough drug that may bring fame and fortune. It can also be extremely difficult to obtain subjects for postmarketing RABCOT studies. For instance, few cancer patients are willing to risk enrolling in a study that might result in their receiving a placebo. After all, they can easily get an active drug at their oncologist's office.

Because of the poor response by companies to undertake follow-up studies, there were calls for the FDA to reduce the breaks given to manufacturers. There are interest groups on both sides of this issue, but the pleas from those supporting the accelerated approval process dominate. Their position may resonate more with the public at large and legislatures, as well, when they argue that patients may die if there are delays in providing access to life-saving drugs.

Writing in *JAMA*, B. Strom suggested that in order to mitigate the unrecognized harmful effects of a drug, its entry into the marketplace should be slowed. This could be accomplished by introducing a new phase called a "conditional approval." When a drug was initially approved, its use would be restricted (e.g., no direct-to-consumer advertising and a statement added to the drug's label that the drug had been studied in only a limited number of patients). This condition would not be removed until the number of exposed patients reached a predetermined limit (e.g. 30,000) and all safety questions raised from the pre-approval clinical trials were addressed. In essence, drug availability would be restricted until there was adequate evidence of safety. There would be plenty of opposition to this approach led by the pharmaceutical manufacturers. Plus it would only work if, for the given indication, there were alternative drugs available to patients. Nevertheless, option such as conditional approvals have merit and deserve serious consideration.

Awash in bad publicity once again, the FDA defended itself. The agency argued that for a long time it did not have the power to require postmarketing studies. It was not until 1992, that the FDA received authority to require Phase IV follow-up studies. This authority applied to drugs that received accelerated NDA status and those that could be used in pediatric patients. Prior to that time, if the agency felt a Phase IV trials was required, it included a statement in the letter approving the drug asking the sponsor to conduct such studies. Without enforcement powers, however, the stipulation was in reality a "gentleman's agreement". This latter condition still applied to the post marketing Phase IV trials that were approved by the customary rather than the accelerated process.

The FDA also faced a legitimate resource problem that affected Phase IV studies, the PMS program and almost all its other functions. The one activity in which adequate resources were assured was reviewing and approving NDAs. Under the

1992 user-fee agreement, the industry promised to give the agency millions of dollars to reduce the time it took to conduct new drug application reviews. However, the agency could spend the money only on functions related to new drug approvals. This stipulation assured the industry that its cash would be spent on evaluating their drugs and not simply doled out to staff assigned other duties. Starting at about 50 percent of the overall budget, new drug approval activities grew to over 80 percent of FDA's budget in the first 10 years of the user-fee program. However, what wasn't anticipated was that Congressional support for the agency as a whole would shrink. As Congress slashed FDA's budget, cuts had to be made somewhere: there were no sacred cows and programs dealing with the safety of marketed drugs were hit.

In response to the cuts, FDA officials eliminated half of the scientists in the agency's drug laboratories and slashed the budget for new equipment. There was more. The agency dropped many projects they had with academics to scrutinize marketed drug problems. Independent scientists had long helped the agency to not only identify possible problems, but also to perform tests to help solve them. The termination of contracts for this valuable kind of scientific detective work did not have to do with performance or need – it simply had to do with the lack of funds. The agency was forced to reduce outside grants, raided money set aside for furniture and cut travel budgets. No question, the many FDA responsibilities focused on the postmarketing period suffered from the Congressional budget cuts.

Former and current FDA officials, outside scientists and patient advocates believed the agency compromised its ability to monitor the harmful effects of marketed drugs because, through the user-fee program, the White House and Congress forced a marriage between the agency and industry. FDA budget restrictions became a bipartisan endeavor as Democratic and Republican administrations happily participated in the financial onslaught.

The FDA was not the only party criticized for the number of drugs that had to be removed from the market. Criticisms was also focused on the pharmaceutical industry. It was assailed for the massive expenditures used to advertise and promote medicines. Drug companies were faulted for their lack of diligence when it came to collecting, evaluating, and reporting data from postmarketing studies. There were charges that drug manufacturers concealed data that could signal the possibility of major drug risks and that they were reluctant to follow-up on the potential risks they uncovered. The behavior by the drug industry motivated a bill in the 2005 Congress that would have sent drug industry CEOs to jail for at least 20 years and pay a fine of up to $2 million if they knowingly concealed serious adverse drug experiences associated with their products. In addition, the CEOs would be required to attest that all evidence of serious adverse effects for an approved drug had been disclosed. The bill was never voted on and never became law.

The Vioxx Saga

Because of lax regulatory enforcement by the FDA and poor supervision of their products by industry, the number of their detractors only increased. The deepening negative image of the FDA and the drug industry it regulated, was heightened by the astonishing downfall of a hugely successful pharmaceutical product – Vioxx.

Vioxx, a drug used in the treatment of rheumatoid arthritis and other conditions in which pain relief was important, was considered a breakthrough when it came onto the market in 1999. Produced by Merck, a prominent manufacturer and one of the most successful companies in the industry, the filing to gain approval was a large one by FDA standards. Over 5,000 patients had been studied. Almost 400 subjects had been on the drug for at least one year and some had been on it for up to 86 weeks. In spite of this impressive résumé, the dangerous problem that would demolish Vioxx was not detected at the time the NDA was approved.

Vioxx belonged to a class of drugs, called Cox 2 inhibitors, that offered a great deal of promise. However, once on the market, Vioxx would be up against a set of well-entrenched pain drugs – aspirin, Aleve, ibuprofen, etc. – and they had been around a long time and could be purchased at a very low price. In addition, the consumer could buy these cheaper drugs without a prescription. As a class, these over-the-counter agents were quite effective, but there was a chance that they could cause gastrointestinal side effects. Research showed that the Cox drugs would not be more effective, but they would be better tolerated, and that was a promising marketing advantage.

The already crowded pain relief market became very heated by the introduction of Vioxx. Contributing to the calamity that was about to unfold was the fact that prescription drugs were advertised directly to the consumer. Because Vioxx had no efficacy advantage over the older drugs on the market – it would require a lot of promotion to make it more attractive. In addition, Vioxx had no recognized advantage over other Cox 2 drugs that were entering the market, (Celebrex and Bextra) so there was another incentive to promote the drug heavily. By 2003, the aggressive marketing of the drug appeared to be well worth the cost. Worldwide sales reached an impressive $2.5 billion. The company estimated that 20 million patients took Vioxx.

Not all the news, however, was good. A year after gaining approval, a red flag appeared based on a study the company itself designed to show Vioxx was better tolerated than an older drug. The comparison drug for the study, referred to as VIGOR, was naproxen but, better known by one of its trade names, Aleve. Although the study demonstrated that Vioxx had a lower incidence of serious gastrointestinal events, there was a higher rate of cardiovascular problems with Vioxx. But the trial did not include a placebo group and, as a result, it was very hard to interpret. You could conclude that Vioxx was risky or that naproxen had a protective cardiovascular effect. Without a placebo control group, it was impossible to tell whether Vioxx was hazardous or naproxen was beneficial. The makers of Vioxx chose to believe that naproxen protected the heart – a choice that allowed them to continue to promote their product vigorously.

In 2001, in response to the cardiovascular problem exposed by VIGOR, an FDA advisory panel convened by the agency recommended that a warning be included in the labeling for Vioxx that mentioned the cardiovascular problems. However, it took over a year before the FDA and Merck agreed on labeling changes that incorporated a cardiovascular warning.

In 2002 and 2004, exploratory studies had found a higher rate of cardiovascular problems with Vioxx. One of the trials was led by researchers from Harvard and the other involved over a million patients from the health maintenance organization, Kaiser Permanente. However, Merck maintained that these case-control studies were too vulnerable to error and only evidence from a RABCOT could be trusted. The possibility of conducting such a trial was investigated and rejected by the company. Any such trial would have to be extremely large and a definitive answer would not be forthcoming for many years. After the fact, a FDA representative also questioned if such a study would even be ethical. Giving subjects a drug to see if they contract heart and blood vessel abnormalities places subjects at a risk for harm with too few offsetting benefits.

In September, 2004 the company found out that once again one of their own RABCOT studies, an attempt to find a new indication for the drug, had backfired. A trial, started in 2000, set out to determine whether Vioxx could prevent nodules in the colon of patients that could lead to colon cancer. This trial was stopped prematurely because twice as many subjects on Vioxx, this time compared to placebo, developed heart problems. In fact, out of 2,600 subjects enrolled in the trial relatively few experienced a stroke or heart attack, so although there was a two-fold difference (estimated to be 15 on Vioxx versus 7.5 on placebo) the risk that an individual patient would suffer a heart attack or stroke related to Vioxx was very small. However, the two-fold difference was a crippling finding given the millions of patients taking the drug. One week after ending the trial, the company withdrew Vioxx from the U.S., and more than 80 other countries where it was marketed. The company maintained that they had acted responsibly – they withdrew Vioxx voluntarily as soon as it was clear that the drug was harmful.

The ramifications from the withdrawal were stunning – thousands of lawsuits were filed against Merck, possibly costing the company billions of dollars. In addition, Congress stirred by the plethora of negative stories in the press held hearings about the case. Hearings by the powerful Senate Finance Committee produced harsh criticism of the FDA. Witnesses and committee members charged the FDA with delaying too long to add a cardiovascular warning and allowing Merck too much control over what was stated in the Vioxx labeling. There were also claims that the original approval for Vioxx was rushed and the agency's reluctance to act on safety problems was because it didn't want to cast doubts on its original approval decision.

An article in the *New England Journal of Medicine*, by H. Waxman, a leading U.S. Congressman, reported results from hearings in the House on why drugs such as Vioxx could remain popular in spite of a serious safety issue. The hearings contained a litany of deceptive marketing devices used by Merck to bolster the sales of Vioxx. Merck was chastised for giving physicians, their sales staff called on, misleading and incomplete information about Vioxx's risk. In addition, selective evidence and biased presentations, were use to get doctors to ignore potential harms associated with Vioxx.

Critics saw the saga of Vioxx as a case of overly vigorous marketing by a company and negligent regulation on the part of the FDA. Major medical figures and Congressional leaders faulted the FDA, claiming the agency was passive and simply didn't do enough to discover and remedy the cardiovascular problem. Merck, critics said, was overly promoting the drug not only by its manipulation of information given to doctors, but through its aggressive consumer advertising campaign as well. Merck countered, no, its consumer advertising campaigns were created to heighten consumer awareness about drugs, not to manipulate them so more drug could be sold. The exchange only reinforced a question about the way drugs are marketed, raising fears that the public doesn't receive clear and balanced information.

Ironically, the Vioxx case offers a good example of how a catastrophic side effect can go undiscovered with the present approval and post-approval systems. Although there is ample evidence to fault Merck in this case, it's also true that the FDA failed. It's also relevant to ask: without the clinical trial that convinced all the players that there was a cardiovascular problem, how long would it have taken the PMS operation to find the problem and then FDA to act?

The Vioxx collapse led to a flurry of criticism by the some of the same members of Congress who had cut the FDA budget. An internal FDA whistleblower, D. Graham who was a physician in the FDA's Office of Drug Safety, and prominent medical journals made news when they accused the agency for the Vioxx mess alluding to the possibility that the FDA was too cozy with drug makers. Graham became a media favorite and his criticisms of the FDA received a great deal of press. For example, he appeared on 60 Minutes where he lamented the fact that drug approval personnel received all the attention and had all the power at FDA and those like himself, who were in a different unit that worried about safety, received little notice and had no power.

FDA Revitalization

Thankfully, Congress took a good hard look at the FDA. Particular help was clearly needed to improve regulatory control in the postmarketing period. Congress responded – in September, 2007 the House and Senate past major regulatory legislation, the FDA Revitalization Act, which was signed into law by President George W. Bush. It gave the FDA the power to deal with many of the concerns its critics raised, such as:

• Order warnings on drug labels
• Require a review of drug ads before they air on television
• Register and make results of drug clinical trials publicly available
• Reduce the number of FDA expert advisers who have industry ties
• Require studies of a new drugs' performance
• Probe patient databases for early signs of side effects

This law is a step in the right direction, providing the agency is also given the funds to conduct these important duties. However, more needs to be done. The programs described in the last chapter: improving the collection and utilization of case reports, using cohort trial to monitor newly approved drugs and insisting on comparative clinical trials are needed to truly protect the public from harmful products.

Chapter 26
Journey's End – A Call for Action

Abstract The book ends with a call for readers to become more informed and engaged in the clinical research enterprise. We live in a society in which medical science frequently decrees not only whether we live or die, but how we live and die. The public has as much right to participate in these decisions as any medical expert. Professionals and non-professionals may clash on what the best path for medical research is, but deliberation and dispute enriches both parties. The public's lack of knowledge means it is excluded from any debate about improving how medical research is done or used. Healthcare professionals should lead the way in becoming better informed about clinical trials and the public will follow their lead. It's ironic that people, in spite of their complacency, believe they should have a lot of influence on how governmental funds for medical research are spent. One poll found that only scientists were considered more important than the public. And this new role for the citizenry is absolutely legitimate – after all it's their health that is at stake

Keywords Healthcare professionals · health research priorities · medical research funding · medical research goals · public participation.

The National Institutes of Health should focus on educational strategies to help patients and communities better understand clinical research. This will help scientists because educating the public will empower and prepare individuals to be informed partners in the clinical research process. (National Institutes of Health Director's Council of Public Representatives)

If you remember only one thing from this book, let it be that reliance on a single study is unreasonable for no study can be comprehensive enough to provide answers to the multitude of questions that need to be answered. Researchers must explore questions about drug efficacy and safety in different ways, never relying on the findings from a single trial. The answers generated from a series of investigations cumulate and interact to give us more complete knowledge about how a human being will respond to a new medical intervention. The more drug research conducted, the better perspectives and understanding we will have.

You should come also away with something else. That something else requires action on your part. Currently clinical research is an enterprise in which the vast majority of people have little or no knowledge. It may not be surprising that pharmaceutical companies and even many researchers like it that way. How could anyone without scientific training understand medical research? However, the public's lack of knowledge means it is rightfully excluded from any debate about improving how medical research is done or used.

It doesn't have to stay that way. The American public does not have to remain an innocent under-educated and defenseless bystander. Healthcare professionals should lead the way in becoming better informed about clinical trial and the public will follow their lead. When that happens citizens no longer will have to play a passive role in how drugs enter and leave the marketplace. Remember the AIDS activists who essentially forced the FDA to change its standards for approving drugs.

Obviously, public participation does not mean the average citizen will play a role in the design, conduct or analysis of medical research investigations – those functions must be done by the talented and competent researchers that now carry out these activities. But healthcare workers and the other influential members of society should become contributing players when it comes to deciding things like (1) the diseases and medical conditions that require the most attention and (2) the best place to assign responsibility for doing postmarketing research and (3) the need to do comparative trials.

We live in a society in which medical science frequently decrees not only whether we live or die, but how we live and die. You and I, our parents and our children have as much right to participate in these decisions as any medical expert. Medical institutions and bureaucratic organizations shouldn't be allowed to exclude us. We should join in the decision-making dialogue. Professionals and non-professionals may clash on what the best path for medical research is, but deliberation and dispute enriches both parties. Regardless of the final resolution, there will be growth and better understanding when there is interaction.

In our lifetime, support for medical research has reached unprecedented levels. It devours over 10 percent of the annual federal budget. On top of that is the billions of dollars spent by the private sector. University research centers, pharmaceutical companies and governmental medical institutions all promote acceleration in spending. Furthermore, these same groups also dominate the regulation of research, the ethical standards for research and the policy issues surrounding research. Under this arrangement, it is imperative to ask: is medical research serving us as well as it should? And to demand that the answer to that question does not come from these same groups who have the most to gain by the present system. Unfortunately, out of complacency too few speak up, but now and then a maverick raises a voice and challenges the medical research establishment. For example, the medical ethicist D. Callahan, argues that it is acceptable to support research that preserves and restores health, but it is not acceptable to simply lengthen a person's life. We need more mavericks to join the debate. We also need to hear from more citizens in and out of the healthcare field.

Medical research is everybody's business. The impact from research is not confined to one area – medical science. The outcomes from medial research touch social, environmental, technological and behavioral arenas as well. Therefore, it makes sense to have more than one core discipline participate in setting priorities and making decisions. Other specialists also should have a role, the practicing doctors, healthcare teachers, nurses, social workers, pharmacists and above all the patients who in the end are the ones that matter most. A greater opportunity for input from all these sectors leads to more robust debate and a more responsible research policy.

Indeed, the involvement of a broad-based public in any debate about clinical research can and should expand. Informed citizens should have a say in the formulation of the research agenda, but that voice is rarely heard. It's ironic that people, in spite of their complacency, believe they should have a lot of influence on how governmental funds for medical research are spent. One poll found that 41 percent of the public say patients should have the most influence in how funds are spent. Only scientists had a higher percent (50) and elected officials came in with a dreary 5 percent. It's true, knowledgeable consumers can make a valuable contribution in assessing research studies, establishing the standards for drug approvals and insisting on studies that have more practical value. But to play those roles they first have to become knowledgeable.

On a personal level, each person should feel free to ask about treatments their doctor decides they should take. This is especially critical when new drugs become available. Is the doctor familiar with the research that supports the use of the drug? As a nation, we believe in technology and always want to be among the first to benefit from the most recent advances. This attitude carries over to the choice of medicines where Americans and their doctors want access to any new treatment that comes along, even though the data to support the treatment's efficacy may be tenuous and its safety profile woefully incomplete. Patients need to take a greater role in educating themselves about the uncertainties associated with drugs, especially the newest ones. Citizens who get more involved in their medical care will be healthier citizens. Informed citizens through social pressure, their elected officials, and direct communications can help in the drive to have the pharmaceutical industry provide better, more complete, and relevant evidence about the clinical trial results they sponsor. A truly informed public can extend their scope and encourage clinical researchers to focus their assessments on outcomes that are crucial to them and their health care.

I now close our exploration into medical research. I hope you have enjoyed your journey. As an educator, my aim in writing this book is to give people information, but more than that, to cultivate an awareness about the process through which medical advances are studied and brought to needy patients. When asked – what do you want from medical research? – we all need to give a confident answer. There are a variety of measures to judge that goal. For the medical professional it may be the number of lives saved. For the person with an incurable disease it may be the quality of life that's left. For the sick child it may be curing a disease. For the public health official it may be reducing costs through innovation. In coming to an answer you too have a legitimate role to play – after all it is your health that is at stake.

Notes/Bibliography

The Information, ideas and recommendations presented in this book come from many sources. In some cases the text contains a specific references (e.g. to a journal article), but in many discussions the material is derived from a variety of general sources which can serve as a reading list. Consequently, these notes, contain "cited references" and "general references" with a separate listing provided for each chapter.

Chapter 1 – Medical Research

Cited References

Association of Clinical Research Organizations. Phase III trials most costly, survey finds. http://www.acrohealth.org/KeyIssues.php?id=1&page=4 Oct 26, 2006.

Fisher R. *Smoking: the cancer controversy*. Edinburgh, UK: Oliver & Boyd, 1959.

Kaprio J, Koskenvuo M. Twins, smoking and mortality: a 12 year prospective study of smoking discordant for cigarette smoking. *Soc Sci Med* 1989:29;1083–1089.

Kripke D, Garfinkel L, Wingard D, et al. Mortality associated with sleep duration and insomnia. *Arch Gen Psychiat* 2002:59;131–136.

General References

Brown B. Statistics, scientific method, and smoking. in Tansur J. (ed). *Statistics: a guide to the unknown*. Oakland, CA: Holden-Day, 1978.

California HealthCare Foundation. *Snapshot healthcare costs* 2006:101. http://72.14.205.104/search?q=cache:pxyMqUxMgQsJ:www.chcf.org/documents/insurance/HealthCareCosts06.pdf + health + care + spending + breakdown&hl=en&ct=clnk&cd=1&gl=us#23 Jan 15, 2006.

Carmelli D, Page W. Twenty-four year mortality in World War II male veteran twins discordant for cigarette smoking. *Int J Epidemiol* 1996:25;554–559.

Center for Science in the Public Interest. US: how Dr. Weil, Dr. Phil, and Larry King turn your trust into cash. http://www.corpwatch.org/article.php?id=13159 Jan 25, 2006.

Charlton B. Mega-trials: Methodological issues and clinical implications. *J R Coll Physicians Lond* 1995:29;96–100.

Doll R. Uncovering the effects of smoking. *Stat Methods Med Res* 1998:7;87–117.

Gehlbach S. *Interpreting the medical literature*. New York: McGraw-Hill, 2002.

Simon H, Controversies and clear thinking. *Newsweek* June 16, 2003:61.

Mann C. Observational research methods. Research design II: cohort, cross sectional, and case-control studies. *Emerg Med J* 2003:20;54–60.

Medical Research Council. Streptomycin in Tuberculosis Trials Committee. Streptomycin treatment for pulmonary tuberculosis. *Br Med J* 1948:ii;769–782.

Meyer J. How cigarettes became a national craze; and lung cancer, once rare, emerged as the leading cancer killer. *Washington Post* May 11, 1993:Z14.

Ornstein R, Sobel D. *The healing brain: breakthrough discoveries about how the brain keeps us healthy*. New York: Simon & Schuster, 1989.

Pearl R. Tobacco smoking and longevity. *Science* 1938:87;216–217.

Vandenbroucke J. In defense of case reports and case series. *Ann Intern Med* 2002:134;330–334.

Chapter 2 – The Case-Control Method

General References

Brody J. A study guide to scientific studies. *New York Times* Aug 11,1998:7F.

Grimes D, Schulz K. Compared to what? Finding controls for case-control studies. *Lancet* 2005:365;1429–1433.

Herman J. Experiment and observation. *Lancet* 1994:344;1209–1211.

Hill G, Connelly J, Hebert R, et al. Neyman's bias re-visited. *J Clin Epidemiol* 2003:56;293–296.

Nelson N. *Epidemiology in a nutshell*. National Cancer Institute. http://www.cancer.gov/newscenter/benchmarks-vol2-issue7/page2 Jul 8, 2002.

Schulz K, Grimes D. Case control studies: research in reverse. *Lancet* 2002:359;431–434.

Wynder E, Stellman S. Artificial sweetener use and bladder cancer: a case-control study. *Science* 1980:207;1214–1216.

Chapter 3 – The Cohort Study

Cited References

Cannon C, Braunwald E, McCabe C, et al. Intensive versus moderate lipid lowering with statins after acute coronary syndromes. *New Engl J Med* 2004:350;1495–1504.

Grodstein F. Stampfer M, Manson J, et al. Postmenopausal estrogen and progestin use and the risk of cardiovascular disease. *New Engl J Med* 1996:335;453–461.

Kaiser Permanente Division of Research. DOR in the news. http://www.dor.kaiser.org/dors/ news/ newshomepage.shtml#TopOfPage Mar 15, 2007.

National Institutes of Health. *Framingham heart study*. http://www.nhlbi.nih.gov/about/ framingham/index.html Dec 21, 2002.

Stampfer M, Willett W, Colditz G, et al. A prospective study of postmenopausal estrogen therapy and coronary heart disease. *New Engl J Med* 1985:313;1044–1049.

Vaccarino V, Krumholz H. Risk factors for cardiovascular disease: one down, many more to evaluate. *Ann Intern Med* 1999:131;62–63.

General References

Black N. Why we need observational studies to evaluate the effectiveness of health care. *Br Med J* 1996:312;1215–1218.

Brody J. A study guide to scientific studies. *New York Times* Aug 11, 1998:7F.

Colditz G, Hankinson S, Hunter D, et al. The use of estrogens and progestins and the risk of breast cancer in postmenopausal women. *New Engl J Med* 1995:332;1589–1593.

Colditz G, Rosner B, Speizer F. Risk factors for breast cancer according to family history of breast cancer. *J Natl Cancer I* 1996:88;1003–1004.

Felson D, Kiel D, Anderson J, et al. Alcohol consumption and hip fractures: the Framingham study. *Amer J Epidemiol* 1988:128;1102–1110.

Grady D, Hulley S. Hormones to prevent coronary disease in women: when are observational studies adequate evidence? *Ann Intern Med* 2000:133;999–1001.

Hankinson S, Manson J, Speizer F, et al. (eds). *Healthy women, healthy lives: a guide to preventing disease, from the landmark Nurses' health study.* New York: Simon & Schuster. 2001.

Harvard Medical School. *Nurses' health study.* http://www.channing. harvard.edu/nhs/index.html Feb 1, 2005.

Hu F, Bronner L, Willett W, et al. Dietary fat intake and the risk of coronary heart disease in women. *New Engl J Med* 1997:337;1491–1499.

Kolata G. New conclusions on cholesterol. *New York Times* Mar 9, 2004a:A1.

Kolata G. Scientists begin to question benefit of 'good' cholesterol. *New York Times* Mar 14, 2004b:A1.

National Institutes of Health. National cholesterol education program. http://www.nhlbi.nih. gov/ guidelinescholesterol/atp3xsum.pdf/May 15, 2001.

Stampfer M, Colditz G, Willett W, et al. Postmenopausal estrogen therapy and cardiovascular disease. Ten-year follow-up from the nurses' health study. *New Engl J Med* 1991:325;756–762.

Szalavitz M. Risk: how HRT went from miracle therapy to health risk. STATS at George Mason University. http://www.stats.org/index.jsp Feb 27, 2006.

Szczcech L, Coladonato J, Owen W. Study designs and their potential influence on conclusions. *Semin Dial* 2002:15;207–211.

Talk of the Nation: Science Friday. *Framingham heart study.* http://www.sciencefriday.com/ pages/1998/Sep/hour2_092598.html Sep 25, 1998.

Chapter 4 – The Clinical Trial

Cited References

Brown D. Clinical trials fighting blindness. *The Braille Monitor.* http://209.85.165.104/ search?q=cache:1XDyrlEpgewJ:www.nfb.org/Images/nfb/Publications/bm/bm05/bm0507/ bm050711.htm + oxygen + blind + children + premature + babies + prevalence&hl=en&ct=c lnk&cd=3&gl=us July 15, 2005

Hill A. The clinical trial. *Br Med Bull* 1951:7;278–282.

General References

Gottlieb S. Bone marrow transplants do not help in breast cancer. *Br Med J* 1999:318;1093.

Grimes D, Schulz K. An overview of clinical research: the lay of the land. *Lancet* 2002:359; 57–61.

National Cancer Institute. Breast cancer transplant trials continue to show no benefit.
    http://72.14.205.104/search?q=cache:27y2QcQ9SLkJ:www.cancer.gov/asco2001/highlights +
    2001 + asco + transplant + breast + cancer + Breast + Cancer + Transplant + Trials + Continue
    + to + Show + No + Benefit&hl=en&ct=clnk&cd=2&gl=us May 12, 2001.
Shaywitz D, Ausiello D. The necessary risks of medical research. *New York Times* July 29, 2001:4.4.
Twyman R. *A brief history of clinical trials.* Wellcome Trust. http://genome. welcome.ac.uk/
    doc_WTD020948.html. Sep 22, 2004.

Chapter 5 – Comparing the Methods

Cited References

Sackett D, Wennberg J. Choosing the best research design for each question. *Br Med J*
    1997:315;1636.

General References

Barton S. Which clinical studies provide the best evidence? *Br Med J* 2000:321;255–256.
Benson K, Hartz A. A comparison of observational and randomized clinical trials. *New Engl J
    Med* 2000:342;1878–1886.
Concato J, Shah N, Horowitz R. Randomized, controlled trials, observational studies and the
    hierarchy of research designs. *New Engl J Med* 2000:342;1887–1892.
Giacomini M, Cook D. User's guides to medical literature: XXII. Qualitative research in health
    care. *JAMA* 2000:284;357–362.
Green J, Britten N. Qualitative research and evidence based medicine. *Br Med J*
    1998:316;1230–1232.
Nelson N. Epidemiology in a nutshell. National Cancer Institute. http://www.cancer.gov/ news-
    center/benchmarks-vol2-issue7/page2 Jul 8, 2002.
Sackett D. The competing objectives of randomized trials. *New Engl J Med*
    1980:303;1059–1060.

Chapter 6 – The Protocol

Cited References

Baker K, Brand D, Hen J. Classifying asthma: disagreement among specialists. *Chest*
    2003:124;2156–2163.
Bellomo R, Ronco C, Kellum J, et al. Acute renal failure – definition, outcome measures, animal
    models, fluid therapy and information technology needs: the Second International Consensus
    Conference of the Acute Dialysis Quality Initiative (ADQI) Group. *Crit Care*
    2004:8;R204–R212.
Blum A, Chalmers T. The Lugano statements on controlled clinical trials. *J Int Med Res*
    1987:15;2–22.
Cummings S, Chapurlat R. What PROOF proves about calcitonin and clinical trials. *Am J Med*
    2000:109;330–331.

Fredrickson D. The field trial: some thoughts on the indispensable ordeal. *Bull NY Acad Med* 1968:44;985–993.

Hennekens C, Peto R, Hutchison G, et al. An overview of the British and American aspirin studies. *New Engl J Med* 1988:318;923–924.

Horwitz R. Complexity and contradiction in clinical trials research. *Am J Med* 1987:82;498–510.

Pincus T. Rheumatoid arthritis: disappointing long-term outcomes despite successful short-term clinical trials. *Clin Epidemiol* 1988:41;1037–1041.

Sackett D. Bias in analytical research. *J Chronic Dis* 1979:32;51–63.

Shelton D. Patients in clinical trials don't always follow the program. *Am Med News* Sep 11, 2000:28.

Quitkin F. Placebos, drug effects, and study design: a clinician's guide. *Am J Psychiat* 1999:156;829–836.

General References

Flick S. Managing attrition in clinical research. *Clin Psychol Rev* 1988:8;499–515.

Liu M, Davis K. *Lessons from a horse named Jim: a clinical trials manual from the Duke Clinical Research Institute*. Durham, NC: Duke Clinical Research Institute, 2001.

Vogelson C. Signing on and staying in. *Mod Drug Discov* 2001:4;24–25.

Chapter 7 – The Control Groups

Cited References

Chalmers I, Toth B. Thomas Graham Balfour's 1854 report of a clinical trial of belladonna given to prevent scarlet fever. The James Lind Library. http://www.jameslindlibrary.org/trial_records/19th_Century/balfour/balfour_commentary.html Apr 12, 2007.

Food and Drug Administration. Center for Drug Evaluation and Research. http://www. fda.gov/CDER/GUIDANCE/4155fnl.htm#P222_10018 May 15, 2001.

Gotzsche P. Methodology and overt and hidden bias in reports of 196 double blind trials of non-steroidal antinflamatory drugs in rheumatoid arthritis. *Control Clin Trials* 1989:10;31–56.

Horwitz R. Complexity and contradiction in clinical trials research. *Am J Med* 1987:82;498–510.

Hrobjartsson A, Gotzsche P. The controlled clinical trial turns 100 years: Fibiger's trial of serum treatment of diphtheria. *Br Med J* 1998:317;1243–1245.

Sacks H, Chalmers T, Smith H. Randomized versus historical controls for clinical trials. *Am J Med* 1982:72;233–240.

Tramer M, Reynolds D, Moore R, et al. When placebo controlled trials are essential and equivalence trials are inadequate. *Br Med J* 1998:317;875–880.

General References

Beecher H. The powerful placebo. *JAMA* 1955:159;1602–1606.

Brooks M. 13 things that do not make sense. *New Scientist*. http://www.newscientist.com/ article.ns?id=mg18524911.600 Apr 21, 2007.

Brown W. The placebo effect. *Sci Am* 1998:278;90–95.

Chalmers I. Comparing like with like: some historical milestones in the evolution of methods to create unbiased comparison groups in therapeutic experiments. *Int J Epidemiol* 2001:30;1156–1164.

Hrobjartsson A, Gotzsche P. Is the placebo powerless? An analysis of clinical trials comparing placebo with no treatment. *New Engl J Med* 2001:344;1594–1602.

Lamb G. If placebos work, should doctors use them? *Christian Sci Monit* Apr 17, 2005:13.

Rothman K, Michels K. The continuing unethical use of placebo controls. *New Engl J Med* 1994:331;394–398.

Simon R. Are placebo-controlled clinical trials ethical or needed when alternative treatment exists? *Ann Intern Med* 2000:133;474–475.

Talbot M. The placebo prescription. *New York Times* Jan 9, 2000:34.

Temple R, Ellenberg S. Placebo-controlled trials and active-control trials in the evaluation of new treatments. Part 1 Ethical. *Ann Intern Med* 2000:133;455–463.

Wager T, Rilling J, Smith E, et al. Placebo-induced changes in fMRI in the anticipation and experience of pain. *Science* 2004:303;1162–1167.

Chapter 8 – Measurements

Cited References

Cardiac Arrhythmia Suppression Trial (CAST) II Investigators. Effect of the antiarrhythmic agent moricizine on survival after myocardial infarction. *New Engl J Med* 1992:327;227–233.

Freemantle N, Calvert M, Wood J, et al. Composite outcomes in randomized trials: greater precision but with greater uncertainty? *JAMA* 2003:289;2554–2559.

Gotzsche P. Methodology and overt and hidden bias in reports of 196 double blind trials double-blind trials of nonsteroidal antiinflammatory drugs in rheumatoid arthritis. *Control Clin Trials* 1989:10;31–56.

McIntosh V, Jordan J, Carter F, et al. Three psychotherapies for anorexia nervosa: a randomized, controlled trial. *Am J Psychiat* 2005:162;741–747.

Rothman K. Significance questing. *Ann Intern Med* 1986:105;445–447.

Rothwell P. External validity of randomised controlled trials: "To whom do the results of this trial apply?" *Lancet* 2005:365;82–93.

Thornley B, Adams C. Content and quality of 2000 controlled trials in schizophrenia over 50 years. *Br Med J* 1998:317;1181–1184.

General References

Editorial. Measurement imprecision. *Lancet* 1992:339;587–588.

Fleming T, Demets D. Surrogate end points in clinical trials: are we being misled? *Ann Intern Med* 1996:125;605–613.

Fogg L, Gross D. Threats to validity in randomized clinical trials. *Res Nurs Health* 2000:23;79–87.

Furberg C. To whom do the research findings apply? *Heart* 2002:87;570–574.

Guyatt G, Naylor C, Juniper E, et al. How to use articles about health-related quality of life. *JAMA* 1997:277;1232–1237.

Harris G. New drug points up problems in developing cancer cures. *New York Times* Dec 21, 2005:A37.

Montori V, Permanyer-Miralda G, Gonzalez I, et al. Validity of composite end points in clinical trials. *Br Med J* 2005:330;594–596.

Simon S. *Statistical evidence in medical trials.* Oxford: Oxford University Press, 2006.
Welsford M, Morrison L. Defining the outcome measures for out-of-hospital trials in acute pulmonary edema. *Acad Emerg Med* 2002:9;983–988.

Chapter 9 – Bias Control

Cited References

Bigby M, Gadenne A. Understanding and evaluating clinical trials. *J Am Acad Dermatol* 1996:34;555–590.
Bingel A. Über Behandlung der Diphtherie mit gewöhnlichem Pferdeserum. *Deutsch Arch Klin Med* 1918:125;284–332.
Fisher S, Greenberg R. How sound is the double-blind design for evaluating psychotropic drugs? *J Nerv Ment Dis* 1993:181;345–350.
Gluud L. Bias in clinical intervention research. *Am J Epidemiol* 2006:163;493–501.
Greenberg R, Bornstein R, Zborowski M, et al. A meta-analysis of Fluoxetine outcome in the treatment of depression. *J Nerv Ment Dis* 1994:182;547–551.
Hewitt C, Hahn S, Torgerson D, et al. Adequacy and reporting of allocation concealment: review of recent trials published in four general medical journals. *Br Med J* 2005:330;1057–1058.
Horgan J. Placebo nation. *New York Times* Mar 21,1999:15 section 4.
Ioannidis J, Anna-Bettina H, Maroudia P, et al. Comparison of evidence of treatment effects in randomized and nonrandomized studies. *JAMA* 2001:286;821–830.
Klotter J. Double blind clinical trials. *Townsend Letter for Doctors and Patients.* June 2002:27–28.
Kodish E, Eder M, Noll R, et al. Communication of randomization in childhood leukemia trials. *JAMA* 2004:291;470–475.
National Cancer Institute. Introduction to clinical trials. www.nci.nih.gov/clinicaltrials/learning/ Oct 12, 2004.
Schulz K. Subverting randomization in controlled trials. *JAMA* 1995:274;1456–1468.
Walizer M. *Research methods and analysis searching for relationships.* New York: Harper & Row, 1978.

General References

Altman D. Comparability of randomised groups. *Statistician* 1985:34;125–136.
Altman D, Schulz K, Moher D, et al. The revised CONSORT statement for reporting randomized trials: explanation and elaboration. *Ann Intern Med* 2001:134;663–694.
Chalmers I. Comparing like with like: some historical milestones in the evolution of methods to create unbiased comparison groups in therapeutic experiments. *Int J Epidemiol* 2001:30;1156–1164.
Day S, Altman D. Blinding in clinical trials and other studies. *Br Med J* 2000:321;504.
Even C, Siobud-Dorocant E, Dardennes R. Critical approach to antidepressant trials. *Br J Psychiat* 2000:177;47–51.
Gill T. Blinded by science. *Lancet* 1994:343;553–554.
Gluud L. Bias in clinical intervention research. *Am J Epidemiol* 2006:163;493–501.
Gotzsche P. Blinding during data analysis and writing of manuscripts. *Control Clin Trials* 1996:17;285–290.
Horgan J. Placebo nation. *New York Times* Mar 21,1999:15.
Kaptchuk T. Intentional ignorance: a history of blind assessment and placebo controls in medicine. *B Hist Med* 1998:72;389–433.

Roberts C, Torgerson D. Understanding controlled trials. Baseline imbalance in randomised controlled trials. *Br Med J* 1999:319;185.

Schulz K, Grimes D. Allocation concealment in randomised trials: defending against deciphering. *Lancet* 2002:359;614–618.

Schulz K, Chalmers I, Altman D. The landscape and lexicon of blinding in randomized trials. *Ann Intern Med* 2002:136;254–259.

Chapter 10 – Utility

Cited References

Hlatky M, Califf R, Harrell F, et al. Comparison of predictions based on observational data with the results of randomized controlled trials of coronary artery bypass surgery. *J Am Coll Cardiol* 1988:11;237–245.

Horton R. Common sense and figures: the rhetoric of validity in medicine. *Stat Med* 2000:19;3149–3164.

Paasche-Orlow M, Taylor H, Brancati F. Readability standards for informed-consent forms as compared with actual readability. *New Engl J Med* 2003:348;721–726.

Patel M, Doku V, Tennakoon L. Challenges in recruitment of research participants. *Adv Psychiat Tr* 2003:9;229–238.

Pieters M, Jennekens-Schinkel A, Schoemaker H. Self-selection for personality variables among healthy volunteers. *Br J Pharmacol* 1992:33;101–106.

Sackett D, Wennberg J. Choosing the best research design for each question. *Br Med J* 1997:315;1636.

Tishler C, Bartholomae S. Repeat participation among normal healthy research volunteers. Professional guinea pigs in clinical trials? *Perspect Biol Med* 2003:46;508–520.

Woods S, Ziedonis D, Sernyak M, et al. Characteristics of participants and nonparticipants in medication trials for treatment of schizophrenia. *Psychiat Serv* 2000:51;79–84.

General References

Alger A. Trials and tribulations. *Forbes* May 17, 1999:316.

Avorn J. *Powerful medicines: the benefits, risks and costs of prescription drugs.* New York: Knopf, 2004.

Black N. Why we need observational studies to evaluate the effectiveness of health care. *Br Med J* 1996:312;1215–1218.

Blum A, Chalmers T. The Lugano statements on controlled clinical trials. *J Int Med Res* 198:15;2–22.

Centerwatch. Clinical trials—a very human enterprise. http://www.centerwatch.com/patient/ifcn_01.html#Section5 May 15, 2007.

Chalmers T. Ethical implications of rejecting patients for clinical trials. *JAMA* 1990:263;825–830.

Ferriman A. Medical ethics: trials and errors. Are doctors being forced to inflict unwanted information. *The Guardian* May 13, 1998:T008.

Furberg C. To whom do the research findings apply? *Heart* 2002:87;570–574.

Horton R. The clinical trial: deceitful, disputable, unbelievable, unhelpful, and shameful—what next? *Control Clin Trials* 2001:22;593–604.

Ridker P, Cook N, Lee I, et al. A randomized trial of low-dose aspirin in the primary prevention of cardiovascular disease in women. *New Eng J Med* 2005:352;1293–1304.

Rothwell P. Can overall results of clinical trials be applied to all patients? *Lancet* 1995:345;1616–1619.

Rothwell P. External valSidity of randomised controlled trials: "To whom do the results of this trial apply?" *Lancet* 2005:365;82–93.

Rothwell P. Factors that can affect the external validity of randomised controlled trials. *PLoS Clin Trials* 2006:1;e9.

Chapter 11 – Research Discrimination

Cited References

Chalmers T. Ethical implications of rejecting patients for clinical trials. *JAMA* 1990:263;825–830.

Groopman J. The pediatric gap. *The New Yorker* Jan 10, 2005:32.

Peterson E, Lytle B, Biswas M, et al. Willingness to participate in cardiac trials. *Am J Geriatr Cardiol* 2004:13;11–15.

Ridker P, Cook N, Lee I, et al. A randomized trial of low-dose aspirin in the primary prevention of cardiovascular disease in women. *New Eng J Med* 2005:352;1293–1304.

Rochon P, Berger P, Gordon M. The evolution of clinical trials: inclusion and representation. *Can Med Assoc J* 1998:159;1373–1374.

Sternberg S. A bitter pill for older patients; excluded from drug trials, the elderly face unknown risks. *USA Today* May 5, 2005:D1.

General References

Baker B. Assessing the risks, benefits of clinical trials. *AARP Bull Online.* http://www.aarp.org / bulletin/yourhealth/Articles/a2003-07-11-clinicaltrials.html June 30, 2006.

Blum A, Chalmers T. The Lugano statements on controlled clinical trials. *J Int Med Res* 1987:15;2–22.

Caschetta M, Chavkin W, McGovern T. FDA policy on women in drug trials *New Engl J Med* 1993:329;1815–1816.

Centerwatch. Clinical trials—a very human enterprise. http://www.centerwatch.com/patient/ifcn _ 01.html#Section5 Feb 15, 2005.

Christie B. Doctors revise declaration of Helsinki. *Br Med J* 2000:321;913.

Food and Drug Administration. Drug research and children. http://www.fda.gov/fdac/special/ test-tubetopatient/children.html Feb 1, 2003.

Food and Drug Administration. Medication and older people. http://www.fda.gov/fdac/features /1997/697_old.html Sept 15, 2003.

Friedman M. Women and minorities guidance requirements. Food and Drug Administration. Center for Drug Evaluation and Research http://www.fda.gov/CDER/guidance/ women.pdf July 20, 1998.

Gauch R. *Statistical methods for researchers made very simple.* Lanham, MD: University Press of America2000.

Greeley A. Concern about AIDS in minority communities. Food and Drug Administration. http:// www.fda.gov/fdac/features/095_aids.html Dec 15, 1995.

Lowe C. Pediatrics: proper utilization of children as research subjects. *Ann NY Acad Sci* 1970:169;337–344.

Lurie P, Wolfe M. Unethical trials of interventions to reduce perinatal transmission of the human immunodeficiency virus in developing countries. *New Engl J Med* 1997:337;853–856.

Mastroianni A, Faber R. *Women and health research: ethical and legal issues of including women in clinical studies.* Washington, DC: National Academic Press. 1994.

Merkatz R, Temple R, Sobel S, et al. Women in clinical trials of new drugs -- a change in food and drug administration policy. *New Engl J Med* 1993:329;292–296.

Merton V. The exclusion of pregnant, pregnable and once-pregnant people (a.k.a. women) from biomedical research. *Am J Law Med* 1993:19;369–451.

Okie S. Minorities less likely to be in HIV trials. Study finds divide in treatment access. *Washington Post* May 2, 2002:A3.

Pickering T. Why is hypertension more common in African Americans? *J Clin Hypertension* 2001:3;50–52.

Society for Women's Health Research. Sex difference in response to pharmaceuticals, tobacco and illicit drugs. http://www.womenshealthresearch.org/site/PageServer?pagename=hs_ facts _dat Aug 30, 2006.

Stein R. A gap in knowledge about kids' medication. *Washington Post* Nov 23, 2007:A1.

Stolberg S. U.S. AIDS research in poor nations raises outcry on ethics. *New York Times* Sep 18, 1997:A1.

Stotland N. Gender-based biology. *Amer J Psychiat* 2001:158;2093–2094.

Strom B, Melmon K, Miettinen O. Post-marketing studies of drug efficacy: why? *Am J Med* 1985:78;475–480.

Studdert D, Brennan T. Clinical trials in developing countries: scientific and ethical issues. *Med J Australia* 1998:169;545–548.

Wenger N. Exclusion of the elderly and women from coronary trials: is their quality of care compromised? *JAMA* 1992:268;1460–1461.

Chapter 12 – Seven Deadly Flaws

Cited References

Blum A, Chalmers T. The Lugano statements on controlled clinical trials. *J Int Med Res* 1987:15;2–22.

Carey B. Study pursues a genetic link to depression. *New York Times* Dec 10, 2004:A36.

Cochrane A. Effectiveness and efficiency: random reflections on health services. Abingdon, UK: *The Nuffield Provincial Hospitals Trust,* 1972.

Editorial. Cranberg L (ed). Evaluating new treatments. *Br Med J* 1998:317;1260.

Freiman J, Chalmers T, Smith H, et al. The importance of beta, the type II error and sample size in the design and interpretation of the randomized control trial. Survey of 71 "negative" trials. *New Engl J Med* 1978:299;690–694.

Furukawa T, Streiner D, Hori S. Discrepancies among megatrials. *J Clin Epidemiol* 2000:53;1193–1199.

Halpern S, Karlawish J, Berlin J. The continuing unethical conduct of underpowered clinical trials. *JAMA* 2002:288;358–362.

Hemminki E. Quality of clinical trials - a concern of three decades. *Methods Inf Med* 1982:21;81–85.

Ioannidis J. Why most published research findings are false. *PLoS Med* 2005:2;e124.

General References

Baum M. Contribution of randomised controlled trials to understanding and management of early breast cancer. *Br Med J* 1999:319;568–571.

Ely J. Confounding bias and effect modification in epidemiologic research. *Fam Med* 1992:24;222–225.

Peto R, Baigent C. Trials: the next 50 years: large scale randomized evidence of moderate benefits. *Br Med J* 1998:317;1170–1171.

Chapter 13 – Statistics

Cited References

Alderson P, Chalmers I. Research pointers: survey of claims of effect in abstracts of Cochrane reviews. *Br Med J* 2003:326;475.

Marks H. *The progress of experiment: science and therapeutic reform in the United States.* Cambridge: Cambridge University Press, 1997.

Moher D, Dulberg C, Wells G. Statistical power, sample size, and their reporting in randomized controlled trials. *JAMA* 1994:272;122–124.

Rothstein J. Much ado about probability. *Phys Ther* 1990:70;535–536.

General References

Altman D. *Practical statistics for medical research.* London: Chapman & Hall, 1990.

Altman D, Bland J. Absence of evidence is not evidence of absence. *Br Med J* 1995:311;485.

Beyea S, Nicoll L. An overview of statistical and clinical significance in nursing research. *AORN J* 1997:65;1129–1130.

Fisher R. *Statistical methods for research workers.* New York: Macmillan, 1970.

Gauch R. *Statistical methods for researchers made very simple.* Lanham, MD: University Press of America, 2000.

Willenheimer R. Statistical significance versus clinical relevance in cardiovascular medicine. *Prog Cardiovasc Dis* 2001:44;155–167.

Chapter 14 – Analysis Issues

Cited References

Altman D. The scandal of poor medical research. *Br Med J* 1994:308;283–284.

CONSORT Handbook. 12. Statistical methods. http://www.consort-statement.org/index.aspx?o=1029 Jan 3, 2003.

Djulbegovic B, Iztok H. When should potentially false research findings be considered acceptable? *PLoS Med* 2007:4;e26.

Goodman S, Greenland S. Why most published research findings are false: problems in the analysis. *PLoS Med* 2007:4;e168.

Hollis S, Campbell F. What is meant by intention to treat analysis? Survey of published randomised controlled trials. *Br Med J* 1999:319;670–674.

Ioannidis J. Why most published research findings are false. *PLoS Med* 2005:2;e124.

Ioannidis J. Evolution and translation of research findings: from bench to where? *PLoS Clin Trials* 2006:1;e36.

Johansen H, Gøtzsche P. Problems in the design and reporting of trials of antifungal agents encountered during meta-analysis. *JAMA* 1999:282;1752–1759.

Pauker S. The clinical interpretation of research. *PLoS Med* 2005:2;e395.

PLoS Medicine Editors. Minimizing mistakes and embracing uncertainty. *PLoS Med* 2005:2;e272.

Shaywitz D. Science and shams. *Boston Globe*. http://www.boston.com/news/science/articles/2006/07/27/science_and_shams/ July 27, 2006.

Shrier I. Power, reliability, and heterogeneous results. *PLoS Med* 2005:2;e386.

Wren J. Truth, probability, and frameworks. *PLoS Med* 2005:2;e361.

Yusuf S, Wittes J, Probstfield J, et al. Analysis and interpretation of treatment effects in subgroups of patient. *JAMA* 1991:266;93–98.

General References

Assmann S, Pocock S, Enos L, et al. Subgroup analysis and other (mis)uses of baseline data in clinical trials. *Lancet* 2000:355;1064–1069.

Cochrane Handbook. 8.4 Intention to treat issues. http://www.cochrane.dk/cochrane/handbook/8_analysing_and_presenting_results/8.4_intention_to_treat_issues.htm Sep 7, 2004.

Ellenberg JH. Intent-to-treat analysis versus as-treated analysis. , Newport Beach, CA: Drug Information Association, Jan 30, 1994.

Ioannidis J. Author's reply. *PLoS Med* 2005:2;e398.

Johansen H, Gøtzsche P. Problems in the design and reporting of trials of antifungal agents encountered during meta-analysis. *JAMA* 1999:282;1752–1759.

Science Daily. Is most published research really false? http://72.14.205.104/search?q=cache:FEm9qpS9llcJ:www.sciencedaily.com/releases/2007/02/070227105745.htm + %22Is + most + published + research + really + false%3F%22&hl=en&ct=clnk&cd=1&gl=us Feb 27, 2007.

Simon S. *Statistical evidence in medical trials*. Oxford: Oxford University Press, 2006.

Chapter 15 – The Meta Analysis

Cited References

Egger M, Smith G. Misleading meta-analysis. *Br Med J* 1995:310;752–754.

Egger M, Smith G. Meta-analysis: potentials and promise. *Br Med J* 1997:315;1371–1374.

Egger M, Smith G. Meta-analysis bias in location and selection of studies. *Br Med J* 1998:316;51–66.

Grady D. Medical journal cites misleading research. *New York Times* Nov 10, 1999:A18.

LeLorier L, Grégoire G, Benhaddad A, et al. Discrepancies between meta-analyses and subsequent large randomized, controlled trials. *New Engl J Med* 1997:337;536–542.

Simon S. *Statistical evidence in medical trials*. Oxford: Oxford University Press, 2006.

Smith G, Egger M. Meta-analysis: unresolved issues and future developments. *Br Med J* 1998:316;221–225.

General References

Clarke M, Stewart L. Obtaining data from randomised controlled trials: how much do we need for reliable and informative meta-analyses? *Br Med J* 1994:309;1007–1010.

Egger M, Smith G, Phillips A. Meta-analysis: principles and procedures. *Br Med J* 1997:315;1533–1537.

Egger M, Smith G, Altman D. (eds). *Systematic reviews in health care: meta-analysis in context.* London: British Medical Journal Publishing Group, 2001.

Egger M, Smith G, Sterne J. Uses and abuses of meta-analysis. *Clinl Med* 2001:1;478–484.

Gerbarg Z, Horwitz R. Resolving conflicting clinical trials: guidelines for meta-analysis. *J Clin Epidemiol* 41:5;503–509.

Naylor C. Meta-analysis and the meta-epidemiology of clinical research. *Br Med J* 1997:15;617–619.

Chapter 16 – Research Results that Clashed

Cited References

Mammography References

Alexander F, Anderson T, Brown H, et al. The Edinburgh randomised trial of breast cancer screening: results after 10 years of follow-up. *Br J Cancer* 1994:70;542–548.

Commentary. Letters to the editor. Cochrane review on screening for breast cancer with mammography. *Lancet* 2001:358;2164.

Gotzsche P, Olsen O. Is screening for breast cancer with mammography justifiable? *Lancet* 2000:355;129–134.

Kerlikowske K, Grady D, Rubin S, et al. Efficacy of screening mammography: a meta-analysis. *JAMA* 1995:11;149–154.

Mayor S. Swedish study questions mammography screening programmes. *Br Med J* 1999:318;621.

Miller A, Baines C, To T, et al. Canadian national breast screening study: 1. Breast cancer detection and death rates among women aged 40 to 49 years. *Can Med Assoc J* 1992:147;1459–1476.

Nystrom L, Rutqvist L, Wall S, et al. Breast cancer screening with mammography: overview of Swedish randomised studies. *Lancet* 1993:341;973–978.

Nystrom L, Andersson I, Bjurstam N, et al. Long-term effects of mammography screening: updated overview of the Swedish randomised trials. *Lancet* 2002:359;909–919.

Shapiro S, Venet W, Strax P, et al. Ten- to fourteen-year effect of screening on breast cancer mortality. *J Natl Cancer Inst* 1982:69;349–355.

Dalkon Shield References

Burkman R. Association between intrauterine device and pelvic inflammatory disease. *Obstet Gynecol* 1981:57;269–276.

Christian C. Maternal deaths associated with intrauterine device. *Am J Obstet Gynecol* 1974:119;441–444.

Collaborative Group of the Primary Prevention Project. Low-dose aspirin and vitamin E in people at cardiovascular risk: a randomised trial in general practice. *Lancet* 2001:357;89–95.

Farley T, Rosenberg M, Rowe P, et al. Intrauterine devices and pelvic inflammatory disease: an international perspective. *Lancet* 1992:33;785–788.

Gareen I, Greenland S, Morgenstern H. Intrauterine devices and pelvic inflammatory disease meta analysis of published studies, 1974–1990. *Epidemiol* 2000:11;589–597.

Kromal R, Whitney C, Mumford S. The intrauterine device and pelvic inflammatory disease: the women's health study reanalyzed. *J Clin Epidemiol* 1991:44;109–122.

Mumford S, Kessel E. Was the Dalkon Shield a safe and effective intrauterine device? The conflict between case-control and clinical trial study findings. *Fertil Steril* 1992:57;1151–1176.

Ory H. A review of the association between intrauterine devices and acute pelvic inflammatory disease. *J Reprod Med* 1978:20;200–204.

Aspirin References

Boston Collaborative Drug Surveillance Program. Regular aspirin intake and acute myocardial infarction. *Br Med J* 1974:1;440–444.

Hammond E, Garfinkel L. Aspirin and coronary heart disease: findings of a prospective study. *Br Med J* 1975:2;269–271.

Hansson L, Zanchetti A, Carruthers A, et al. Effects of intensive blood-pressure lowering and low-dose aspirin in patients with hypertension: principal results of the Hypertension Optimal Treatment (HOT) randomised trial. *Lancet* 1998:351;1755–1762.

Hennekens C, Karlson L, Rosner B. A case-control study of regular aspirin use and coronary deaths. *Circulation* 1978:58;35–38.

Jick H, Miettinen O. Regular aspirin use and myocardial infarction. *Br Med J* 1976:1;1057.

Paganini-Hill A, Chao A, Ross R, et al. Aspirin use and chronic diseases: a cohort study of the elderly. *Br Med J* 1989:299;1247–1250.

Peto R, Gray R, Collins R, et al. Randomized trial of prophylactic daily aspirin in British male doctors. *Br Med J* 1988:296;13–16.

Steering Committee of the Physicians' Health Study Research Group. Preliminary report: findings from the aspirin component of the ongoing Physicians' Health Study. *New Engl J Med* 1988:318;262–264.

Steering Committee of the Physicians' Health Study Research Group. Final report on the aspirin component of the ongoing Physicians' Health Study. *New Engl J Med* 1989:321;129–35.

The Medical Research Council's General Practice Research Framework. Thrombosis prevention trial: randomised trial of low-intensity oral anticoagulation with warfarin and low-dose aspirin in the primary prevention of ischaemic heart disease in men at increased risk. *Lancet* 1998:351;233–241.

General References

Mammography References

Farmer C, Kane K. Screening decreases breast cancer-specific deaths but not all-cause mortality. *J Fam Pract* 2002:51;513.

Freedman D, Petitti D, Robins J. On the efficacy of screening for breast cancer. *Int J Epidemiol* 2004:33;43–55.

Goodman S. The mammography dilemma: a crisis for evidence-based medicine. *Ann Intern Med* 2002:137;363–365.

Gotzsche P. Mammographic screening: no reliable supporting evidence? *Lancet* 2002:359;706.

Gotzsche P, Olsen O. Screening mammography reevaluated. *Lancet* 2000:355;752.

Juffs H, Tannock I. Screening trials are even more difficult than we thought they were. *J Natl Cancer Inst* 2002:94;167–173.

Mocharnuk R. Mammography: the screening controversy continues. *38th Annual Meeting of the Am Soc Clin Oncol* 2002 May 18–21, Orlando, FL.

Olsen O, Gotzsche P. Cochrane review on screening for breast cancer with mammography. *Lancet* 2001:358;1340–1342.

Woolf S. Taking critical appraisal to extremes: the need for balance in the evaluation of evidence. *J Fam Pract* 2000:49;1081.

Wright C, Mueller C. Screening mammography and public health policy: the need for perspective. *Lancet* 1995:346;29–32.

Dalkon Shield References

Barron T. IUDs struggle to shake off legacy of past. *Family Plan World* 1992:2;10–11.

Burkman R, Lee N, Ory H, et al. Response to "The intrauterine device and pelvic inflammatory disease: the Women's Health Study reanalyzed." *J Clin Epidemiol* 1991:44;123–125.

Cheng D. Intrauterine device: still misunderstood after all these years. *South Med J* 2000:93;859–864.

Goodhue P. The Dalkon Shield debate. *Conn Med* 1983:47;138–141.

Women's Resource Health Center. What was the Dalkon Shield? http://health.yahoo.com/birth control-overview/what-was-the-dalkon-shield/pdr--Women_wmn_art_00018535.html Jan 1, 2003.

Aspirin References

Agency for Healthcare Research and Quality. U.S. Preventive Services Task Force urges clinicians and patients to discuss aspirin therapy. http://72.14.205.104/search?q=cache:JVcNc OfrpMUJ:www.ahrq.gov/news/press/pr2002/aspirpr.htm + U.S. + Preventive + Services + Task + force + aspirin + use + heart + attack&hl=en&ct=clnk&cd=1&gl=us Jan 14, 2002.

Altman L. New questions on aspirin and heart; two studies produce seemingly contrasting results. *New York Times* Nov 18, 1989:8.

Hennekens C. Update on aspirin in the treatment and prevention of cardiovascular disease. *Am J Manag Care* 2002:22 (Suppl);S691–S700.

Hennekens C, Peto R, Hutchison G, et al. An overview of the British and American aspirin studies. *New Engl J Med* 1988:318;923–924.

Squires S. More confusion over benefits of aspirin use. *Los Angeles Times* Nov 23, 1998:5.

Steinbrook R. Elderly warned about aspirin use medicine: findings in a USC study seem sure to stir controversy. *Los Angeles Times* Nov 18, 1989:32.

Chapter 17 – Hormone Replacement Therapy

Cited References

Bath P, Gray L. Association between hormone replacement therapy and subsequent stroke: a meta-analysis. *Br Med J* 2005:330;342–345.

Bergkvist L, Adami H, Persson I, et al. Risk of breast cancer after estrogen and estrogen-progestin replacement. *New Engl J Med* 1989:321;293–297.

Bush T, Whiteman M. Hormone replacement therapy and risk of breast cancer. *JAMA* 1999:281;2140–2141.

Bush T, Whiteman M, Flaws J. Hormone replacement therapy and breast cancer: a qualitative review. *Obstet Gynecol* 2001:98;498–508.

Centers for Disease Control Cancer and Steroid Hormone Study. Long-term oral contraceptive use and the risk of breast cancer. *JAMA* 1983:249;1591–1595.

Colditz G, Hankinson S, Hunter D, et al. The use of estrogens and progestins and the risk of breast cancer in postmenopausal women. *New Engl J Med* 1995:332;1589–1593.

Coronary Drug Project Research Group. The coronary drug project: findings leading to discontinuation of the 2.5-mg/day estrogen group. *JAMA* 1973:226;652–657.

Ettinger B, Friedman G, Bush T, et al. Reduced mortality associated with long-term postmenopausal estrogen therapy. *Obstet Gynecol* 1996:87;6–12.

Finucane F, Madans J, Bush T, et al. Decreased risk of stroke among postmenopausal hormone users. Results from a national cohort. *Arch Intern Med* 1993:153;73–79.

Grodstein F, Stampfer M, Manson J, et al. Postmenopausal estrogen and progestin use and the risk of cardiovascular disease. *New Engl J Med* 1996:335;453–461.

Grodstein F, Manson J, Colditz G, et al. A prospective, observational study of postmenopausal hormone replacement therapy and primary prevention of cardiovascular disease. *Ann Intern Med* 2000:133;933–941.

Grodstein F, Clarkson T, Manson J. Understanding the divergent data on postmenopausal hormone therapy. *New Engl J Med* 2003:348;645–650.

Hays J, Ockene J, Brunner R, et al. Effects of estrogen plus progestin on health-related quality of life. *New Engl J Med* 2003:348;1839–1854.

Henderson B. The cancer question: an overview of recent epidemiologic and retrospective data. *Am J Obstet Gynecol* 1989:161;1859–1895.

Hoover R, Gray L, Cole P, et al. Menopausal estrogens and breast cancer. *New Engl J Med* 1976:295;401–405.

Hulley S, Grady D, Bush T, et al. Randomized trial of estrogen plus progestin for secondary prevention of coronary heart disease in postmenopausal women. *JAMA* 1998:280;605–613.

Hulley S, Furberg C, Barrett-Connor E, et al. Noncardiovascular disease outcomes during 6.8 years of hormone therapy: Heart and Estrogen/Progestin Replacement Study follow-up (HERS II). *JAMA* 2002:288;58–64.

Humphrey L, Chan B, Sox H. Postmenopausal replacement therapy and the primary prevention of cardiovascular disease. *Ann Intern Med* 2002:137;273–284.

Ioannidis J. Contradicted and initially stronger effects in highly cited clinical research. *JAMA* 2005:294;218–228.

Kittner S, Bousse M. Post-menopausal hormone replacement therapy and stroke risk. *Cephalalgia* 2000:20;208–213.

Kolata G. Scientists debating future of hormone replacement. *New York Times* Oct 23, 2002:A20.

Kolata G. In public health, definitive data can be elusive. *New York Times* Apr 23, 2002:F1.

Kolata G. Hormone therapy, already found to have risks, is now said to lack benefits. *New York Times* Mar 18, 2003:A30.

Kolata G. Health risk to older women is seen in hormone therapy. *New York Times* Apr 4, 2007:A10.

McDermott M, Schmitt B, Wallner E. Impact of medication nonadherence on coronary heart disease outcomes. A critical review. *Arch Intern Med* 1997:157;1921–1929.

Rossouw J, Prentice R, Manson J. Postmenopausal hormone therapy and risk of cardiovascular disease by age and years since menopause. *JAMA* 2007:297;1465–1477.

Sackett D. Hormone relacement therapy: the arrogance of preventive medicine. *Can Med Assoc J* 2002:167;363–364.

Shumaker S, Legault C, Rapp S, et al. Estrogen plus progestin and the incidence of dementia and mild cognitive impairment in postmenopausal women. *JAMA* 2003:289;2651–2662.

Stampfer M, Colditz A. Estrogen replacement therapy and coronary heart disease: a quantitative assessment of the epidemiologic evidence. *Prev Med* 1991:20;47–63.

Stampfer M, Grodstein F. Cardioprotective effect of hormone replacement therapy is not due to selection bias. *Br Med J* 1994:309;808–809.

Stampfer M, Willett W, Colditz G, et al. A prospective study of postmenopausal estrogen therapy and coronary heart disease. *New Engl J Med* 1985:313;1044–1049.

The National Women's Health Network. *The truth about hormone replacement therapy: how to break free from the medical myths of menopause.* Roseville, CA: Prima Publishing, 2002.

U.S. Preventive Services Task Force. Postmenopausal hormone replacement therapy for the primary prevention of chronic conditions: recommendations and rationale. http://www.aafp. org/ afp/20030115/us.html Jan 15, 2003.

Wilson P, Garrison R, Castelli W. Postmenopausal estrogen use, cigarette smoking, and cardiovascular morbidity in women over 50: the Framingham study. *New Engl J Med* 1985:313;1038–1043.

Wilson R. *Feminine forever.* New York: Pocket Books, 1968.

Writing Group for the Women's Health Initiative Investigators. Risks and benefits of estrogen plus progestin in healthy postmenopausal women: principal results from the women's health Initiative randomized controlled trial. *JAMA* 2002:288;321–333.

General References

Barrett-Connor E, Grady D. Hormone replacement therapy, heart disease, and other considerations. *Annu Rev Publ Health* 1998:19;55–72.

Coronary Drug Project Research Group. Influence of adherence to treatment and response of cholesterol on mortality in the coronary drug project. *New Engl J Med* 1980:303;1038–1041.

Garbe E, Suissa S. Issues to debate on the Women's Health Initiative (WHI) study. Hormone replacement therapy and acute coronary outcomes: methodological issues between randomized and observational studies. *Hum Reprod* 2004:19;8–13.

Grady D, Hulley S. Hormones to prevent coronary disease in women: when are observational studies adequate evidence? *Ann Intern Med* 2000:133;999–1001.

Grady D, Rubin S, Petitti D, et al. Hormone therapy to prevent disease and prolong life in postmenopausal women. *Ann Intern Med* 1992:117;1016–1037.

Grady D, Herrington D, Bittner V, et al. Cardiovascular disease outcomes during 6.8 years of hormone therapy: Heart and Estrogen/progestin Replacement Study follow-up (HERS II). *JAMA* 2002:288;49–57.

Hankinson S, Manson J, Speizer F, et al. (eds). *Healthy women, healthy lives: a guide to preventing disease, from the landmark Nurses' Health Study.* New York: Free Press, 2001.

Hemminki E, McPherson K. Impact of postmenopausal hormone therapy on cardiovascular events and cancer: pooled data from clinical trials. *Br Med J* 1997:315;149–153.

Horwitz R. Complexity and contradiction in clinical trials research. *Am J Med* 1987:82;498–510.

Klaiber E, Vogel W, Rako S. A critique of the Women's Health Initiative hormone therapy study. *Fertil Steril* 2005:6;1589–1601.

Manson J, Hsia J, Johnson K, et al. Estrogen plus progestin and the risk of coronary heart disease. *New Engl J Med* 2003:349;523–534.

Michels K. The Women's Health Initiative — curse or blessing? *Int J Epidemiol* 2006:35;814–816.

Persson I, Adami H, Bergkvist L, et al. Risk of endometrial cancer after treatment with estrogens alone or in conjunction with progestogens: results of a prospective study. *Brit Med J* 1989:298;147–151.

Posthuma W, Westendorp R, Vandenbroucke J. Cardioprotective effect of hormone replacement therapy in postmenopausal women: is the evidence biased? *Br Med J* 1994:308;1268–1269.

Rifkind B, Rossouw J. Of designer drugs, magic bullets, and gold standards. *JAMA* 1998:279;1483–1485.

Rothenberg C. The rise and fall of estrogen therapy: the history of HRT. http://leda.law.harvard. edu/leda/data/711/Rothenberg05.pdf Apr 25, 2005.

Tanner L. Hormone heart risks overstated for some. US News and World Reports. http://hosted. ap.org/dynamic/stories/H/HORMONE_RISKS?SITE=DCUSN&SECTION=HEALTH&TE MPLATE=DEFAULT Apr 4, 2007.

Taubes G. Do we really know what makes us healthy? *NY Times Mag* Sep 16, 2007:52.

Chapter 18 – Publishing

Cited References

Altman D, Goodman S, Schroter S. How statistical expertise is used in medical research. *JAMA* 2002:287;2817–2820.

Chan A, Altman D. Identifying outcome reporting bias in randomised trials on PubMed: review of publications and survey of authors. *Br Med J* 2005:330;753.

Chan A, Hróbjartsson A, Haahr M, et al. Empirical evidence for selective reporting of outcomes in randomized trials: comparison of protocols to published articles. *JAMA* 2004:291;2457–2465.

Diamond G, Bax L, Kaul S. Uncertain effects of Rosiglitazone on the risk for myocardial infarction and cardiovascular death. *Ann Intern Med.* Epub http://www.annals.org/cgi/content/abstract/0000605-200710160-00182v1 Aug 7, 2007.

Home P, Pocock S, Beck-Nielsen H. Rosiglitazone evaluated for cardiovascular outcomes — an interim analysis. *New Engl J Med* 2007:357;28–38.

Kassirer J. Reflections on medical journals: has progress made them better? *Ann Intern Med* 2002:137;46–48.

May G, DeMets D, Friedman L, et al. The randomized clinical trial: bias in analysis. *Circulation* 1981:64;669–673.

Nissen S, Wolski K. Effect of Rosiglitazone on the risk of myocardial infarction and death from cardiovascular causes. *New Engl J Med* 2007:356;2457–2471.

Science and technology: sloppy stats shame science. *The Economist* June 5, 2004:371;79.

Smith R, Roberts I. Patient safety requires a new way to publish clinical trials. *PLoS Clin Trials* 2006:1;e6.

General References

Altman D. Poor-quality medical research: what can journals do? *JAMA* 2002:287;2765–2767.

Altman L. When peer review produces unsound science. *New York Times* June 11, 2002:F6.

Altman L. The doctor's world: for science's gatekeepers, a credibility gap. *New York Times* May 2, 2006:F1.

De Angelis C, Drazen J, Frizelle F, et al. Clinical trial registration: a statement from the International Committee of Medical Journal Editors. *New Engl J Med* 2004:351;1250–1251

Editorial. For truth in drug trial reporting. *New York Times* June 20, 2004:412.

Editorial. Manipulating a journal article. *New York Times* Dec 11, 2005 p 4.11.

Fontanarosa P, Flanagin A, DeAngelis C. Reporting conflicts of interest, financial aspects of research, and role of sponsors in funded studies. *JAMA* 2005:294;110–111.

Gorner P. Medical studies make news, worthy or not; researchers see flaws in coverage. *Chicago Tribune* June 5, 2002:110.

Harris G. New York State official sues drug maker over test data. *New York Times* June 3, 2004:A1.

Jefferson T. Effects of editorial peer review: a systematic review. *JAMA* 2002:287;2784–2786.

Korn D, Ehringhaus S. Principles for strengthening the integrity of clinical research. *PLoS Clin Trials* 2006:1;e1.

Meier B. Contracts keep drug research out of reach. *New York Times* Nov 29, 2004;A1.

Meier B. Two studies, two results, and a debate over a drug. *New York Times* June 3, 2004:C1.

Rennie D. Fourth international congress on peer review in biomedical publications. *JAMA* 2002:287;2759–2760.

Specter M. Quality control of published medical studies debated. *Washington Post* May 15, 1989:A20.
Steinbrook R. Registration of clinical trials — voluntary or mandatory? *New Engl J Med* 2004:351;1820–1822.

Chapter 19 – Communicating

Cited References

Moynihan R, Bero L, Ross-Degnan D, et al. Coverage by the news media of the benefits and risks of medications. *New Engl J Med* 2000:342;1645–1650.
Schwartz L, Woloshin S, Baczek L. Media coverage of scientific meetings: too much, too soon. *JAMA* 2002:287; 2859–2863.
Woloshin S, Schwartz L. Translating research into news. *JAMA* 2002:287;2856–2858.

General References

Altman L. When peer review produces unsound science. *New York Times* June 11, 2002:F6.
American College of Physicians. Direct to consumer advertising for prescription drugs. http://72.14.205.104/search?q=cache:zdn-iwZYPbcJ:www.acponline.org/fcgi/search%3 Fq% 3Dnt%26num%3D10%26site%3Ddefault_collection%26start%3D30 + %22American + College + of + Physicians%22 + Direct + to + Consumer + Advertising + For + Prescription + Drugs+ Oct+ 9,+ 1998&hl=en&ct=clnk&cd=3&gl=us Oct 9, 1998.
American College of Physicians. Direct to consumer advertising for prescription drugs. http://www.acponline.org/hpp/pospaper/dtcads.htm Oct 9, 1998.
Brody J. Separating gold from junk in medical studies. *New York Times* Oct 22, 2002:F7.
Cassels A. The media-medicine mix: quality concerns in medical reporting. *Open Medicine.* http://www.openmedicine.ca/article/viewArticle/54/4 Aug 1, 2007.
Eggner S. The power of the pen: medical journalism and public awareness. *JAMA* 1998:279;1400.
Fishman J, Casarett D. Mass media and medicine: when the most trusted media mislead. *Mayo Clin Proc* 2006:81;291–293.
Goldin R. Are Aleve's problems due to chance? Media ignores statistical significance in evaluating risk. Stats at George Mason University. http://www. stats.org/stories/are_aleve's _probs_ jan12_05.htm Jan 12, 2005.
Gorner P. Medical studies make news, worthy or not; researchers see flaws in coverage. *Chicago Tribune* June 5, 2002:110.
Grady D. Medical journal cites misleading research. *New York Times* Nov 10, 1999:A18.
Horton R. The clinical trial: deceitful, disputable, unbelievable, unhelpful and shameful. *Control Clin Trials* 2001:22;593–604.
Picard A. How can we improve medical reporting? Let me count the ways. *Int J Health Serv* 2005:35;603–605.
Schwartz L, Woloshin S. The media matter: a call for straightforward medical reporting. *Ann Intern Med* 2004:140;226–228.
Stamm K, Williams J, Noël P, et al. Helping journalists get it right. A physician's guide to improving health care reporting. *Gen Intern Med* 2003:18;138–145.
Stats at George Mason University. Relative risk and causation. http://www.stats.org/in_depth/ evaluate_healthrisks/health_risks_page5.htm Mar 1, 2002.

Voss M. Why reporters and editors get health coverage wrong. *Nieman Reports* 2003:57;46.

Zukerman D. Hype in health reporting "checkbook science" buys distortion of medical news. National Center for Policy Research for Women & Families. http://www.center4research. org/ hypehlthrpt902.html. Oct 30, 2002.

Chapter 20 – Product Development

Cited References

Horn J, de Haan R, Vermeulen M, et al. Nimodipine in animal model experiments of local cerebral ischemia: a systematic review. *Stroke* 2001:32;2457–2465.

General References

Americans for Medical Advancement. Nonhuman primates are not furry-looking humans. http://64.233.179.104/search?q=cache:EfK206XuT_AJ:www.curedisease.com/article1.html+ monkey+ research+ cost&hl=en&gl=us&ct=clnk&cd=8 July 25, 2007.

Bukaty R. MSNBC. Mice play a critical role in medical research. http://www.msnbc.msn.com/ id/11700807/ Mar 6, 2006.

Calabrese E. *Principles of animal extrapolation.* New York: Wiley, 1983.

Centers for Science in the Public Interest. Saccharin still poses cancer risk, scientists tell federal agency. http://www.cspinet.org/new/saccharn.htm Oct 28, 2005.

DiMasi J. Risks in new drug development: approval success rates for investigational drugs. *Clin Pharmacol Ther* 2001:69;297–307.

FDA Consumer Magazine. The FDA's drug review process: ensuring drugs are safe and effective. http://www.fda.gov/Fdac/features/2002/402_drug.html July 30, 2003.

Szalavitz M. The stats guide to evaluating health risks. Statistical Assessment Center. http://www. stats.org/index.jsp Feb 19, 2006.

Chapter 21 – Medical Innovation

Cited References

DiMasi J. Risks in new drug development: approval success rates for investigational drugs. *Clin Pharmacol Ther* 2001:69;297–307.

Harris Interactive. FDA gets good marks for ensuring new drug safety and efficacy but not for getting new drugs to market quickly. *Wall Street Journal Online.* http://harrisdealerpoll.com/ news/allnewsbydate.asp?NewsID=803 May 25, 2004.

Harris Interactive. Confidence in FDA hits new low, according to WSJ.com/Harris Interactive study. http://www.harrisinteractive.com/news/allnewsbydate.asp?NewsID=1301 Apr 22, 2008.

Lexchin J, Bero L, Djulbegovic B, et al. Pharmaceutical industry sponsorship and research outcome and quality: systematic review. *Br Med J* 2003:326;1167–1170.

Sinclair U. *The Jungle.* New York: Doubleday, 1906.

General References

Association of American Medical Colleges. 2001 medical school graduation questionnaire. http://
www.aamc.org/data/gq/allschoolsreports/2001.pdf June 21, 2002.
Berenson A. Pricey drug trials turn up few new blockbusters. *New York Times* Dec 18, 2004:A1.
Congressional Research Service. The Prescription Drug User Fee Act (PDUFA). http://opencrs.
cdt.org/document/RL33914 Mar 13, 2007.
Davis M, Manning A, Schmid G. Chapter 3: The Food and Drug Administration. Institute for the
Future. Regulation: a fragmented future. http://www.iftf.org/system/files/deliverables/
SR-775_Regulation_AFragementedFuture.pdf Nov 30, 2002.
DiMasi J, Hansen R, Grabowski H. The price of innovation: new estimates of drug development
costs. *J Health Econ* 2003:22;151–185.
Kermani F. The future is pharmacogenomic. Pharmaceutical Technology. http://www.ptemag.
com/pharmtecheurope/article/articleDetail.jsp?id=464310&pageID=1&sk=&date=The future
is pharmacogenomic Oct 1, 2007.
Food and Drug Administration. Milestones in U.S. Food and Drug law history. http://www.fda.
gov /opacom/backgrounders/miles.html May 3, 2002.
Food and Drug Administration. 2004 FDA accomplishments. http://64.233.161.104/
search?q=cache:AJSHq_CBT7wJ:www.fda.gov/bbs/topics/ANSWERS/2005/ANS01346.
html+ drugs+ number+ approved+ fda+ 2004&hl=en Mar 22, 2005.
Food and Drug Administration. Innovation or stagnation. http://www.fda.gov/oc/initiatives/criti-
calpath/whitepaper.pdf Mar 25, 2005.
Food and Drug Administration. Fast track, accelerated approval and priority review. http://www.
fda.gov/oashi/fast.html May 21, 2006.
Lowrance W. The promise of human genetic databases. *Brit Med J* 2001:322:1009–1010.
Merrill R. Modernizing the FDA: an incremental revolution. *Health Affair* 1999:18;96–111.
Nathan D. Careers in translational clinical research—historical perspectives, future challenges.
JAMA 2002:287;2424–2427.
Nathan D, Wilson J. Clinical research and the NIH – a report card. *New Engl J Med*
2003:349;1860–1865.
Service R. Surviving the blockbuster syndrome. *Science* 2004:202;1796–1799.
Thompson C. Antibacterial research and development in the 21st century – an industry perspective
of the challenges. *Curr Opin Microbiol* 2004:7;445–450.

Chapter 22 – Science and Politics

Cited References

Harris Interactive. Health-care professionals, pharmacies, hospitals gain the public's top
trust. http://www.harrisinteractive.com/news/allnewsbydate.asp?NewsID=749 Jan 28,
2004.
Harris Interactive. FDA gets good marks for ensuring new drug safety and efficacy but not for
getting new drugs to market quickly. *Wall Street Journal Online*. http://harrisdealerpoll.com/
news/allnewsbydate.asp?NewsID=803 May 25, 2004.
Harris Interactive. Reputation of pharmaceutical companies, while still poor, improves sharply for
second year in a row. http://www.harrisinteractive.com/news/allnewsbydate.asp?NewsID=1051
Apr 25, 2007.

The ALLHAT Officers and Coordinators for the ALLHAT Collaborative Research Group. Major outcomes in high-risk hypertensive patients randomized to angiotensin-converting enzyme inhibitor or calcium channel blocker vs diuretic: the Antihypertensive and Lipid-Lowering Treatment to Prevent Heart Attack Trial (ALLHAT). *JAMA* 2002:288;2981–2997.

Winer R, Hughes J, Feng Q, et al. Condom use and the risk of genital human papillomavirus infection in young women. *New Engl J Med* 2006:354;2645–2654.

General References

Advocate.com. FDA proposes condom labeling that warns of risk. http://www.advocate.com/news_detail_ektid22486.asp Nov 12, 2005.

Alliance for Human Research Protection. Another deadly drug recalled - FDA asks congress for power to dictate warnings. http://www.ahrp.org/infomail/05/03/01a.php Mar 1, 2005.

Baldwin J. Demand grows for early access to promising cancer drugs. *J Natl Cancer I* 2002:94;1668–1670.

Berenson A. Sending back the doctor's bill. *New York Times* July 29, 2007:WK3.

Coburn T. Dr. Coburn says new FDA condom regulations make inconclusive, exaggerated claims about condom effectiveness. http://coburn.senate.gov/public/index.cfm?FuseAction=LatestNews. PressReleases&ContentRecord_id=7602b477-6536-4c3c-a715-bb40fb9752ec Nov 10, 2005.

Collins D. Doctors to reassess antibiotics for 'chronic Lyme' disease. Associated Press. http://hosted.ap.org/dynamic/stories/L/LYME_DISEASE?SITE=AP&SECTION=HOME&TEMPLATE=DEFAULT May 3, 2008.

Daemmrich A, Bowden M. A rising drug industry. *Chem Eng News* 2005:83;51.

Drinkard J. Drugmakers go furthest to sway Congress. *USA Today* http://72.14.205.104/search?q=cache:ehhLBh1JjOEJ:www.usatoday.com/money/industries/health/drugs/2005–04–25-drug-lobby-cover_x.htm+drinkard+pharmaceutical+lobbying+2004&hl=en&ct=clnk&cd=1&gl=us Apr 4, 2005.

Editorial. Politicizing the FDA. *Washington Post* Aug 30, 2005:A16.

Food and Drug Administration. HIV and AIDS. http://www.fda.gov/oashi/aids/expanded.html Oct 7, 1998.

Gale E. Lessons from the Glitazones: a story of drug development. *Lancet* 2001:357;1870–1875.

Harris G. 2 cancer drugs, no comparative data. *New York Times* Feb 26, 2004:C1.

Harris G. Bush picks F.D.A. chief, but vote is unlikely soon. *New York Times* Mar 16, 2006:A8.

Henderson D. FDA chief quits; tenure marked by turmoil. *Boston Globe* Sep 24, 2005:A3.

Henry D, Hill S. Comparing treatments: comparison should be against active treatments rather than placebos. *Br Med J* 1995:310;1279.

Institute for OneWorld Health. Turning the tide. http://www.oneworldhealth.org/global/global_tide.php?PHPSESSID=555baa29b33ba487030b20975df3d79f June 1, 2007.

Kaufman M. 2 FDA officials urged to resign over Plan B. *Washington Post* May 13, 2004:A3.

Kaufman M. FDA official quits over delay on Plan B. Women's health chief says Commissioner's decision on contraceptive was political. *Washington Post* Sep 1, 2005:A8.

Lerner B. No shrinking violet: Rose Kushner and the rise of American breast cancer activism. *West J Med* 2001:174;362–365.

Lerner B. Ill patient, public activist: Rose Kushner's attack on breast cancer chemotherapy. *B Hist Med* 2007:81;224–240.

National Pharmaceutical Council. Issue area - value of pharmaceuticals. http://www.npcnow.org/resources/issuearea/valueofpharmaceuticals.asp Dec 1, 2006.

Pollack A. F.D.A. panel weighs fate of a drug for cancer. *New York Times* Mar 5, 2005:A8.

Rados C. The FDA speeds medical treatments for serious diseases. Food and Drug Administration. http://209.85.165.104/search?q=cache:mEJvXREy1iYJ:www.fda.gov/fdac/features /2006/206_

treatments.html+ fda+ accelerated+ approval+ cancer+ groups+ criticism&hl=en&ct=clnk&c
d=11&gl=us Apr 25, 2006.
Roehr B. FDA seeks to ease burden on trial review boards. *Br Med J* 2005:330;748.
Rusnak E. Center for Clinical Research. http://www.ccrp.com Feb 19, 2006.
Schaffer A. Viral effect: the campaign for abstinence hits a dead end on HPV. http://www.slate.
com/id/2144903/ July 3, 2006.
Smith R, Birnbaum J. Drug bill demonstrates lobby's pull. *Washington Post* Jan 12, 2007:A1.
Szabo L. 'Accelerated' drugs raise concern. *USA Today* http://www.usatoday.com/news/
health/2005–03–09-fda-drugs_x.htm Mar 10, 2005.
Willman D. How a new policy led to seven deadly drugs. *Los Angeles Times* Dec 20, 2000:A1.
Wood S. FDA action will harm women's health. Sound science and responsible decisions are
being trampled by politics. *St. Louis Post Dispatch* Oct 24, 2005:B9.

Chapter 23 – Research Misconduct

Cited References

Beecher H. Ethics and clinical research. *New Engl J Med* 1966:274;1354–1360.
Davidoff F, DeAngelis C, Drazen J, et al. Sponsorship, authorship, and accountability. *Ann Int
Med* 2001:135;463–465.
Joyce C. Congress slams misconduct in medical research. *New Scientist.* http://www. newscientist.com/
article/mg12717340.300-congress-slams-misconduct-in-medical-research-.html 15 Sep 30, 1990.
Krimsky S, Rothenberg L, Stotte P, et al. Scientific journals and their authors' financial interests:
a pilot study. *Psychother Psychosom* 1998:67;194–201.
Martinson B, Anderson M, de Vries R. Scientists behaving badly. *Nature* 2005:435;737–738.
McCarty M. Perspectives. Book. Lies, damn lies, and scientific research. *Lancet* 2004:364;
1657–1658.
Quick J. Maintaining the integrity of the clinical evidence base. *B World Health Organ* 2001:79;1093.
Ranstam J, Buyse M, George S, et al. Fraud in medical research: an international survey of bio-
statisticians. ISCB subcommittee on fraud. *Control Clin Trials* 2000:21;415–427.
Willman D. Stealth merger: drug companies and government medical research. *Los Angeles Times*
Dec 7, 2003:A1.

General References

Angell M. Is academic medicine for sale? *New Engl J Med* 2000:342;1516–1518.
DeAngelis C, Fontanarosa P, Flanagin A. Reporting financial conflicts of interest and relation-
ships between investigators and research sponsors. *JAMA* 2004:286;89–91.
Eichenwald K. U.S. officials are examining clinical trials. *New York Times* July 14, 1999:C1.
Eichenwald K, Kolata G. Research for hire. A doctor's drug studies turn into fraud. *New York
Times* May 17, 1999:A1.
Emanual E, Wood A, Fleishman A, et al. Oversight of human participants research: identifying
problems to evaluate reform proposals. *Ann Intern Med* 2004:141;282–291.
Health and Human Services. Hearing: avoiding conflicts of interest at the National Institutes of
Health. Statement by Ruth Kirchstein, M.D. http://www.hhs.gov/asl/testify/t040122a.html Jan
22, 2004.
Health and Human Services. Code of Federal Regulations. Part 46 Protection of human subjects.
http://www.hhs.gov/ohrp/humansubjects/guidance/45cfr46.htm#46.107 June 23, 2005.

Ioannidis J, Lau J. Completeness of safety reporting in randomized trials: an evaluation of 7 medical areas. *JAMA* 2001:285;437–443.

Judson H. *The great betrayal: fraud in science*. New York: Harcourt, 2004.

Lurie P, Almedia C, Stine N, et al. Financial conflict of interest disclosure and voting patterns at Food and Drug Administration drug advisory committee meetings. *JAMA* 2006:295; 1921–1928.

Miller F, Rosenstein D, DeRenzo E. Professional integrity in clinical research. *JAMA* 1998:280; 1449–1454.

National Institutes of Health. Conflict of interest information and resources. http://www.nih.gov/about/ethics/evaluationslides.pdf Oct 26, 2006.

National Institutes of Health. NIH history. http://www.nih.gov/about/history.htm Aug 1, 2006.

Schneider W. The establishment of institutional review boards in the U.S. http://www.iupui.edu/~histwhs/G504.dir/irbhist.html Jan 3, 2006.

Sontag D. Abuses endangered veterans in cancer drug experiments. *New York Times* Feb 6, 2005:A1.

Warlow C. Clinical research under the cosh again. *Brit Med J* 2004:329;241–242.

Weiss R. U.S. researchers reach deal in '99 gene therapy case. *Washington Post* Feb 10, 2005:A3.

Chapter 24 – Postmarketing Surveillance

Cited References

Bennett C, Nebeker J, Lyons E, et al. The research on adverse drug events and reports (RADAR) project. *JAMA* 2005:293;2131–2140.

Committee on the Assessment of the US Drug Safety System. The Future of drug safety. Institute of Medicine. http://www.iom.edu/CMS/3793/26341/37329.aspx Sep 22, 2006.

Editorial. Half a step on drug safety. *New York Times* Feb 17, 2005:A28.

Food and Drug Administration. The Future of drug safety — promoting and protecting the health of the public FDA's response to the Institute of Medicine's 2006 Report. http://www.fda.gov/oc/reports/iom013007.html Jan 30, 2007.

Furberg C, Levin A, Gross P, et al. The FDA and drug safety. A proposal for sweeping changes. *Arch Intern Med* 2006:166;1938–1942.

General Accounting Office. Drug safety improvements needed in FDA's postmarketing oversight process. http://209.85.165.104/search?q=cache:537MckWKkJIJ:www.gao.gov/ Mar 25, 2006.

Health and Human Services, Office of Inspector General. FDA review process for New Drug Applications (OEI-01-01-00590) Mar 2003.

Lasser K, Allen P, Woolhandler S. Timing of new black box warnings and withdrawals for prescribing medicines. *JAMA* 2002:287;2215–2220.

Mangano D, Tudo J, Dietzel C. The risk associated with Aprotinin in cardiac surgery. *N Engl J Med* 2006:54;353–365.

Moore T, Psaty B, Furberg C. Time to act on drug safety. *JAMA* 1998:279;1571–1573.

Olson M. Pharmaceutical policy change and the safety of new drugs. *J Law and Econ* 2002:45; 615–616.

Shah R. Can pharmacogenetics help rescue drugs withdrawn from the market? Pharmacogenomics 2006:7;889–908.

Smith S. Sidelining safety – the FDA's inadequate response to the IOM. *New Engl J Med* 2007:357;960–963.

Union of Concerned Scientists. FDA scientists pressured to exclude, alter findings; scientists fear retaliation for voicing safety concerns. http://www.ucsusa.org/news/press_release/fda-scientists-pressured.html. July 20, 2006.

Vlahakes G. The value of phase 4 testing. *N Engl J Med* 2006:54;413–415.

Willman D. How a new policy led to seven deadly drugs. *Los Angeles Times* Dec 20, 2000:A1.

Wood A, Stein C, Woosley R. Making medicines safer — the need for an independent drug safety board. *N Engl J Med* 1998:339;1851–1855.

General References

Agency for Healthcare Research and Quality. CERTS overview. http://www.ahrq.gov/clinic/certs-ovr.htm Feb, 2007.

Centers for Education and Research on Therapeutics (CERTs). Risk assessment of drugs, biologics and therapeutic devices: present and future issues. *Pharmacoepidemiol Drug Saf* 2003:2;653–662.

Fontanarosa F, Rennie D, DeAngelis C. Postmarketing surveillance – lack of vigilance, lack of trust. *JAMA* 2004:292;2647–2650.

Food and Drug Administration. Postmarketing surveillance programs. http://www.fda.gov/cder/regulatory/applications/postmarketing/surveillancepost.htm Apr 9, 2004.

Gardner A. Experts urge major FDA overhaul. *Live Science*. http://www.livescience.com/health-day/535418.html Oct 10, 2006.

Gottlieb S. Opening pandora's pillbox: using modern information tools to improve drug safety. *Health Affair* 2005:24;938–948.

Harris G. F.D.A. to create advisory board on drug safety. *New York Times* Feb 16, 2005:A1.

Harris G. F.D.A. widens safety reviews on new drugs. *New York Times* Jan 31, 2007:A17.

Kaufman M. Many workers call FDA inadequate at monitoring drugs. *Washington Post* Dec 17, 2004:A8.

Kramer B, Wilentz J, Alexander D, et al. Getting it right: being smarter about clinical trials. *PLoS Med* 2006:3;e144.

MacPherson K. MDs ring the alarm on safety of drugs. *The Newark Star Ledger* Oct 10, 2006:2C.

Psaty B, Furberg C, Ray W, et al. Potential for conflict of interest in the evaluation of suspected adverse drug reactions. *JAMA* 2004:292;2622–2631.

Ray W, Stein C. Reform of drug regulation – beyond an independent drug-safety board. *New Engl J Med* 2006:354;94–201.

Siebenaler J. FDA postmarketing commitment studies. *Regulatory Affairs Focus Magazine Archives*. http://www.raps.org/s_raps/rafocus_article.asp?TRACKID=&CID=61&DID=27043 Apr 15, 2006.

Trontell A. Expecting the unexpected-drug safety, pharmacovigilance, and the prepared mind. *New Engl J Med* 2004:351;1385–1387.

World Health Organization. The importance of pharmacovigilance - safety monitoring of medicinal products. http://www.who.int/medicinedocs/en/d/Js4893e/#Js4893e.1 Dec 21, 2002.

Chapter 25 – Regulatory Reform

Cited References

Food and Drug Administration. Report to Congress on postmarketing studies (FDAMA 130) Apr, 2002.

Health and Human Services. Office of Inspector General. Postmarketing studies of prescription drugs (OEI-03-94-00760) May, 1996.

Health and Human Services. Office of Inspector General. Monitoring of postmarketing study commitments (OEI-01-04-00390) June, 2006.

Health and Human Services. Office of Inspector General. The Food and Drug Administration's oversight of clinical trials (OEI-01-06-00160) Sep, 2007.

Markey E. Conspiracy of silence: how the FDA allows drug companies to abuse the accelerated approval process. Staff Summary of Responses by the Food and Drug Administration and the Securities and Exchange Commission to Correspondence from Rep. Edward J. Markey (D-MA). Executive Summary (pp 5–7). http://markey.house.gov/docs/health/iss_health_rep050601.pdf Mar 9, 2007.

Waxman H. The lessons of Vioxx — drug safety and sales. *New Engl J Med* 2005:352;2576–2578.

General References

Alliance for Human Research Protection. Another deadly drug recalled - FDA asks Congress for power to dictate warnings. http://www.ahrp.org/infomail/05/03/01a.php Mar 1, 2005.

Belknap S, Lyons E, McKoy J, et al. Report card for accelerated FDA approval oncology drugs (1995–2003): is it time for a make-up test? *J Clin Oncol* 2004:22;6002.

Bombardier C, Laine L, Reicin A, et al. Comparison of upper gastrointestinal toxicity of rofecoxib and naproxen in patients with rheumatoid arthritis. *New Engl J Med* 2000:343;1520–1528.

Bombardier C, Laine L, Burgos-Vargas R, et al. Response to expression of concern regarding VIGOR study. *New Engl J Med* 2006:354;1196–1199.

CBS News. 60 Minutes. FDA: harsh criticism from within. http://www.cbsnews.com/stories/2005/02/15/60II/main674293.shtml Feb 16, 2005.

Editorial. Manipulating a journal article. *New York Times* Dec 11, 2005:411.

Editorial. Reforming the F.D.A. *New York Times* May 3, 2007:A22.

Graham D, Campen D, Hui R, et al. Risk of acute myocardial infarction and sudden cardiac death in patients treated with cyclo-oxygenase 2 selective and non-selective non-steroidal anti-inflammatory drugs: nested case-control study. *Lancet* 2005:365:475–481.

Harris G. F.D.A. leader says study tied to Vioxx wasn't suppressed. *New York Times* Nov 18, 2004:C7.

Harris G. Strong drug ties and less monitoring at F.D.A. *New York Times* Dec 6, 2004:A1.

Harris G. Report assails F.D.A. oversight of clinical trials. *New York Times* Sep 28, 2007:A1.

Kelly J. Harsh criticism lobbed at FDA in Senate Vioxx hearing. *Medscape Medical News.* http://www.medscape.com/viewarticle/538021 Nov 23, 2004.

Kweder S. U.S. Senate Committee on Finance. Statement of Sandra Kweder. http://64.233.161.104/search?q=cache:ZWFzcfcI3qcJ:www.fda.gov/ola/2004/vioxx1118.html+ vioxx+ ispe+ kaiser&hl=en Nov 10, 2004.

Rockoff J. Congress acts to improve drug safety. *Baltimore Sun.* http://www.baltimoresun.com/news/nation/bal-te.fda21sep21,0,2275298 Sep 21, 2007.

Rubin R. How did Vioxx debacle happen? *USA Today* Oct 12, 2004:D1.

Rubin R. Merck halts Vioxx sales; pain reliever linked to heart attack, stroke. *US Today* Oct 1, 2004:A1.

Solomon D, Schneeweiss S, Glynn R, et al. Relationship between selective cyclooxygenase-2 inhibitors and acute myocardial infarction in older adults. *Circulation* 2004:109:2068–2073.

Strom B. How the US drug safety system should be changed. *JAMA* 2006:295;2072–2075.

Szabo L. 'Accelerated' drugs raise concern. *USA Today* http://www.usatoday.com/news/health/2005-03-09-fda-drugs_x.htm Mar 10, 2005.

U.S. Senate Committee on Finance. Testimony of David J. Graham. http://www.senate.gov/~finance/hearings/testimony/2004test/111804dgtest.pdf. Nov 18, 2004.

Chapter 26 - Journey's End

Cited References

Callahan D. *What price better health? Hazards of the research imperative.* Berkeley, CA: University of California Press, 2003.
National Institutes of Health. Report and recommendations on public trust in clinical research. Director's Council of Public Representatives. http://copr.nih.gov/reports/public_trust.asp Dec 2, 2004.

General References

Research!America. Americans say more funding for medical research vital to U.S. economic health. http://www. research america.org/polldata/2006/NationalPoll2006.pdf Jan 26, 2006.

Glossary

Absolute Difference	The difference between two measurements obtained by subtracting one measurement from the other. If the risk of a heart attack is 2 in 100 (2%) in one group of patients and 1 in 100 (1%) in a comparison patient group, the absolute difference is derived by simply subtracting the two risks (2 − 1) and getting an absolute change of 1 percent. See Relative Difference.
Accuracy	A determination of how close a measurement comes in respect to its true value.
Adverse Effect	See Side Effect.
Adverse Reaction	See Side Effect.
Applied Research	Scientific investigations that are directed at real world problems. See Basic Research.
Baseline Measurement	A measurement made at the beginning of a trial. Most baseline measurements will be repeated during and at the end of the trial to determine what kind of change occurred.
Basic Research	Scientific investigations that advances scientific knowledge, but is not directed at commercial objectives. See Applied Research.
Bias	An error in the design or conduct of a medical investigation that leads to a wrong conclusion. For instance, study groups that are not equivalent may cause one group to end up with a more positive or negative treatment result. See Publication Bias and Selection Bias.
Blinding	The process by which the treatments used in a clinical trial are disguised so subjects and researchers cannot identify one treatment from another.
Case Report	A description of a patient or group of patients who have an unusual condition or response

that a health professional believes should be brought to the attention of others. The case report is considered the lowest level of the primary medical research methods.

Case-Control Study A research method that starts with an outcome and looks retrospectively for a cause. In a case-control study, the histories of a group of patients with a disease or condition of interest (the cases) are compared to another group (the controls) who do not have the disease or condition.

Categorical Scale A way of classifying variables that are mutually exclusive and cannot be arranged in any kind of hierarchy. Examples include gender (male or female) and outcome (lived or died). Statisticians commonly call this kind of scale a nominal scale. See Ordered Scale and Numerical Scale.

Causation See Cause and Effect.

Cause and Effect A relationship in which one event produces a change in another factor and there is no other explanation for that change. If you do X then the direct consequence is an alteration in Y.

Clinical Relevance The minimal treatment difference that is medically meaningful. A clinically significant difference should be sufficiently large to have a practical benefit for patients.

Clinical Trial A research study in humans who receive an experimental or control treatment in order to assess treatment safety and/or effectiveness. Randomization, blinding and a controlled experimental setting are generally employed to control for bias in a clinical trial. See RABCOT.

Cohort Study A research investigation that records the health status of subjects who are followed over a period of time. Typically, two sets of people (those with and those without a disease or medical problem) are compared to see how the groups differ in terms of health factors collected in the study.

Comparative Trial See Equivalence Trial.

Composite Endpoint A medical outcome that combines multiple endpoints together to make a single measurement.

Confidence Interval A range of values that is likely to include the true difference between treatments. A given 95 percent confidence interval will either include or exclude

	the true population value, but 95 percent of the time the true value is included.
Control Group	The group of subjects participating in a medical study who do not receive the experimental treatment. The treatment results from the control group are compared to the results from the experimental group.
Controlled Trial	A study that includes an experimental treatment and a control treatment (usually a placebo).
Cost Benefit Analysis	An evaluation technique in which expected costs are compared to expected benefits to determine the most profitable course of action.
Cross Sectional Study	A survey of people that usually is used to determine prevalence of a disease or other medical factor. A cross-sectional study can be completed in a relatively short period of time, but cannot guarantee that the finding is a cause and effect relationship. See Exploratory Research Method.
Database	A collection of information that is organized so that it can easily be accessed, managed, and updated.
Data Mining	Searching a database and looking for every kind of a relationship between variables that have not been previously discovered.
Declaration of Helsinki	A series of guidelines adopted by the World Medical Association in Helsinki, Finland in 1964. The Declaration addresses ethical issues for physicians conducting medical research involving human subjects.
Double-Blind Study	A clinical trial in which neither the participants nor the research staff know if a subject is in the experimental or control group.
Efficiency	Ability to obtain reliable results from a medical investigation in terms of minimizing time, cost and resources (e.g. number of subjects required).
Endpoint	An outcome in a medical investigation.
Epidemiology	The study of factors affecting the health and illness of people.
Equivalence Trial	A clinical trial designed to evaluate whether an experimental treatment is similar to a standard treatment.
Experiment-Wise Error	The probability that at least one statistical test will yield a positive result (e.g. produce a p-value of .05 or less) when statistical tests are used repeatedly in the same study.

Experimental Setting	The environment in which a clinical trial takes place where researchers try to keep extraneous factors from biasing the trial results. For example, researchers want all experimental conditions except for the treatments being administered, to be the same for all study groups.
Experimental Research Method	A research technique in which subjects are usually assigned to a treatment group or control group by a randomized method. Assessments are made at the start and repeated at the end of a study to determine what differences exist between the study groups. Investigators are able to intervene and control to some extent a subject's behavior during the study. See Clinical Trial Randomization and RABCOT.
Exploratory Research Method	A class of research studies in which the subject's treatment is chosen by the patient or his/her physician and other medications the subjects took or is taking were also selected in the same manner. Furthermore, the behavior of the subject is not restricted to any extent. See Cohort, Cross Sectional, and Case-Control studies which are examples of exploratory studies.
False Negative	A test result that indicates that a person does not have a specific disease or condition when the person actually does have the disease or condition.
False Positive	A test result that indicates that a person has a specific disease or condition when the person actually does not have the disease or condition.
Generalizability	See Usefulness.
Historical Controls	The use of data from the medical records of subjects who were treated some time in the past. Their information is compared to the data for subjects who participated in a current clinical trial.
Informed Consent	The principle that potential subjects are given adequate, accurate and understandable information about a research study before they agree to participate in the study.
Institutional Review Board (IRB)	A specially constituted review body established to protect the welfare of human subjects recruited for a clinical trial.

Intention-to-Treat Analysis	The evaluation of study results in which all subjects who were assigned to a treatment group are included in the analysis whether they completed or even started treatment.
Interim Analysis	A statistical analysis that compares the treatment groups at any time before the formal completion of the trial.
Investigational New Drug Application (IND)	The document by which a drug sponsor requests the FDA to allow human testing of its experimental product.
Margin of Error	A range of values reflecting the amount of error in the result of a poll or survey. A margin of error is actually a 95 percent confidence interval. See Confidence Interval.
Mathematical Model	An abstract representation of a process that uses mathematical language and relationships to describe its behavior.
Measurement	Refers to all the data collected on the subjects in a medical study including qualitative and quantitative assessments. Measurements include responses to questions ("how do you feel"), making elementary observations (noting eye color) or recording results from sophisticated medical equipment.
Measurement Validity	The extent to which an assessment instrument or test accurately measures what it is supposed to measure.
Meta Analysis	A statistical method that combines the results from a number of studies investigating the same research question and provides an overall assessment by integrating the findings from the individual studies.
Multicenter trial	A clinical trial conducted at multiple sites using a common protocol.
Multiple Testing	Performing multiple statistical tests in a single study. Typical situations that cause multiple tests are analyzing many variables, doing subgroup analyses and conducting interim analyses.
New Drug Application (NDA)	The submission to the FDA of all the chemical, production and scientific information that the sponsor has gathered about a new drug. Approval of an NDA allows the drug to be marketed.
Null Hypothesis	A contention used when conducting statistical tests that there is no difference between the

	treatments being compared. Investigators usually hope that the experimental treatment is better than the control treatment thereby allowing them to reject the null hypothesis.
Numerical Scale	A way of classifying variables in which uniform mathematical units make up the measurement scale. Examples include age and blood pressure. Statisticians commonly call this kind of scale an interval scale. See Categorical Scale and Ordered Scale.
Objective Measurement	An assessment based on observable and measurable attributes that are not distorted by personal judgments and interpretations. Examples include height and weight measurements. See Subjective Measurement.
Ordered Scale	A way of classifying variables that can be ranked and placed in an ordered sequence, but they cannot be distinguished in terms of the size of the difference between the ranked items. An example is pain that can be classified as no pain, mild pain, moderate pain and severe pain, but the differences between the rankings are not numeric. Statisticians commonly call this kind of scale an ordinal scale. See Categorical Scale and Numerical Scale.
Outcome Measurement	An assessment used to measure the safety or efficacy of a treatment. The primary outcome is the assessment of greatest importance.
Peer Review	The process by which journal editors solicit evaluations of submitted articles from outside experts who remain anonymous to the authors.
Phase I Study	The initial set of clinical trials in humans that are usually conducted on small numbers of healthy subjects to learn about a drug's toxicity, absorption, distribution and metabolism.
Phase II Study	The early clinical trials of patients with the disease or condition that an experimental drug is expected to help. These trials provide additional information about the relative safety of the new drug and begin the assessment of its effectiveness.
Phase III Study	Large clinical trials designed to generate the data needed to gain marketing approval.
Phase IV Study	Clinical trials that are carried out after a drug has been approved by the FDA. Phase IV studies

	may be required by the FDA to confirm an efficacy or safety claim, explore additional patient populations or new conditions in which the drug may be of value, compare the drug to a competitor's product or study a serious safety issue that was not recognized earlier.
Placebo Effect	An explanation of how placebos work. There are many theories, but no general agreement on why and how people respond to placebos.
Placebo	A chemically inert substance (e.g. sugar pills) often given to control groups.
Population	The entire group of people with the disease, illness or condition who will potentially be treated with the experimental treatment.
Probability Level	The likelihood that the results of a statistical test could be due to chance. A .05 probability level means there is a 5 percent chance (i.e. a .05 probability) that the result obtained in a trial could be due to chance. See Significance Level and Statistical Significance.
Probability Standard	The probability value selected to determine whether a treatment difference is or is not associated with statistical significance. In medical research, that standard is almost always .05.
Protocol	The formal plan for the conduct of a clinical trial that includes a description of the research design or methodology to be employed, the eligibility requirements for prospective subjects and controls, the treatment regimen(s), and the clinical measurements that will be assessed.
Protocol Deviation	A failure to adhere to the conditions and restriction specified in the protocol.
Publication Bias	The increased likelihood that studies will be published if there are positive results (e.g. the treatment differences were statistically significant).
P-Value	The probability that a treatment difference could have occurred by chance. In medical research, a p-value of .05 or lower has become the acceptable level needed to claim that there is a statistically significant treatment effect.
Qualitative Research	Investigations that attempts to provide insight into social, emotional, and experiential phenomena in health care. Examples include inquiry about the meaning of illness to patients

or evaluating how counseling influences the medication taken by the elderly.

Quality of Life
An evaluation of a person's ability to enjoy normal life activities. The components that measure quality of life vary depending on the patient's age, expectations, and physical and mental capabilities.

RABCOT
A clinical trial that randomizes study treatments to subjects, is blinded and includes a control group.

Randomization
A process used to assign study treatments to subjects in which the treatment allocated to a subject is determined by chance. The treatment assignment is not influenced in any way by the researcher(s) conducting the trial.

Relative Difference
The ratio of one statistic compared to a second statistic. If the risk of a heart attack is 2 in 100 (2%) in one group of patients and 1 in 100 (1%) in a comparison patient group, the relative change is derived by calculating the ratio of the two risks (1/2 = 50) and getting a relative change of 50%. See Absolute Difference.

Reliability
The degree to which repeated assessments of a measurement gives consistent, stable, and uniform results.

Risk Factor
A characteristic or condition that increases a person's chance of getting a disease.

Sample
A subset of the population. In medical research, the members of a sample should be representative of the population of interest. See Population.

Sample Size
The number of patients or subjects selected for a research study.

Scientific Method
The systematic pursuit of knowledge used by scientists that involves, identifying an issue or problem, forming a hypothesis, testing the hypothesis by conducting an experiment and drawing conclusions based on the experimental results.

Selection Bias
An incorrect result in a medical investigation because the treatment group assignments produced dissimilar groups in respect to factors that influenced the treatment evaluations.

Side Effect
An undesired effect from a treatment. Common side effects include nausea, headache, dry mouth and insomnia. However, side effects can be serious resulting in permanent harm or death.

Significance Level	The probability level set by a researcher to determine whether or not to declare that the result of a treatment comparison is statistically significant. In medical research the probability level is almost always .05. See Probability Level and Statistical Significance.
Sponsor	A company, institution, or organization that initiates, manages, and/or finances a clinical trial.
Standard Treatment	The currently accepted treatment considered to be effective in the treatment of a specific disease or condition.
Statistical Association	The presence of a relationship between two variables, but one that is not necessarily a cause and effect relationship.
Statistical Assumption	Suppositions about the characteristics of the data used in a statistical test. If the study data are inconsistent with the suppositions then the test result can be inaccurate.
Statistical Significance	A declaration made by researchers when the probability, that the treatment difference they found could be due to chance, is .05 or less. The .05 probability standard is routinely used in medical research, but in unique situations it made by more liberal (e.g. .10) or conservative (e.g. .01).
Study Validity	Refers to the rigor in which a medical study has been designed and executed so that the study ends up with correct and accurate conclusions.
Subgroup Analysis	Conducting statistical tests to see if treatment difference exists among patients with particular characteristics (e.g. performing tests to see if treatment effects are the same for male and female subjects). Subgroup analyses should be specified at the start of the trial with an appropriate adjustment incorporated in the analysis for the additional testing required.
Subjective Measurement	An assessment that takes place primarily in one's mind and is heavily influenced by individual bias and personal experiences. An example is an assessment of a subject's degree of happiness. See Objective Measurement.
Trial Monitoring	The process of overseeing the way a trial is performed and determining whether the results in a double blind study require early study termination. Monitoring committees, independent

	from the study researchers, review and analyze the data on a periodic basis to make certain that the level of risk incurred by participants remains acceptable.
Type 1 Error	The mistake that occurs when an investigator concludes that there is a treatment difference when, in fact, there isn't one.
Type 2 Error	The mistake that occurs when an investigator concludes that there is no treatment difference when, in fact, there really is one.
Usefulness	The extent to which the results and conclusions from a clinical investigation can be applied to other groups or situations than the one studied. Usefulness is frequently called external validity in the medical literature.
Validity	See Measurement Validity and Study Validity.
Variance	A measure of the degree to which the values for a given variable are dispersed. The greater the dispersion, the greater the variance.

Index

Printed in the United Kingdom
by Lightning Source UK Ltd.
134802UK00008B/276/P